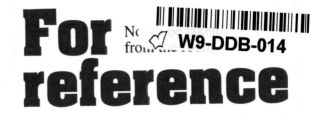
A DICTIONARY OF

Medical
Derivations

THE **REAL** MEANING OF MEDICAL TERMS

DATE DUE

Dedication

For my friend Barry Fisher Dickson

A DICTIONARY OF
Medical Derivations

THE **REAL** MEANING OF MEDICAL TERMS

William Casselman

The Parthenon Publishing Group

International Publishers in Medicine, Science & Technology

NEW YORK   LONDON

Published in the USA by
The Parthenon Publishing Group Inc.
One Blue Hill Plaza
PO Box 1564, Pearl River
New York 10965, USA

Published in the UK and Europe by
The Parthenon Publishing Group Ltd
Casterton Hall, Carnforth
Lancs. LA6 2LA,UK

Library of Congress Cataloging-in-Publication Data
Casselman, Bill, 1942–
Dictionary of medical derivations: the real meaning of medical words/ by
William Casselman
      p. cm.
    ISBN 1-85070-771-5
      1. Medicine—Terminology—Dictionaries. 2. English language—
Etymology—Dictionaries. I. Title.
     [DNLM: 1. Nomenclature—dictionaries.   W 13 C344d 1997]
R123.C33 1997
610.1'4—dc21
DNLM/DLC
for Library of Congress

97-26856
CIP

British Library Cataloguing in Publication Data
Casselman, William
Dictionary of medical derivations: the real meaning of medical words
1. Medicine – Terminology – Dictionaries
I. Title
610.1'4

ISBN 1-85070-771-5

Typeset by Martin Lister Publishing Services, Carnforth, UK
Printed and bound by The Bath Press, Bath, UK

Foreword

Medical terminology conjures up the image of a strange and mysterious discipline, one to which the uninitiated have but limited access. It would even appear that the communication system was devised to intimidate those outside of the field and thus to contribute in some obscure way to the worth of those who are practitioners of the art. Those of us who have daily exposure to this bizarre and fascinating system of communication are usually unaware that we have acquired a different language. We still recall, however, the sense of bewilderment that it presented in the earlier phases of our education as we were introduced to a barrage of words that were completely foreign. There is little doubt that language is deeply embedded in the culture of medicine. How helpful it would have been to have had available a compendium of medical derivations, one which would demystify the linguistic jargon which is apparently so important in medical communication!

Dissection of the derivation of words, authoritatively and accurately done, provides instant insight into their actual meaning. Identification of the components from which the words are derived allows associations which are easily recognizable and in many cases eliminate the need for rote memorization. This is particularly important in today's world, with increasing specialization, accompanied by a greater and greater diversity among the subsets of fields of medicine. This compendium provides definitions of the basic building block terms derived from Latin and Greek, coupled with an explanation of the systems which combine them to form precise medical meanings. In this way it provides instantaneous insight and contributes greatly to the demystification of commonly-used words and phrases. Over and above its utilitarian aspect, it serves as a source of bemused entertainment for those of us in medicine who have tried not to take ourselves too seriously. What was designed to appear complicated and mysterious suddenly becomes straightforward and sensible when we return to its very roots.

Luigi Mastroianni Jr
William Goodell Professor of
Obstetrics and Gynecology
University of Pennsylvania
School of Medicine

THE AUTHOR

William Casselman

William Casselman is the author of four previous books about the etymology of English words – and has written regularly about technical vocabulary and its origins for the past 20 years. He currently lives near Toronto, Canada.

The author would like to acknowledge with thanks the advice of:

Ronald Casselman

Dr Casselman graduated from the University of Western Ontario with an MD, and served for three years with the Canadian Armed Forces. He received a fellowship in Urology from the Royal College of Physicians and Surgeons of Canada.

Dr Casselman practices in St. Catharines, Ontario, where he is the Chief of Surgical Services at the Hôtel Dieu Hospital. He is married to Judy Casselman and they have a son and daughter.

Judith Casselman

Judith Casselman graduated with an RN from the Victoria Hospital School of Nursing in London, Ontario. She received a Diploma in Public Health Nursing from Dalhousie University. Judy has practiced nursing across Canada, and is presently a nursing consultant in St. Catharines.

Introduction

What this book does

Medical words can be daunting when they are first encountered. Large poly-syllabic jaw-breakers such as cholecystectomy are not part of everyday English. What is colloquially referred to as a black eye, in medical literature may be described as a bilateral circumorbital hematoma!

There is, however, a way to solve the mystery of medical jargon by using a logical system to understand the terminology, which lessens the need for the grind of memory work. This book uses the following approach:

1. Break the long medical words up into their very simple Greek and Latin root parts;
2. Learn what these root elements mean;
3. See how root parts are combined to make old and new medical terms.

By learning the most frequently used roots of English medical words, the reader will be able to make an educated guess when presented with an unfamiliar medical term. Before long, it will be possible to access instantly the general meaning of more than 50 000 medical words!

Why Latin and Greek?

Ninety per cent of all scientific words in English are derived from Latin and Greek. In medical English, 98% of all technical terms have Latin or Greek roots.

In origin, English is a Germanic language based on the Germanic dialects of the Angles, Saxons and Jutes who conquered Britain. However, further invasions, and migrations to the British Isles of peoples speaking other languages, such as Latin, Old Norse and French, added foreign terms to the basic Anglo-Saxon vocabulary. The English language now contains more words than any other language, with a larger vocabulary even than Chinese, French, Russian or Arabic. Our simple words are still of Anglo-Saxon origin: 'give', 'man', 'father', for example, but almost all our technical words have been borrowed from Latin and Greek.

Western medicine was taught in Latin and, to a lesser extent, Greek, for 2000 years. The Greek word *asphyxia* is 3000 years old. Its meaning has changed slightly, but it is still used in English and also in most European languages. Until the end of the 17th Century, medical textbooks were written in Latin. A student at the Sorbonne, or at Oxford or Bologna, would learn anatomy and physiology from books written in Latin and based on the writings of famous Roman physicians such as Galen, who lived from AD 129 to 199. As late as AD 1542, the influential anatomist Vesalius assembled his personal knowledge of anatomy based on his own dissections and observations, thus changing the course of medical inquiry from superstition to science. Vesalius wrote his famous book in Latin, but included an index of all the Greek names for parts of the body – because the medical students who would use his textbook were required to have a knowledge of both Latin and Greek. The first American medical textbooks used at Harvard University were written in Latin.

Roman physicians largely obtained their medical knowledge from the ancient Greeks. The earliest extant Greek medical texts were written by a Greek doctor named Hippocrates and physicians who had been his students in the 5th Century BC. On the tiny, peaceful Greek island of Cos, Hippocrates ran a school for doctors. Here he formulated the famous Hippocratic Oath, still sworn today by some medical students. Its most famous rule is 'First, do no harm'.

Those so-called 'dead' languages, Latin and Classical Greek, however, are used to form scientific and technical terms for the following reasons. First, it is traditional – as described above. Second, in a 'dead' language, the meaning of a word does not change: it is consistent. *Callus* will always mean 'hard skin' in Latin. In a living language, words acquire new meanings. For example, in 1930, 'acid' meant a chemical such as the acetic acid in vinegar. Nowadays 'acid' is English slang for LSD, a dangerous hallucinogenic drug.

Because precise meaning and precise use of words can be crucial in all forms of medical communication, it helps to be able to make new medical terms from Latin and Greek roots whose meanings do not alter with time. The Greek root *akro-* will always mean 'high' and *phobos* will always mean 'fear', so acrophobia will always mean 'morbid fear of heights'. Classical Greek is a dead language also in the sense that the root meanings cannot change, as they can in modern English. (It should be noted here that modern Greek is a vibrant language, still very much alive in Greece and wherever in the world Greek people gather.) Additionally, knowing roots such as *akro-* helps to understand the origins of many other commonly used English words. An acrobat was first a highwire walker, on ropes strung across a room or a street. The Greek adjective *akrobatos* literally meant 'walking on tiptoe'. The high, defended part of an ancient Greek city was an acropolis, from the Greek *polis*, 'city'. Athens had the most famous acropolis, but it is easy to guess what and where the Acrocorinth was.

One final reason Latin and Greek roots are used to form medical words, although perhaps hard to believe, is that they result in terms that are shorter and more convenient than long descriptions in English. Cholecystostomy is much quicker and easier to write than its definition in English, namely, the surgical making of a mouth-like opening (Greek *stoma*) in the wall of the gall (Greek *chole*) bladder (Greek *cysto-*) to introduce a catheter for the purpose of draining excess fluid accumulation. Greek and Latin terms provide a method of shorthand for the description of complex objects and procedures in medicine. Also, a knowledge of the simple Greek roots can even help in spelling a word more easily.

Eponyms: to be avoided

Of course, alternative forms of medical nomenclature exist. Instead of Latin and Greek roots which actually denote something about a medical procedure, medical eponyms are sometimes used. An eponym is a name for a structure, disease or syndrome based on the surname of a physician or medical researcher, often associated with the discovery or first clinical description of the object or disorder. Although it is pleasant to remember and honor pioneers like James Parkinson, which name is more helpful and descriptive: Parkinson's disease or paralysis agitans? The expressions Parkinsonism and Parkinsonian syndrome only add to the confusion.

Also, for example, consider the term Zinn's zonula. Johann Gottfried Zinn (1727–1759), a German anatomist, was the author of a classic treatise on the eye, but it is debatable how many first-year medical students know the whereabouts of Zinn's zonula. A more appropriate label is the ciliary zonula. *Zonula* means 'little belt, little girdle' in Latin. The ciliary zonula is a group of hair-like (*cilium*, Latin, fine hair, eyelash) fibers that connect the lens of the eye to the ciliary body. Eponyms are not practical, not efficient and not scientific labels and should be discouraged. Wherever possible a scientific name and not an eponym should be used. It takes decades, sometimes centuries, to eradicate such meaningless honorific terms, which in fact do no honor to the pioneering physicians and researchers. Most of them would be appalled to know that their surnames have been applied to clumsy and impractical medical terms that make learning medical nomenclature more difficult for students.

As long ago as 1955, at a conference in Paris, the International Congress of Anatomy adopted a new official list of anatomical names, the Nomina Anatomica, abbreviated *NA* in many medical dictionaries. All eponyms and proper names were eliminated, so that terms like 'the foramen of Winslow', 'Scarpa's fascia', 'Hunter's canal' and others were abandoned. The *NA* list is updated and revised regularly. These new terms speed the learning of medical nomenclature, improve the clarity of journal research articles and medical literature in general, and make easier international and interlingual medical communications. Perhaps the most salient criticism of eponyms is that research into their origins leads to the sobering discovery that, in anatomy at least, many of the surnames attached to structures are false or incorrect. The men and women honored by having their names attached to some anatomical part were in fact not the first to describe them or discover them! So, even as honorifics, eponyms fail. They should be avoided: the *NA* term is the one to use.

A little Latin trivia

There is an old schoolboy rhyme:

O Latin is a dead tongue, as dead as it can be
It killed the ancient Romans, and now it's killing me!

However, Latin must not be too quickly dismissed as a 'dead' language. Roman numerals, for example, are frequently used, not least as page numbers for the 'Introduction' to this book. In the United States, most people carry Latin on their person every day in the form of three Latin phrases on an American one-dollar bill. For those that are interested in trivia, the three phrases on the dollar bill are:

1. *Annuit coeptis*   He (God) has approved our actions;
2. *Novus ordo seclorum*   A new order of ages (i.e. a new era has begun with the founding of the USA); motto of the Great Seal of the United States;
3. *E pluribus unum*   One nation from many states.

Who is the *Dictionary of Medical Derivations* for?

The *Dictionary of Medical Derivations* is an excellent way for a student of any course within the health professions to learn how medical words are formed from Latin and Greek roots. It will enable the reader to construct a medical vocabulary by learning to identify the common word roots from which medical words were created in the past. New medical words, which arise every month, are created using these same roots. It will help nursing students, those in pre-med and medical courses, dental students and paramedic students, as well as any word lover who wants to master medical vocabulary in English. The *Dictionary of Medical Derivations* will prove useful to any writer or teacher who is planning introductory courses in the technical language of the medical sciences.

The definitions are brief and simple. The purpose of this book is to acquaint the reader with Latin and Greek word-forming elements as found in medical terms. For full definitions, a large medical dictionary should be consulted.

The word examples are hyphenated only to show the word roots, *not* for pronunciation. The pronunciation of medical words varies from country to country, and from region to region within a country. Harvard medical English does not sound at all like Louisiana medical English, for example. Correct pronunciation should be learned from a standard medical dictionary, and from teachers.

Because of the sheer weight of facts to be learned, medicine is often studied in isolation from other fields of knowledge, in particular from the humanities. However, the advancement of medical knowledge has affected and illuminated history, culture and literature. The reader will find pertinent references, both historical and cultural, added to the explanations of the origin of medical words. For example, the false but very ancient theory of humors is mentioned in the entry on *abscess*, because the theory helps explain the origin of the word. Such references make the root words easier to remember, and make medical etymology a fuller, richer experience.

Any suggestions for improving the book should be forwarded to the authors through the publisher.

How to read an entry

❶	chole-
❷	*chole* Greek, bile or gall
❸	chole-ster-ol
❹	*chole* ❺Greek, bile, gall + *stereos* Greek, solid + *ol* meaning alcohol
❺	Cholesterol, now the bane of dieters, is a solid alcohol of animal fats, which was first isolated in gall stones. Early doctors thought it was solidified bile.

(1)   At the top left of each entry is the root word.

(2)   The root is shown in its original form and its language identified, followed by its basic meaning in that ancient language, and its modern medical meaning if that is different from the ancient meaning.

(3)   The medical word with the pertinent root is presented, divided by hyphens to show its parts. Note that the hyphens do *not* indicate pronunciation.

(4)   Each root in the word is listed in *italics*.

(5)   The language to which each root belongs comes next, followed by the basic meaning of each root.

(6)   A definition of the word, and possibly other related words, concludes the entry.

A few peculiarities of the *Dictionary of Medical Derivations* style

This section clarifies the methods that have been used in presenting the etymologies. For example, occasionally strict alphabetical order is over-looked so that related words, or words derived from the same root, can be grouped together. Also, alphabetical order has sometimes not been strictly observed when introducing a word root in a place deemed proper by the authors.

What do < and > mean in linguistic descriptions?

Linguistics has borrowed the above two arithmetical operator signs. As a mathematical symbol, > means 'greater than', and < means 'less than'. But in language study, > means 'develops into, is the root of'; and < means 'stems from, derives from'. For example, consider the following *Dictionary of Medical Derivations* entry:

---

lateral

lateralis Latin, of a side, on the side < *latus* side

Lateral as an anatomical position means on the side, toward the side, or more away from the center of a body.

The second line may be read to mean: *lateralis* is Latin and means 'of a side, on the side', and *lateralis* derives from the earlier noun *latus* which means 'side'.

Or consider the following entry:

---

pneum-

pneumon Greek, the lungs < *pneuma* air, gas, spirit < *pnein* to breathe

---

Seen in our word *pneumonia*, the root *pneum-* is from *pneumon*, the Greek word for lung or the lungs, which comes from an earlier Greek word *pneuma* which meant 'air, gas, spirit', which itself derives from the ancient Greek verb *pnein* 'to breathe'.

Now, consider the following entry:

> ## lacrimal apparatus
>
> *lacrimalis* Latin, pertaining to structures that secrete, hold, or transport tears. *ad* > *ap* to + *paratus* Latin, ready > *apparatus* Latin, literally 'something prepared for a special purpose', like a medical instrument. Compare the motto of the Boy Scouts: *Semper Paratus*, 'always prepared'.

The third line may be read as follows: the prefix *ad* assimilates to the *p* of *paratus* to become *ap-*, to which is added *paratus* which is Latin for 'ready', and these two roots develop into the word *apparatus*.

Repeating some information

The reader will find some derivations deliberately repeated in the text. For example, palatoschisis is defined under its initial component, *palato-* and later under its terminal component, *-schisis*. Repetition is permissible and a necessary part of memory work. Writing down and repeatedly speaking aloud the roots and parts of medical words is, in fact, the best possible way to memorize them.

Why so many forms of some Latin and Greek words?

The simple or nominative case of a Latin or Greek noun is not always the form used to make an English medical term. For example, many Latin and Greek nouns do not contain the full root form in the nominative case, but do show the full root form in the genitive. Thus, it is traditional in learning Latin and Greek nouns to quote a noun in the nominative and genitive cases. This is frequently seen in dictionaries, and will occasionally be seen here in the *Dictionary of Medical Derivations*. For example, the following is the main entry for the common root *chrom-*:

> ## chrom-
>
> *chroma chromatos* Greek, color of the skin, then any color; combining form signifying 'color'

The Greek is given as *chroma, chromatos* because English has borrowed both the nominative and the following genitive of the Greek word for color to make new scientific words. In medicine – particularly in histology, the microscopic study of body cells and tissues – chromatic is the term used for a substance or tissue able to be stained or colored by a dye. However, chromosome uses only the nominative stem; and the English scientific word *chroma* uses the Greek nominative in its original form.

Like all languages whose nouns have declensions of different case endings, and whose verbs have many conjugational endings, Latin and Greek words have many forms. Different parts of Latin and Greek nouns and verbs have been used over the centuries to make new scientific words. That is why the *Dictionary of Medical Derivations* sometimes shows a classical word in several forms.

What can the *Dictionary of Medical Derivations* offer that other introductory texts on medical vocabulary cannot?

The *Dictionary of Medical Derivations* offers correct and helpful etymologies. For example, the word *cataract* from *kata* Greek, down + *rrhaktes* something that rushes, drops quickly. Several contemporary medical dictionaries state that this term comes from the Greek word for waterfall. Medically, a cataract is a loss of transparency in the lens of the eye and it is difficult to perceive in what way this progressive opacity of the lens might be related to a waterfall. The word *cataract*, in fact, derives from a Greek noun whose prime meaning was sluice gate, portcullis or dense iron grating over a window, that is, something that obstructed a view – as a cataract may be said to do. In only one of the current dictionaries of medical English is this explanation offered. Instead, what the reader often finds are Latin and Greek roots apparently just copied from older dictionaries, with no research into the validity of the etymology, suggesting that the compilers have little real knowledge of Latin and Greek medical literature; indeed astounding mistakes abound in some dictionaries. In one well-known current text, for example, it states that the medical word *inoculum*, the substance injected into a body during an inoculation, derives from a Latin word *inocuus*, 'harmless'. However, there is no such Latin word. The compiler presumably mistook the spelling of *innocuus*, 'harmless'; from the same root came the English word *innocent*. Obviously inoculate has no connection with *innocuus*. Inoculate was borrowed from Medieval Latin gardening vocabulary, where *inoculare* meant literally 'to put an eye-like opening in something', and later was used for a certain method of grafting plants. The main root of the word *inoculare* is *oculus*, Latin for 'eye'. The medical doctor who first borrowed the gardening term was using *inoculare* because it is a good verb to mean 'make an eye-like, pin-prick injection in'. It has nothing to do with harmless or innocent.

As for programmed text manuals designed to teach medical terms, some are excellent; but surprising errors can be found in others. For example, in a new edition of a well-known text we find the following comment. 'The Greek word tomos means 'cutting'. From this word we build many suffixes that refer to cutting: ectomy (to cut out), tomy (to cut into), tome (an instrument that cuts), stomy (to form a new opening)'. There are two errors here. First, the noun ending *-stomy* comes from the Greek word *stoma* which means 'mouth'. It has no relationship whatsoever with the Greek root *-tom* 'cut'. The Greek word *tomos* means 'a slice, an individual cut'. It is not a gerund; it does not mean 'cutting'. A few pages further on in the same text, the reader sees this: 'Emia is a suffix from the Greek word *hema*, for blood'. The Greek word for blood is *haima*. Hema is what happened to the spelling as it came through Latin into French and English. *-Emia* is not a suffix: *-ia* is a suffix. The *-em* is a root, a contracted form of *haima* Greek, blood.

These are just some examples of the many irritants which prompted the writing of the present volume in which the reader will discover clear, accurate and helpful derivations of common medical terms. There is no better short-cut to a vast medical vocabulary than learning the Latin and Greek roots from which most medical words have evolved. Finally, the reader will find a review printed at the end of this book.

Bill Casselman, Scientific Writer

Ronald Casselman, MD, FRCS, Consultant to the Author
Judith Casselman, RN, DPHN, Consultant to the Author

a-, an-

a, an Greek, not
This very common negative prefix *a* (*an* before a vowel) appears at the beginning of many medical words. It was the usual Greek negative prefix. This *a* is called alpha privative, because alpha is the Greek name of the letter *a*, and because of the negative force of this privative *a*, because of its de*priv*ing of the root which follows it; thus:
asexual means 'involving no sexual act';
asymptomatic means 'with no symptoms';
atypical means 'not typical'.

a-mnes-ia

a not + *mnesis* Greek, remembering + *ia* medical condition
Amnesia is the pathological loss of memory. It is not forgetting for a moment where you have mislaid the keys to the car.

an-aero-bic

an not + *aer* Greek, air + *bi(ot)ikos* living < *bios* Greek, life
Anaerobic bacteria do not 'live in air', do not require molecular oxygen. Some anaerobic bacteria are killed by oxygen. Some species live with or without O_2. Anaerobic infections caused by such bacteria are, for example, tetanus and gangrene.

an-em-ia

an not + *em* short for *haima* Greek, blood + *ia* medical condition
Anemia originally meant any blood deficiency; now the general meaning of anemia is a reduced concentration of red blood cells.

an-esthet-ic

an not + *esthetikos* Greek, pertaining to feeling or sensation
General and local anesthetics are drugs that produce temporary insensitivity to pain. General anesthesia is induced before major surgery by an anesthesiologist.

an-hydr-ous

an not + *hydros* of water + *ous* English adjective ending
Anhydrous crystals contain no water molecules. Related English words from the Greek word *hydor, hydros,* 'water' are: hydro-power, hydrometer.

an-odyne

an no + *odyne* pain
Anodyne is a general term for any drug that eases pain. One may also encounter in medical literature the rarer term anodynia, 'freedom from pain'.

an-omal-y

an not + *homalos* normal, regular + *y* noun ending
Anomaly means 'abnormality'. A fetus stillborn with no heart is a fetal anomaly or fetal monster. An anomalous structure might be an extra toe.

an-orex-ia

an no + *orexis* appetite + *ia* medical condition
Anorexia is loss of normal appetite. When it leads to emaciation and is caused by emotional disorders, it is called anorexia nervosa, 'nervous appetite loss'.

an-ox-ia

an no + *oxy-* oxygen + *ia* medical condition
Anoxia is loss or deficiency of oxygen in the tissues of the body. The physiology of anoxia concerns divers, climbers, aviation scientists and doctors.

a-path-y

a no + *pathos* Greek, normal feeling + *y* noun ending
Apathy means 'lack of emotion, listless indifference to ordinary concerns of living'. *Pathos* in Greek first meant 'deep feeling', then 'disease'. See the entry for '*pathology*'.

a-phas-ia

a not + *phasis* Greek, power of speech + *ia* medical condition
Aphasia is a defect in or loss of the power of speaking, writing, or comprehending spoken or written language. Specific brain lesions cause aphasia.

a-pnea

a no + *pnoe* Greek, breathing
Apnea is stopped or interrupted breathing, due to physical imperfections of the respiratory system or to disease. Sleep apnea may be of medical significance.

a-prax-ia

a not + *praxis* Greek, action, doing something + *ia* medical condition
Apraxia is a general term for inability to perform movement for a purpose, but motor and sensory damage is not present; most apraxic episodes are due to lesions of the cerebral cortex. Motor apraxia may be illustrated by a psychiatric patient who recognizes a cup of coffee but can't raise the cup and take a sip. In amnesic apraxia, a patient might not remember how to turn on a radio, even after he is repeatedly shown the procedure.

a-rrhythm-ia

a not + *rrhythmos* Greek, timed beat in music + *ia* medical condition
A cardiac arrhythmia is a variation from the normal rhythm of the heartbeat. The read-out of an electrocardiograph visualizes such arrhythmias. An antiarrhythmic is a chemical agent or physical force that prevents or controls cardiac arrhythmias. See *anti-* entry.

a-septic

a not + *septikos* rotten, so aseptic is literally 'not rotten', hence 'not infected'
Aseptic means free of infection by micro-organisms, sterile, not contaminated. Asepsis is exclusion of bacteria from surgical sites and wound dressings.

ab, abs

ab is a Latin preposition used as a prefix to mean 'away from, out of, off of'. It adds *s* before *t* in words like abstract, abstain, abstruse. *Ab* may be shortened to *a* in words like averse. Something abnormal is 'away from the normal'. To abuse is 'to use in a manner away from what is proper'. Latin phrases used in scientific writing include:
ab ovo, from the egg, from the very beginning;
ab initio, from the beginning, initial;
ab origine, from the beginning, aboriginal.

ab-ducens

ab away from + *ducens* Latin, leading
The abducens muscle is the lateral rectus muscle of the eye, that abducts, or leads the eye away from the midline of the body, that is, it contracts to rotate the eyeball outward to the side. There is also a pair of motor nerves called the abducens nerves, the sixth cranial nerves, which arise in the brain stem and innervate the abducens muscles of the eyes.

ab-duct-or

ab away from + *duct* lead, draw + *or* agent noun ending in Latin, so that abductor is literally 'thing that leads away from'
An abductor muscle abducts or leads a body part away from the median plane of the body. The human thumb has two abductor muscles that help move the thumb away from the hand. A duct is a tube that leads or carries fluids.

ab-errant

ab away from + *errans, errantis* Latin present participle, wandering, deviating
Aberrant behavior 'wanders away' from normal behavior. *Errare* is a Latin verb that means 'to wander, to err, to make a mistake or an error'. In medieval times, a knight errant was one who travelled and wandered in search of good deeds to do.

ab-lact-ation

ab away from + *lact* milk + *ation* noun ending
-Ation is a very common suffix, in Latin, in the Romance languages, and in English, whose function is to make the root into an abstraction (condition of,

quality of, state of, manner of) or to label an action or the result of an action, or to name a process, as it does here in the word *ablactation*.

Ablactation means weaning, getting an infant used to taking solid food instead of breastfeeding. Ablactation also means cessation of maternal milk secretion.

> *Lac, lactis* is Latin for milk.
> *Lactatio* is a Latin noun that means 'secreting milk'.
> Lactose is the sugar found in milk.
> Lactase is an enzyme found in the small intestine that converts lactose into simpler sugars used by the body.
> Lactiferous ducts carry milk from the lobes of the breast to the nipple.

ab-ortion

ab away from + *ortio, ortionis* Latin, disappearing

Induced abortion is termination of a pregnancy before the fetus is viable, that is, can live on its own. Spontaneous abortion occurs due to natural disorders.

ab-rasion

ab off + *rasio, rasionis* Latin, a scraping

Abrasion is the scraping off of an area of skin or mucous membrane either due to injury or for medical reasons. To abrade means 'to scrape off'. A razor scrapes off a man's beard. To scrape or rub something out is to erase (*e, ex* away, out) it, perhaps with an eraser, in an act of erasure.

ab-reaction

ab un + reaction

Abreaction in psychiatry means emotionally reliving an experience that earlier caused anxiety and so was repressed. The word is a loan translation into English from Sigmund Freud's German coinage *abreagieren*. So the *ab* here is influenced by one way the prefix is used in German, to mean 'un' in English, for example, doing and undoing. Abreaction is unreacting, undoing the original reaction by re-experiencing it. Psychiatry calls the process catharsis, Greek for purging, in this case, cleansing the mind of the unpleasant experience.

ab-rupt

ab off + *ruptus* broken

The same root appears in rupture, 'a breaking', in corrupt, 'thoroughly broken', and in interrupt, 'break between'.

Abruptio placentae is a Latin phrase used in medicine that means 'a breaking off of the placenta'. This premature detachment of the placenta is a serious disorder of pregnancy. The placenta nourishes the fetus. If detached, blood supply to the fetus is cut off, leading to fetal death and possibly fatal maternal hemorrhage.

abs-cess

abs off + *cessus* thrown

An abscess is a collection of pus, as in the abscessed root of a tooth. The Roman medical writer Celsus, in his famous textbook *De Medicina*, published about AD 30, believed in the theory of humors. This now discredited and disproved theory of humoralism, at least 3000 years old, claimed that the body's health was regulated by four juices or humors, namely blood, phlegm, black bile and yellow bile. When these secretions were in balance, the body was healthy. If there was too much of one humor, illness resulted. Celsus and other ancient physicians thought pus was a throwing off by the body of bad humor, in this case yellow bile. So he translated into Latin a Greek word that meant a throwing off of humors. The discovery of the circulation of the blood, and later of oxygen and its role in human metabolism, put an end to the belief in humors, although the theory persisted until the end of the 18th Century. This abandoned theory lies behind many words and phrases in Western languages. It is the origin of 'bad humor' and 'good humor' and of international words like melancholy (sadness supposedly due to an excess of black bile), which in Greek was *melancholia* (melanos *black* + chole *bile*).

We now know that an abscess is the result of infection by bacteria in which a cavity of purulent, liquified material forms. It causes pain and fever and urgently needs surgical drainage if spontaneous drainage does not occur.

ab-sorb

ab away from + *sorbere* to suck up

To absorb is to take up substances into or across tissues. A familiar medical example is intestinal absorption, in which food fluids, solutes, proteins, fats and other nutrients are taken from the lumen of the intestines up into the epithelial cells lining the intestines and thence into the blood and lymph systems. Absorbent cotton readily sucks up fluids.

abs-tin-ence

abs away from + *tin, ten* Latin root, holding + *entia* noun ending

Abstinence is holding oneself away from an activity, abstaining from it, for example, refraining from the use of certain foods, drugs, or from sexual intercourse. One may choose not to vote. One who does so is an abstainer.

acanth-, ac-antha

ak Greek root, pointed part + *anthos* Greek, flower

In medicine, an acantha is a spiny, bony process of a vertebra. The pointy, prickly part of a plant is the thorn or spine. The root *ak* appears in all languages of the Indo-European family, where it means something with a sharp point. For example, in some English words derived from Latin, the *ak-* stem gives rise to acid, acetic, acne, acrid, acupuncture, acute and exacerbate.

acanth-ion

acanth spine + *ion* Greek, a diminutive suffix, that is, a noun ending meaning 'little'

The maxilla or upper jawbone has a bony crest at the front where it meets some bones of the nose. This crest itself, called the anterior nasal spine, has a tiny tip or point at its base called the acanthion.

acantho-cyte

acantho thorny + *cytos* cell

In certain blood deficiency diseases, the red blood cells or erythrocytes appear distorted by little rays of protoplasm projecting from their surfaces giving the cell a thorny look. The presence in the blood of these thorny blood cells is called acanthocytosis. A common medical suffix is *-osis,* meaning 'diseased or disordered condition'.

acanth-oma

acanth thorny + *oma* common medical noun suffix that means 'tumor, swelling'

The middle layer of the epidermis is called the prickle-cell layer of the skin. An acanthoma is a tumor there, composed of epidermal or squamous cells.

acanth-osis

acanth prickly + *osis* diseased condition

Acanthosis is diffuse thickening of the prickle-cell layer of the epidermis, for example, as seen in psoriasis. Acanthosis nigricans (Latin, *blackening*) is another skin disease with dark gray or black warty lesions in the body folds. In adults, it is often associated with internal cancer; in children, it is often benign and related to disturbance of the endocrine system or to obesity.

the acanthus leaves of classical architecture

Acanthus spinosus is a prickly-leaved plant native to the shores of the Mediterranean. In their most ornate order, Greek architects decorated the capitals of their Corinthian columns with rows of stylized acanthus leaves, which the ancient Greeks considered to be the most elegant of all leaves.

acet-

acetum Latin, vinegar, that is, something that tastes sharp < *ac* Latin root form, pointed, sharp

acet-abulum

acetum vinegar + *-abulum* Latin diminutive suffix meaning small container, thus *acetabulum* = vinegar cup
The Roman encyclopedist Pliny the Elder is the first writer to report the similarity of the pelvic socket to a vinegar cup, hence the name, acetabulum. It forms a ball-and-socket joint with the head of the femur, thus permitting great freedom of movement of the legs.

acet-ic acid

acetum vinegar + *ic* adjectival ending
When wine turns sour, the ethyl alcohol at one stage is converted to acetic acid. Ancient winemakers knew this, and thus acetic acid was the first organic acid known to science. This chemical effect also accounts for the origin of our word *vinegar*. In Latin it was *vinum acetum* 'sour wine', transformed into French as *vin aigre*, which the English in turn borrowed and then wrote as vinegar.

acet-one

acet acetic acid + *one* a Greek suffix meaning in modern chemistry 'ketone'
Acetone CH_3COCH_3 is a ketone used as a solvent and once widely used in medicine as a disinfectant skin swab before injections and vaccinations. Acetone has a unique, sweet odor and is present in normal urine, but it occurs in abnormally large amounts in the urine of those suffering from diabetes mellitus. Thus some diabetics self-test for acetone in the urine by using specially treated paper which turns color.

acetyl-choline

acetyl combining form of acetic acid + *choline* an amine present in body tissues

Acetylcholine is a neurotransmitter in nerve cells that permits such neurons to transmit electro-chemical impulses to one another across synapses. Neurotransmitters work by altering the electrical potential of the membrane of the receiving neuron. Acetylcholine is concentrated in basal ganglia neurons.

acid-

acidus Latin, sharp, sour-tasting

acid

acidus sour-tasting

Early Roman physicians knew some acids. They called vinegar *vinum acetum*, and also called it *acidum*, 'tart'. In modern chemistry, an acid is a substance which forms hydrogen ions in solution, and those ions may be displaced by a metal when a salt is formed. There are thousands of named acids, among the more familiar being acetic acid, amino acids, deoxyribonucleic acid (DNA), and folic, hydrochloric, nitric, ribonucleic (RNA), sulfuric and tannic acids. In current slang, 'acid' is LSD, lysergic acid diethylamide, a dangerous hallucinogenic drug.

acid–base balance

Equilibrium between acids and bases (alkalis) in the tissues of the human body is regulated by blood, lungs and kidneys. Normal blood is slightly alkaline, with a pH of 7.35–7.45.

acid-em-ia

acidus acid + *em* shortened form of *haima*, Greek, blood + *ia* medical condition

Abnormally high acidity of the blood. Any concentration of hydrogen ions producing a pH of less than 7 indicates acidemia.

acid-osis

acidus acid + *osis* suffix meaning 'pathological condition'

Acidosis is too much acid in body tissues due to disorders such as carbon dioxide retention, severe diarrhea, impaired kidney function, diabetes and some poisons. The buildup of excess alkalis or bases in body tissues is alkalosis.

acro-

akros Greek, high; or *akron* extremity of the body such as an arm, leg, hand, finger, toe, foot

acro-a-gnosis

akron Greek, extremity + *a* not + *gnosis* knowing, recognition of. The Greek noun *gnosis* has the same root as *know* in English.
Acroagnosis is the inability to recognize through the senses one's own arm or leg or finger. It is often the result of brain damage suffered in a stroke.

acro-an-esthesia

akron extremity + *an* not + *esthesia* sensing, feeling
Anesthesia is the chemically induced loss of pain sensation to permit performance of surgery. Acroanesthesia is anesthetizing one or more limbs or extremities. See the *esthes, esthet* entry.

acro-megaly

akros extremity + *megale* enlargement, from the Greek adjective *megas* large, big, great
Acromegaly is a growth defect after maturity in which the pituitary gland secretes extra growth hormone, causing gross enlargement of the skeletal extremities: fingers, toes, nose, jaw.

acr-om-ion

akros high + *omos* shoulder + *ion* diminutive ending meaning 'little'
The acromion is the highest point of the scapula or shoulder blade. It can be felt by pressing a finger on the upper distal end of each shoulder. Don't know where that is? See the *distal* entry.

acr-omphalus

akros high + *omphalos* navel, umbilicus

Acromphalus is a bulging or protruding navel, sometimes natural, sometimes a sign of the beginning of an umbilical hernia.

acro-myo-ton-ia

akron extremity + *myo* of muscle + *tonos* tension, stretching + *ia* medical condition
Myotonia is any disorder involving tonic spasm of muscle tissue. Therefore acromyotonia is this abnormal pulling or stretching of the muscles of the hand and foot (extremities). Such abnormal muscular contractions may cause a deformity.

acro-nym

akros high (i.e. spelled with capital letters) + *onyma* Greek, name
An acronym is a word formed from the initial letters of a phrase or compound name, e.g. LASER from 'light amplification by stimulated emission of radiation'. AIDS is an acronym for 'acquired immune deficiency syndrome'. Modern clinical practice abounds with acronyms, like TURP for 'transurethral prostatectomy', or SIDS for 'sudden infant death syndrome'.

acro-phob-ia

akros high + *phobos* fear + *ia* medical condition
Acrophobia is a morbid fear of heights. Most humans exercise reasonable caution in high places, but acrophobics have an utter terror of heights.

actino-

aktis, aktinos Greek, ray

actino-therapy

aktis, aktinos ray + *therapeia* tending the sick, remedy, cure, treatment
Actinotherapy is the treatment of a disease with special rays, for example ultraviolet radiation. Actinic rays such as those of ultraviolet radiation produce a chemical action. An actinogenic source produces actinic rays. See the *gen* entry. The study of radiant energy and the biochemical effects of light is actinology.

ac-

acutus Latin, sharp, pointed or *acus* needle

acute

acutus Latin, sharp or pointed-in-time, hence quick

An acute disease comes to a crisis point quickly, has rapid onset and is of short duration. A chronic disease is the opposite of an acute disease. A chronic disorder persists, or lasts for a long time. Chronic comes from a Greek adjective *chronikos* which means 'of time, enduring'. But neither acute nor chronic necessarily identifies the severity of the disease. The common cold and smallpox are both acute infections. Athlete's foot and leprosy are both chronic.

Acute has another use in clinical or hospital jargon, where it may mean 'requiring immediate surgical attention'. For example, a patient presents with severe abdominal pain, but symptoms may not make it clear whether the patient has a ruptured appendix or a perforated ulcer. It may be said in the emergency room that the patient has an 'acute abdomen'. Urgent surgical exploration of the abdomen is needed to make a precise diagnosis.

acu-puncture

acus Latin, a needle + puncture

Chinese pain control method involving piercing areas of the body along peripheral nerves with fine needles, to relieve pain, for anesthesia, and for therapy.

ad

ad is a Latin preposition seen in English in the phrase, 'an *ad hoc* committee', a committee formed to address a specific problem

Literally, *ad hoc* means 'to this one thing'. Something done *ad nauseam* is done 'to sickness', to such a disgusting extent that it makes one want to vomit. A stand-up comedian may *ad lib* a few jokes, that is, improvize the jokes off the cuff. *Ad lib* is short for the Latin phrase *ad libitum,* 'at one's pleasure' or 'as one wishes'. It is also written in prescriptions where *ad lib* means 'freely' or 'as much and as often as desired'. Naturally the invitation to such pharmacological freedom is rare.

However, *ad* is more frequent in English as a prefix in front of other Latin roots, a few of which are given below. In medicine *ad* is also used as a suffix. See the next entry. When *ad* precedes certain consonants, its *d* is assimilated to the first letter of the following root, for example in words like accept, affix, aggressive, apparatus, arrange and assert. Such assimilation eases pronunciation. A well-known legal document with an assimilated *ad* is affidavit, a Latin verb form that means literally 'one has sworn *to* it on *faith*'. Compare *fides,* 'faith', in Latin.

ad-duct

ad to, toward + *duct* Latin verb root, lead, carry, draw

To adduct is to draw toward the midline of the body. To adduct fingers and toes is to draw them toward the axis line of their limb. Muscles do this. For example, the adductor muscle of the thumb draws the thumb inward toward the palm of the hand. Often adductor muscles are paired with abductor muscles.

ad-hesion

ad to + *haesio, haesionis* Latin, a sticking, a clinging

Adhesion in medicine is the abnormal sticking together of membranes as a result of inflammation caused by injury or surgery. The band of fibers that holds structures together abnormally is also called an adhesion. It is fibrous connective tissue that has grown into clots formed in the fluids produced by inflammation. Thus inflamed parts that should move loosely in, for example, joints, lungs, or abdominal organs may adhere to one another, i.e. get stuck together.

The root shows up in other English words too. Adhesive tape sticks things together. One who sticks to a philosophy or point of view is an adherent. A coherent argument holds (sticks) together. An inherent quality is characteristic of a person or an object. It sticks in the object, is innate.

ad-nexa

ad to + *nexa* Latin, connections, ties, bonds

In anatomy adnexa are adjoining parts of an organ, appendages or accessory structures. The adnexa of the eye include the eyelid, eye muscles, orbit, the tear gland and tear duct. The adnexa of the uterus include the Fallopian tubes and the ovaries. Related words are nexus, a common bond among members of a series, and words like annex and connect.

ad-renal

ad to + *renalis* Latin, pertaining to the kidneys < *ren, renis* kidney

One adrenal gland sits atop each kidney. Each adrenal gland consists of two distinct organs. An outer adrenal cortex surrounds an inner adrenal medulla. The positions are easy to remember if you know that *cortex* means 'outer bark' in Latin, and *medulla* means 'little thing in the middle'. Their being found together however is simply an accident of anatomical evolution.

The adrenal medulla is part of the sympathetic nervous system. When stimulated, it pours adrenaline (also called epinephrine) into the bloodstream. Epinephrine's basic effect is to get organs ready for exertion. Blood is diverted to muscles, the heart pumps more blood, and glucose for fuel is released from the liver into the bloodstream.

The adrenal cortex is an endocrine (ductless) gland that secretes many hormones including the corticosteroids that are important in maintaining a kind of chemical *status quo* in the changing environment of the body, thus protecting living tissue, which does not tolerate extreme chemical ups and downs in its immediate surroundings. These steroid hormones prevent upheaval of body chemistry by forces such as illness, injury, mental stress and great exertion. Without this chemical mediation by the hormones of the adrenal cortex, internal chemical fluctuations might prove lethal.

af-fect

ad (with the *d* assimilated to the following *f*) to + *fectus* a thing done, something made

The great pioneer of psychiatry Sigmund Freud borrowed the Latin word *affectus* and used it in German. Freud's *Affekt* also had a meaning close to that used by the Roman Cicero, for whom *affectus* meant 'a state of body or mind produced in one by some influence'. Today affect can have a general meaning of emotion, feeling, or mood. But in psychiatry, affect means the emotional tone of an individual's response to a particular situation. Schizophrenic patients may exhibit a lack of appropriate affect. Most of us don't laugh when we accidentally burn ourselves. A schizophrenic person might do so.

ag-glutin-ate

ad > *ag* (with the *d* assimilated to the following *g*) to + *gluten* Latin, glue + *ate* verb ending

In medicine, to agglutinate is to cause to stick together, for example, in the agglutination or clumping together of certain cells like bacteria or red blood cells. An agglutinin is an antibody that causes clumping of a specific antigen-carrying cell. Part of determining blood types involves an agglutination test which identifies unknown antigens. The same test is part of tissue matching and also sometimes helps determine a patient's susceptibility to certain disorders. When incompatible blood types of different groups are mixed, agglutination of blood cells occurs. Sometimes such cell clumping is fatal.

-ad

Here *-ad* is a suffix, a particle tacked on the end of the root to extend its meaning. In anatomical description, one finds words like dorsad, ventrad, cephalad and orad.

cephal-ad

kephale Greek, head + *ad* toward

Cephalad in anatomical description means 'toward the head', or 'toward the topmost aspect of a structure'.

dors-ad

dorsum Latin, the back + *ad* toward

Dorsad means 'toward the back'. *Dorsum* is the back in Latin. A dorsal fin protrudes from the back of a fish. One may even encounter the anatomical term dorsocephalad, 'toward the back of the head'. See the *dorsal* entry.

or-ad

os, oris mouth + *ad* toward

Orad is 'toward the mouth'.

ventr-ad

venter Latin, belly, stomach + *ad* toward

Ventrad means 'toward the stomach', 'toward the ventral side', or 'toward the ventral aspect of a structure'. See the *ventral* entry.

adeno-

aden Greek, acorn, gland shaped like an acorn

aden-itis

aden gland + *itis* inflammation of

Adenitis is inflammation (see *i* entry) of a gland or gland-like structure like a lymph node. Acute throat infections in children may be accompanied by cervical adenitis or neck adenitis in which the lymph nodes of the neck are swollen, inflamed and tender. The suffix *-itis* is one of the most common in medicine and has the general meaning of inflammation.

adeno-carcin-oma

aden gland + *karkinos* Greek, crab, cancer + *oma* tumor
Adenocarcinoma is a malignant tumor of glandular tissue or one in which the
tumor cells form glandular structures. See the entry for *cancer* to explain the
'crab' connection.

aden-oids

aden gland + *oid* like, similar, a common English suffix from
the Greek noun *eides* which means 'form, shape'
Adenoids looked to 19th Century physicians 'like glands'. In fact, adenoids are a
mass of lymphoid tissue at the back of a child's throat, which if enlarged due to
inflammation may obstruct breathing, or cause snoring, a nasal voice or mouth
breathing. If inflammation is resistant to antibiotics and stubbornly persistent,
adenoids may be cut out during a now rare adenoidectomy, a surgical procedure
of whose name the component roots are: *aden* gland + *oid* like + *ec* out + *tomy*
cutting.

aden-oma

aden gland + *oma* tumor
Adenoma is a benign epithelial tumor of glandular tissue or one in which the
tumor cells form glandular structures. The Greek suffix *-oma* is very common at
the end of medical words denoting tumors, both benign and malignant. The
occurrence of many adenomas (or adenomata, the formal plural) is termed
adenomatosis where *-osis* is a frequent medical word ending denoting diseased
condition or abnormal increase.

adeno-sine

aden gland
This biochemical name is a blend of two other chemical names, adenine and
ribose. Adenosine is an important compound that is part of DNA, RNA, many
enzymes, and other biochemicals involved in, for example, storing energy and
releasing it to muscles.

AMP or adenosine monophosphate

This biochemical found in muscle tissue is also important in metabolism. Cyclic
adenosine monophosphate or cAMP is a messenger chemical in complex actions
of many hormones.

ATP or adenosine triphosphate

This biochemical is present in all cells and participates in the storage of energy by the cell. It is especially important in muscle cells where it assists in the transfer of energy needed to expand and contract muscle fibers.

adeno-virus

aden Greek, gland, of the adenoids + *virus* Latin, poison, venom; medical meaning: virus

This large group of viruses was so named because specific ones were first discovered in adenoid tissue in the human throat. Adenoviruses cause many infections of the upper respiratory tract, including the common cold. See the *virus* entry.

adipo-

adeps, adipis Latin, lard, hog fat, fatty body tissue

adipose

adipis of fat + *osus* Latin adjectival ending meaning 'full of, abounding in'

Adipose in plain English is now a somewhat outmoded synonym for fat, corpulent, or overweight. But adipose tissue is a current medical term to describe connective tissue rich in fat cells and found chiefly under the skin as a layer of insulation and as a reservoir of cell fuel stored as fat.

adip-osis

adipis of fat + *osis* Greek noun ending meaning 'disease'

Adiposis is fatness or obesity. Hepatic adiposis is a fatty change in liver cells. Cerebral adiposis involves abnormal deposits of fat in brain tissue.

adipo-kinin

adipis of fat + *kinesis* Greek, movement of + *in* noun ending for organic chemical compound

Adipokinin is a pituitary hormone which speeds up adipokinesis, the movement and use of stored body fat. The same Greek root for moving gives us our English word for motion pictures, cinema, from Greek *kinema* 'something that moves'.

adipo-lysis

adipis of fat + *lysis* Greek, a breaking up

Adipolysis is the digestion of fats. A synonym is lipolysis, where the Greek word for fat *lipos* is used as the root instead of its Latin equivalent *adeps, adipis*. See the *lipo-* entry.

-agog, -agogue

agogos Greek adjective, leading, inducing, helping to produce, drawing toward

emmen-agogue

emmenia Greek, the menses < *men* Greek, a month + *agogos* leading, inducing

An emmenagogue is any chemical agent that helps induce menstruation, the monthly discharge of blood from the non-pregnant uterus.

galact-agogue

gala, galactos Greek, milk + *agogos* inducing

A galactagogue is a chemical agent that helps promote the flow of milk in the breasts of nursing mothers.

hypn-agogue

hypnos Greek, of sleep + *agogos* inducing

An hypnagogue helps induce sleepiness or drowsiness.

secret-agogue

secreta Latin, secretions + *agogos* inducing

A secretagogue is any chemical agent that stimulates the production of secretions. Related English words are synagogue, 'a place that leads people together', specifically a Jewish place of worship; demagogue, 'one who leads the people together', from Greek *demos* 'the people', but with the implication of making false claims and appealing to prejudice in order to gain power; and pedagogue or pedagog, 'one who leads the children', that is, a teacher. Pedagogy is the art or profession of teaching. Sometimes pedagogue carries the negative connotation of a dry, boring teacher. In classical Greece a *paidagogos* was the literate slave who accompanied children to a school or taught them at home.

alb-

albus Latin, flat white. Shining white is *candidus*, also used in medical words. See the *candid-* entry.

albino

albino Portuguese 'whitey', 'little white one'

An albino is a person born with a congenital defect that results in less than normal pigment in eyes, hair and skin. Albinism often presents as pale skin, white hair and pink eyes. One interesting suggestion concerning the origin of the word in Portuguese is that 15th Century Portuguese navigators sailing around Africa encountered their first albino persons among negroid peoples. Having never seen a 'white' black person, the sailors thought they must be covered with plaster dust. A Latin word for plasterer is *albinus*.

albumin

albumen Latin noun, whiteness

Albumin is a white protein found in most animal tissues. It is one of the proteins in blood plasma. It is soluble in water, and curdles when heated. Egg white, also called albumen (note the 'e'), contains much albumin. The amount of albumin in blood, urine and other body fluids can be measured and is a useful marker for various disorders.

albumin-uria

albumin + ouron Greek, urine + *ia* medical condition

A constant excess of albumin in the urine may be a sign of kidney disease. A temporary excess can be merely the result of strenuous exercise.

Related words in English from the *alb-* root include the neuter Latin adjective giving a word for a book of blank white pages, an album. A white vestment worn by some Christian priests is an alb. A poetic name for England is Albion, 'little white place', so called because Roman and French invaders noticed the white cliffs of Dover. Albescent is a scientific adjective that means 'whitish'. To daub a wall was originally to whitewash it. Daub derives from an Old French verb *dauber*, which is just the Latin verb *de-albare*, 'to whitewash, to whiten, to plaster', containing the emphatic prefix *de* + *albare* = literally 'to whiten thoroughly'.

-algia, algo-

algos Greek, pain, equivalent to the Latin *dolor*. *Algia* was an irregular plural form

The most common English word containing this root is *nostalgia*, homesickness or any sentimental longing to return to the recent past or for objects of the past. Homer uses the word *nostos,* 'a homeward journey, a return home', constantly in the Odyssey when describing Ulysses' pining for his little native island of Ithaca.

algo-phobia

algos pain + *phobos* Greek, fear + *ia* medical condition

Algophobia is an obsessive or excessive dread of pain, a morbid dwelling on the thought of pain yet to be experienced, far beyond the normal person's distress when specialized nerve endings communicate pain to the brain.

an-algesic

an not + *algesis* Greek, the feeling of pain

An analgesic is a drug that relieves pain while the patient remains conscious, for example, common aspirin. Analgesia is the state thus attained.

hyper-algesia

hyper above, beyond normal + *algesia* feeling pain

Hyperalgesia is an abnormal sensitivity to pain, sometimes abetted by algophobia (see above).

my-algia

mys, myos Greek, muscle + *algia* feeling pain

Myalgia is any muscle pain.

neur-algia

neuron Greek, nerve + *algia* feeling pain

Neuralgia, beloved of the copywriters who compose patent medicine labels is, in medicine proper, any severe, excruciating nerve pain. Migrainous neuralgia, for example, is an older term for cluster headaches.

oste-algia

osteon Greek, bone + *algia* feeling pain
Ostealgia is pain due to any bone abnormality or perceived 'pain in the bones'.

ot-algia

ous, otos Greek, ear + *algia* feeling pain
Otalgia is earache or any ear pain. Some ear pains have specific names, such as geniculate neuralgia, involving the geniculate ganglion with the pain limited to the middle ear and auditory canal.

allo-

allos Greek adjective, akin to the Latin *alius*; both have the basic sense of 'another' and the developed sense of foreign, outside the self, other, different, abnormal

allergen

allergeia allergy + *gen* Greek root form, making, producing, causing
An allergen is any substance able to induce the hypersensitivity of an allergic response. In allergy tests, allergens are purified proteins of suspect substances such as food, pollen, or bacteria.

all-ergy

allos outside the self, external + *ergeia* a working
Although allergic responses were recognized early in medical history, the clinical entity was first named in 1905 by the German doctor Clemens von Pirquet who recognized it as a body's abnormal reaction to foreign proteins. Allergic people form antibodies against substances that are not harmful to normal people. The immune responses of allergy-sufferers are chemically too finely tuned. Pirquet coined the German word *Allergie* on the analogy of *Energie*, taking the very basic meaning of the Greek roots in energy to mean roughly 'work inside the body', so that allergy meant 'something that works first from outside the body', that is, the allergens of pollen and food come from sources external to the patient. It is a clumsy use of Greek, but the word stuck. And English was not immune to borrowing it.

all-esthesia

allos in another place + *esthesia* feeling, sensation
Allesthesia can be simply illustrated. I touch you on the left arm, but you experience the sensation of the touch on your right arm. Allesthesia is seen in certain mental disorders and sometimes in a patient who has suffered a cerebral insult such as a stroke.

allo-eroticism

allos another person + *erotikos* Greek, pertaining to sexual love
This term in psychology labels the focusing of sexuality outward toward other people, and is the opposite of autoeroticism whose classic instance is masturbation. Alloeroticism also expresses itself in sexual fantasies and daydreams.

allo-tropic

allos another person + *tropikos* Greek, turning toward
In psychology, an allotropic person is one who cares about other people and is not self-centered. The allotrope may even be preoccupied with others' well-being to his own personal detriment. A synonyn for allotropic from popular psychology is 'other-directed'.

alve-olus

alveus Latin, a trough, a hollow, a tub, a cell in a honeycomb + *olus* diminutive ending, 'small'
A dental alveolus is a tooth socket, one of the cavities in either jaw in which are embedded the roots of a tooth. The plural is alveoli. The maxilla is the upper jaw. The mandible is the lower jaw. Teeth are arranged in a maxillary arch and a mandibular arch. The bony prominence on each jawbone that holds teeth is called the alveolar ridge.

Pulmonary alveoli are the tiny air sacs of the lungs, found at the end of each bronchiole in clusters like little grapes. The walls of alveoli are one cell thick and surrounded by very small blood vessels called capillaries. During breathing, it is across the alveolar membrane that carbon dioxide leaves capillary blood and is exhaled as a gas, while oxygen inhaled as a gas into the lungs diffuses into capillary blood and bonds with hemoglobin, so that the blood can carry oxygen to other body cells.

ambul-

ambulare Latin, to walk

ambul-ance

ambulantia Late Latin noun, the act of walking

An ambulance was originally any vehicle that helped patients move about. The first *ambulancia* was Spanish. Queen Isabella introduced a special wagon to carry the wounded at the Siege of Malaga in 1487.

ambul-ator-y

ambulare to walk + *ator* agent suffix in Latin equal to 'er' in English, so *ambulator* = walker + *y* adjectival suffix

An ambulatory patient is able to walk, is not confined to a hospital bed. Ambulatory care clinics are popular now, to avoid expensive in-patient services.

somn-ambul-ism

somnus Latin, sleep + *ambul* walk + *ism* noun suffix indicating a condition or a theory

Somnambulism or sleep-walking occurs in the deepest part of sleeping, Stage 4 of non-REM sleep, when there is no rapid eye movement, little dreaming, plenty of delta waves (slow brain waves of large amplitude), rhythmic breathing and good muscle tone. Sleep-walking is only classified as a sleep disorder if it recurs frequently and significantly disrupts the patient's life. A synonyn of the verb somnambulate is noctambulate, to walk at night, with a prefix from the Latin *nox, noctis*, 'night'.

Related words in English from the *ambul-* stem include to amble (to walk at a leisurely gait) and to ramble (to walk idly with no specific goal), from *ambulare* and *re-ambulare*. Circumambient, from *circum*, 'around' and *ambiens*, 'walking', is used in scientific writing to mean 'surrounding, enclosing, nearby'. To circumambulate a park is to walk around it or around in it. A perambulator, the British word for a baby carriage, often shortened to pram, is simply a synonym for stroller, with the roots *per*, 'through' + *ambulator*, 'walker'. A preamble is an introductory statement or preface, but is literally 'a walking in front of', with the Latin prefix *prae*, 'before, in front of'. *Prae* is also part of prefix, of course, from Latin *praefixus*, 'anything set in the front of something else'.

amnio-

amnion Greek, inner sac enclosing fetus < *amnos* Greek, lamb

amnio-cent-esis

amnion sac enclosing fetus + *kent* Greek root form, puncture + *esis* Greek noun ending, action of

Amniocentesis is a diagnostic procedure in which, early in a pregnancy, at about the 16th week, a small sample of amniotic fluid is aspirated through a hollow needle put through the uterine wall. If done late in the pregnancy, the procedure can be performed through the cervix. Chemical analyses of the fluid and genetic analysis of the fetal cellular debris in the fluid may help determine the health of the fetus and the presence of some congenital defects such as Down's syndrome or Tay-Sachs disease.

amnion

amnion Greek, caul, inner sac enclosing fetus < *amnos* Greek, lamb

The amnion is an inner membrane that forms a bag containing the fetus floating in amniotic fluid. In Classical Greek *amnion* meant amniotic sac or caul. If a baby is born with a piece of amnion still on its head, this piece is termed a caul. *Amnos* was a Greek word for lamb, so *amnion* meant 'little lamb-like thing', that is, lambskin. The ancient Greeks named the amniotic sac 'lambskin' because it is, after all, even in humans, a very soft leathery membrane. Latin and then English borrowed amnion directly and with the same meaning.

amnio-rrhexis

amnion + *rrhexis* Greek, a rupturing, a bursting

The natural rupture of the amnion usually occurs in the first stage of labor. Most babies are born head first. In this early stage, muscles of the uterus contract while those of the cervix relax. The baby's head enters the cervix and a pocket of the amniotic sac containing fluid is trapped in front of the baby's head. After more contractions, when this pocket is squeezed, the amnion bursts.

amniotic fluid

amniotikos Greek adjective, pertaining to the amnion

The fluid supports and protects the fetus like a liquid shock-absorber, from the fourth week until birth. It also takes fetal urine, equalizes the pressure around the fetus, and acts as a medium to exchange materials between the mother and her fetus.

amniotic sac

amniotikos + saccus Latin, bag

The amniotic sac comprises an inner membrane, the amnion, and an outer membrane. The outer membrane is the chorion which forms the fetal part of the placenta. A popular name in English is 'the bag of waters'. During childbirth, the amniotic sac or bag of waters ruptures due to forceful uterine contractions. Popular speech reports this as 'her bag of waters broke' or 'my waters broke'.

amnio-tomy

amnion + *tome* Greek, a surgical incision
If the bag of waters does not rupture naturally during the early stages of labor, a doctor may surgically rupture the amnion to facilitate labor.

amyl-

amilum Latin, starch < *amylon* Greek, starch, from *a* not + *myle* a flour mill
The general semantic force of *amylon* was 'not milled'. The ancient Greeks got starch from unmilled wheat. In biochemistry, amyl is an aliphatic hydrocarbon radical whose chemical formula is $C_5 H_{11}$.

amyl-ase

amyl starch + *ase* suffix in biochemistry meaning 'enzyme'
Amylase is a common enzyme in saliva, pancreatic juices and in some foods and bacteria. It acts as a catalyst in reactions that break down starch into simpler carbohydrates. Amylase in saliva begins the breakdown of starches into simple sugars and nutrients in a form the body can metabolize.

amyl nitrite

amyl aliphatic hydrocarbon radical $C_5 H_{11}$ + *nitrite* a salt of nitrous acid
Amyl nitrite is a highly flammable liquid vasodilator (dilates vessels) whose fumes are sometimes inhaled to relieve the pain of angina pectoris. For some patients, it has unpleasant side-effects.

amylo-pectin

amylo starch + *pectin* a polymer of sugar acids < *pektos* Greek, jellied, congealed
Pectin was named from its use in making jam. It forms a gel when cooked with sugar. Amylopectin is the insoluble component of starch. The gel-forming quality of pectins gives starches their 'stickiness'.

25

amylo-psin

amylo starch + *psin* contraction of 'pepsin', an enzyme < *pepsis* Greek, digestion

Amylopsin is the enzyme in pancreatic juice that converts starch to sugars. It is the pancreatic amylase. Certain kinds of enzymes carry the same suffix, e.g. pepsin, trypsin.

amyl-ose

amyl starch + *ose* suffix indicating a carbohydrate, especially a sugar (sucrose, fructose, lactose)

Amylose is the part of starch that is soluble, due to the presence of straight chains of glucose units. Also called amylogen (starch-producing). Amylosuria is the presence of excess amylose in the urine.

amyl-uria

amyl starch + *uria* urine condition

Amyluria is the presence of excess starch in the urine.

ana[1]

ana Greek, up, on, again, against

The Greek preposition *ana* shows up in dozens of common medical words.

ana-bol-ic

ana up + *bole* Greek, the act of building something + *ikos* adjective ending

Anabolic substances help the process of changing nutrients into chemicals that build body cells. For example, controversial anabolic steroids help athletes build muscle, but at the cost to their future health of long-term, deleterious side-effects. Breaking down body cells is catabolism from Greek *kata*, 'down'. The combined processes of anabolism and catabolism are called metabolism from Greek *meta* 'across' with the added semantic hint of 'change'.

ana-chron-ism

ana against + *chronos* Greek, time + *ism* noun ending that indicates action, abstract state, doctrine, moral practice; in medicine, the suffix *-ism* often denotes an abnormal condition brought on by excess, e.g. alcoholism

An anachronism is an error against time. For example, there is a movie in which Julius Caesar is seen wearing a wristwatch! A medical anachronism would be the present-day use of leeches to 'bleed' a patient, a medical practice discredited for more than a century.

ana-log

ana up, near, beside + *logos* Greek adjective, gathered < *legein* to collect; both roots comprised a Greek noun *analogia* which came to mean 'proportion, relation, resemblance'

Analogos in Greek meant originally 'mathematically proportionate', or 'resembling'.

In comparative anatomy, an analog is a part or organ similar in function, but different in origin. The classic examples of analogous organs are lungs and gills. The quality of being similar in function but different in origin is analogy. Analogy also has a more general definition of similarity or correspondence.

But there are also organs and structures that are similar in origin, but different in function. These are said to be homologous; for example, arms and wings are homologous. *Homos* is a Greek adjective that means 'same'.

ana-lysis

ana up + *lysis* Greek, loosening, breaking up

The basic meaning of analysis is breaking something up to determine its component parts. The noun is widespread in all branches of science, and the 'something' broken up may be a chemical, a belief, an emotion, etc.

ana-stom-osis

ana up + *stoma* Greek, mouth, opening + *osis* process of making

An anastomosis is a connection between two body parts, or an opening between two body parts that are naturally separate. Anastomosis may be surgical, or caused by disease or injury. The verb is to anastomose. Blood vessels may be anastomosed for a variety of medical reasons. Side-to-side anastomosis creates an opening between two adjacent body structures. End-to-end anastomosis joins two body structures by their ends. Advanced cancer of the stomach may necessitate a complete gastrectomy. After the entire stomach is removed, the esophagus may be connected to the duodenum in an anastomotic surgical procedure called an esophagoduodenostomy. The plural is anastomoses.

ana·tomy

ana up + *tome* Greek, a slicing, a cutting

The original sense of anatomy persists, the cutting up of a body. More broadly, anatomy now means study of the structure of living organisms. Gross anatomy, subject of the oldest medical-school joke still making the rounds, is anatomical study with the naked eye. Microscopic anatomy uses the full armament of modern medical instrumentation to study bodily structures.

an·eurysm

ana through + *eurysma* Greek, a widening < *eurys* wide + *isma* - ism, which denotes an abnormal condition

An aneurysm is a bulging out in the wall of an artery. The weak spot in the arterial wall is often the result of atherosclerosis in which fatty plaques form in the linings of the artery and so weaken it. High blood pressure, bacterial infection, trauma and genetic predisposition are other causes. Common sites are the lower aorta and the arteries at the base of the brain. Drugs provide certain symptomatic relief but surgical resection of the artery is sometimes called for.

ana²

ana Greek, without. Greek also used *ana* as a negative preposition that meant 'without'. It was a double negative, a combination of alpha privative *an* + another *a* privative.

ana·phylaxis

ana without + *phylaxis* Greek, protection

Anaphylaxis is a severe allergic reaction to a protein or other chemical to which a person has become hypersensitized by previous exposure. You are allergic to shellfish, but you eat clams anyway. Within minutes you suffer a violent reaction. Itching, edema and possibly anaphylactic shock may result. Anaphylactic shock is sometimes fatal, but prompt treatment with epinephrine and other drugs is effective. When Charles Richet studied the phenomenon and coined the term in 1902, he thought in error that the victim's immunity to a specific chemical might have been destroyed by first exposure, and so the victim would be 'without protection'.

anal

The anus is the opening of the rectum on the body surface.
Latin *anus* is probably related to the Roman word *annus*, a ring,
circle, hence a cyclical year. Compare words like annual,
annuity and AD for *anno Domini* 'in the year of our Lord'.

anal fissure

analis modern scientific Latin, of the anus + *fissura* Latin, a rip,
split, groove

An anal fissure is a small rip in the skin of the anus that develops into a painful
groove-like ulcer, usually due to straining at stool during constipation. If it does
not heal after the constipation is corrected, it is reparable by surgery.

However, there are two meanings for fissure in medicine, the pathological
one we have mentioned, and the other, natural one. In the anatomy of the brain,
natural clefts or grooves occur in the cerebral hemispheres. They are deep folds
in the cerebral cortex, the outer covering of the brain. They are named after
early anatomists, e.g. the fissure of Rolando, the fissure of Sylvius.

anal fistula

analis modern scientific Latin, of the anus + *fistula* Latin,
waterpipe, tube

A fistula is an abnormal passage between two internal organs, or between an
organ and the surface of the body. Anal fistula or *fistula in ano* is a pathological
opening from the rectum to the skin near the anus. It begins with a localized
infection of the mucous membranes of the rectum or anus that does not heal but
grows and ulcerates. Surgical correction is effective.

anal impotence

analis modern scientific Latin, of the anus + *im, in* not +
potentia, power to perform

Anal impotence is a term in psychoanalysis to describe the common plight of
being incapable of having a bowel movement when other people are present.
Such modesty is widespread and of no psychoanalytic concern whatsoever –
unless the patient makes it so. All cultures do not share this fecal shyness.
Among the ruins of Roman baths, archaeologists have found three- and four-
seater marble toilets with no partitions. The ancient Romans chatted amiably
with neighboring fellow defecators while at stool. But nowadays we do not.
Who is to say which habit encourages healthier bowels?

anal sphincter

analis + *sphinkter* Greek, squeezer, constrictor

The anal sphincters are two sets of constricting ring muscles, one inside the rectum, the other external, around the rectal tube. These sphincters open and close the anal orifice before and after defecation.

Other English words and medical terms contain a similar root, all of them related to the Greek verb *sphingein* 'to bind tight, to squeeze, to clutch, to pulse'. The sphinx of ancient Greece and Egypt clutched victims in its paws. The pupillary sphincter is composed of circular fibers in the iris that constrict the pupil of the eye. A medical instrument called a sphygmometer is used to measure the pulse. See *sphygmo* 'pulse' entry. A sphygmoscope renders the pulse beat visible. Asphyxia means no oxygen or too little oxygen getting into the blood through the lungs, with possibly fatal results. Asphyxia may be caused by accidents like choking, electric shock, drowning, or inhaling poison gas. Cardiopulmonary resuscitation may revive the victim, and prevent brain damage due to lack of oxygen. But the old meaning of asphyxia was 'no detectable pulse' from the Greek roots *a* not + *sphyxis* pulsing, throbbing, clutching. Because this pulseless state was associated with breathing difficulties, the word gradually acquired its present meaning.

pruritus ani

pruritus Latin, itching + *ani* of the anus

Pruritus ani is known more humbly as itchy asshole, usually neuritic and transient, but it may involve anal skin. It is easily treated. Bathing regularly is a good start.

ano-rectal

anus + *rectum* Latin, straight, from the old medical Latin phrase *rectum intestinum* 'the straight portion of the great intestine'

Anorectal refers to the anus and the rectum considered as a single unit or location.

ano-perineal

anus + (see *perineum* entry)

Anoperineal refers to the anus and the perineum, the area between the anus and the vaginal opening in females, between the anus and the scrotum in males. In anatomy, perineum includes not only the surface structures of this area but also the area below a group of various muscles called the pelvic diaphragm.

andro-

aner, andros Greek, man, male. The root is most familiar in the personal name Andrew, from Greek *andraios,* 'manly'. Because of the Christian Saint Andrew, it takes many international forms like *André, Andrei, Andreas and Andrea.*

andro-gen

andro male + *gen* Greek, producing, making
Androgens are hormones like testosterone and androsterone that maintain secondary male sexual characteristics such as deep voice and facial hair. These hormones are secreted by the adrenal cortex, testes and in small amounts in the female by the ovaries.

andro-gloss-ia

andro male + *glossa* Greek, tongue, speaking + *ia* medical condition
Androglossia is the possession by a female of a deep voice with male qualities.

andro-gyn-y

andro male + *gyne* Greek, female + *y* noun suffix
Androgyny is a condition in which male and female sexual characteristics are present in the same individual. Although the word can apply to both physical and behavioral blending, an androgyne can be labelled as male or female. Unlike such an androgenous individual, an hermaphrodite cannot be so easily assigned as male or female. In the pseudo-hermaphrodite, external genitalia are of one sex and internal organs of the other sex. These terms are not synonyms for bisexual or effeminate. Some psychological literature uses androgyny to describe biological males with female characteristics, and then reverses the roots to form the word *gynandry* in describing biological females with male characteristics. Clear? Why, it's almost as confusing as sex itself!

andr-oid

aner, andros male or human being + *oid* adjectival suffix meaning 'like, similar to'
In science fiction, androids are robots that look like humans. In medicine, android means resembling a male. The term was happily employed in the title of

Phillip K. Dick's novel *Do Androids Dream of Electric Sheep?* on which the 1982 film *Blade Runner* was loosely based.

andro-phobia

andro male + *phobos* Greek, fear of

Androphobia is fear of the male sex, just as gynephobia is fear of the female sex.

mis-andry

misos hatred + *andreia* Greek, masculinity

This word, long lost and buried in early 20th Century psychology texts, is due for revival. Its mate, misogyny (hatred of women) is everywhere in the popular press. But equally ubiquitous is misandry, 'hatred of men'. Its spiteful, misandrous adherents fume and seethe on every media corner. And misandry is an apt label for their pathological hatred of men.

angina, angina pectoris

angina Latin, a choking pain + *pectoris* Latin, of the chest

Angina pectoris is excruciating pain starting in the left chest and shooting down the left arm and sometimes into the neck, caused by low oxygen supply to the muscles of the heart. Two small branches of the aorta called the coronary arteries supply oxygenated blood to heart muscles. *Coronarius* is the Latin adjective meaning 'of or like a corona, a crown', since the coronary arteries encircle the upper area of the heart like a crown. If these coronary arteries become hardened, degenerated and clogged with lipids, as in atherosclerosis, they cannot expand properly to supply increased blood to the heart during times of exertion. The agonizing pain of angina stops the victim from all exertion and tells him something is wrong with the coronary arteries. Diet, drugs like amyl nitrite, reduced exertion and surgery to increase blood supply to the heart all assist in preventing recurrence.

Other English words and foreign terms contain a similar root, all of them related to the ancient Indo-European root *ankh* 'narrow, constricted'.
- Anger was originally felt to be a narrow, tight, choking rage. Anguish is distress of slighter force than anger.
- To angle is to fish with a hook. An angler is such a fisherman. Both words have the Old English or Anglo-Saxon root *angul*, 'fish hook, thing bent and narrowed'.
- Anglo-Saxon recalls the Angles, Germanic invaders of Britain from a narrow angle of land between the peninsula of Denmark and the European mainland. *Angle-land* evolved into the word *England*. Similarly, *ænglisc*, originally a term for the Angles' dialect, became the word *English*.

- Angostura bitters is a digestive tonic made from the bark of a Venezuelan tree. Both tree and tonic are named after the Venezuelan town of Angostura, which means 'the narrows of a river' in Spanish.
- *Angst* in German is an anxious, depressed feeling.
- Ankle, where the leg is slender or narrow, and the joint where the foot 'hooks' to the leg, where the foot forms an angle with the leg, comes from Old English *ancleow*, which has the same *ankh* root.

angio-

angeion Greek, a little box, container, chest, pail, and then a bodily vessel that carried a fluid such as blood or lymph

angio-cardio-gram

angeion blood vessel + *kardia* Greek, heart + *gram* Greek, root form, something written or recorded

An angiocardiogram is the X-ray film taken of the heart and larger vessels after an opaque dye has been introduced into the heart or vessels as a contrast medium. The process is angiocardiography from Greek *grapheia* 'a writing, a recording'. See also the *electrocardiogram* entry.

angio-gram

angeion blood vessel + *gram* something recorded

An angiogram is an X-ray of blood vessels.

digital subtraction angiography (DSA)

DSA is a medical imaging process in which computer graphics software enhances an X-ray picture of blood vessels, providing higher resolution and contrast to produce a clearer view of the vessels.

angio-lith

angeion blood vessel + *lithos* Greek, stone

An angiolith is a chalky deposit in the wall of a blood vessel. An abundance of such deposits is angiolithiasis with the ending *asis/osis,* 'a diseased condition'.

angi-oma

angeion blood vessel + *oma* Greek, tumor

An angioma is a generally benign tumor made of blood vessels. When congenital, it is sometimes called a naevus, Latin 'mole, wart, birthmark', and rather than being true tumors, these naeval angiomata (formal plural) are mere malformations of blood vessels. However, some angiomas may require surgical removal, for example, ones inside the skull. The disease of vessels with multiple angiomas is angiomatosis. *Angio* is found in the names of other tumors too.

- Angio-blast-oma is a brain tumor composed of angioblast, the early, formative tissue from which blood cells and vessels arise. Greek *blastos*, 'bud, sprout'.
- Angio-fibr-oma is a tumor made up of blood or lymph vessels and fibrous tissue.
- Angio-lip-oma is a tumor made up of blood or lymph vessels and fatty tissue. Greek *lipos*, 'fat'.
- Hem-angi-oma is a benign tumor made of newly formed blood cells. Greek *haima-*, 'blood'.
- Lymph-angi-oma is a tumor of newly formed lymph spaces and channels, some filled with lymphatic fluid. And – just so we can take a crack at a good, long, medical word – let's consider lymph-angio-fibr-oma, a tumor with lymphatic tissue and fibrous tissue combined.

angio-necr-osis

angeion blood vessel + *nekros* Greek, dead + *osis* diseased condition

Angionecrosis is the death of cells or localized areas of tissue in the walls of blood vessels, seen for example in the later stages of severe atherosclerosis.

angio-pathy

angeion vessel + *pathos* Greek, disease

Angiopathy is any disease of the arteries, veins or lymph vessels.

angio-plasty

angeion blood vessel + *plastia* new scientific Greek, a shaping, a forming, with later implication of 'forming by means of surgery'

Angioplasty is any surgery of the blood vessels. Balloon angioplasty is a surgical procedure to open an obstructed blood vessel by inserting a catheter with a deflated balloon attached. When the small balloon is inflated, the blood vessel is widened.

angio-spasm

angeion blood vessel + *spasmos* Greek, stretching, convulsing, contracting violently

Angiospasm is sudden, involuntary contraction of the tiny muscles associated with blood vessels.

angio-sten-osis

angeion blood vessel + *stenos* Greek, narrow + *osis* diseased condition

Angiostenosis is the pathological narrowing of blood vessels.

angio-tens-in

angeion blood vessel + *tensus* Latin, stretched out, hence narrowed + *in* noun ending indicating a chemical compound

Angiotensin I and II are blood chemicals that cause natural narrowing of the blood vessels.

ante

Preposition and prefix meaning 'before' (of time or place), hence 'prior to' or 'in front of'

ante cibum (a.c.)

ante before + *cibus* Latin, food

A.c. is a common abbreviation in prescriptions indicating that medication is to be taken 'before meals', the common times of administration in North America being 7 a.m., 11 a.m. and 5 p.m.

ante-flexion

ante before, in front of + *flexio, flexionis* Latin, a bending

Anteflexion is the abnormal forward bending of a body part, for example, the normal forward curving of the uterus may be exaggerated in some instances and may become clinically significant.

ante mortem

ante before + *mors, mortis* Latin, death

A declaration made by a patient on his or her deathbed may be termed an ante mortem statement. Compare the more familiar opposite, *post mortem*, after death.

ante partum

ante before + *partus* birth

When used by itself, the two-word phrase from obstetrics is printed with the words separated. When used as an adjective, as in antepartum hemorrhage, the two words are written together. Antepartum hemorrhage is bleeding from the uterus just before birth. A frequent cause is the placenta lying below the baby, so that the placenta is dislodged at the beginning of labor, instead of its normal release at the end of labor, shortly after the birth of the infant. See the *placenta previa* entry.

Another form of the adjective is antepartal, and both refer to the period between conception and labor. Antepartal care of a pregnant woman continues to the onset of labor. Compare post partum, 'after birth'. See the entries for *par-* and *post*. Note that antepartal refers to care of the mother. Prenatal is used to refer to the unborn child.

anterior

anterior Latin, more in front. Anterior is a Latin comparative adjective from *ante*, so it literally means 'more before, more in front of' something. Anterior means situated in front or on the front surface of a body part. Its opposite is posterior, 'more towards the back'.

For example, the eye has an ocular chamber in front of the lens. This chamber is divided by the iris into an anterior and a posterior chamber. The anterior chamber, in front of the iris, is filled with aqueous humor, a watery liquid.

As a description of anatomical position, one says that the liver is anterior to the right kidney. In surgery, an A&P repair refers to anterior and posterior vaginal repair for cystocele and rectocele. See the *cele, cysto* and *recto* entries.

The anterior nares are the ends of the nostrils, the front openings in the nose that permit air to enter and leave the pharynx during normal breathing. The posterior nares are the openings at the back of the nasal cavity.

anti

anti Greek preposition and prefix, against, working against, effective against, counteracting

anti-bio-tic

anti effective against + *biotikos* pertaining to life

A drug, like penicillin, often produced by a micro-organism, that acts to destroy or limit growth of another disease-producing micro-organism, like *Streptococcus* bacteria.

anti-body

anti against + body (antibody is a loan translation from the German *Antikörper*, coined in 1900)

Part of the body's natural immune system, an antibody is a large protein called an immunoglobulin, produced by lymph tissue in response to viruses, bacteria, or other toxins invading the body. Antibodies neutralize the destructive effects of the invading micro-organisms.

anti-gen

anti against + *gen* Greek, making, producing

An antigen is a virus, bacterium, or other toxin that stimulates production of a specific antibody. The immune reaction is also called an antigen–antibody reaction, in which an antigen produces an antibody that chemically binds to the antigen and makes it harmless to the body.

anti-sepsis

anti against + *sepsis* Greek, rotting, decaying

Sepsis is infection of tissue by micro-organisms like bacteria and their toxins, also contamination introduced by a wound. Therefore antisepsis is destruction of micro-organisms by inhibiting their growth and reproduction. Among the hundreds of antiseptic agents, some may be as simple as soap, others as complex as hexachlorophene.

Many medical words are formed with the prefix *anti*:

antiarthritic	a therapy that relieves the symptoms of arthritis
antibacterial	a chemical agent that destroys or suppresses harmful bacteria
anticoagulant	an agent that delays or prevents the coagulation or clotting of blood, also called an antihemorrhagic
anticonvulsant	an agent that prevents convulsions. Some epilepsy sufferers may use one
antidiabetic	an agent that treats diabetes mellitus
antidiarrheal	controls or stops diarrhea
antidepressant	prevents or relieves depression
antidote	a chemical that counteracts a poison; a Greek word borrowed into Latin where the *dote* is a form of the Greek verb *didonai*, 'to give', so that an *antidotum* was something 'given to act against' the poison
antiemetic	prevents vomiting; in Greek 'to vomit' is *emein*; an emetic induces vomiting
antiflatulent	prevents excessive farting by reducing the amount of intestinal gas produced
anti-inflammatory	counteracts inflammation
antimutagen	drug that reduces spontaneous mutations or counteracts a mutagen; a mutagen is an agent that promotes genetic mutations or increases their rate of occurrence; see the *mut* entry
antipruritic	drugs like corticosteroids and antihistamines that may be used to prevent or relieve itching; *pruritus* is the Latin word for 'itching'
antipyretic	agent that reduces body temperature in a patient with fever, from the Greek *pyretos*, 'fever'
antispasmotic	prevents or relieves muscle spasm
antitubercular	drug that treats tuberculosis
antitussive	a drug like codeine that relieves coughing; *tussis* is Latin for 'a cough'
antiviral	agent that destroys viruses

aorta

aorte Greek, Aristotle's term for the great artery < *aeirein* to raise, lift up; in medicine, the main trunk vessel of the arterial circulatory system

The aorta is the great trunk artery, a muscular tube about one inch in diameter, that rises from the left ventricle of the heart and starts freshly oxygenated blood on its arterial passage through the entire body. The plural may be aortas or aortae.

aortic aneurysm

aortikos adjective, of the aorta + *aneurysma* from *ana* through + *eurysma* Greek, a widening

An aneurysm is a bulging out in the wall of an artery. The aortic wall thins, balloons out, and forms a sac that may burst if not repaired surgically, often by replacing the damaged tissue with a Teflon tube.

aortic stenosis

aortikos of the aorta + *stenosis* a pathological narrowing

Aortic stenosis is a congenital narrowing of the aortic valve (see next entry). Alternatively, the cusps of the valve may fuse due to scars caused by the inflammations of rheumatic fever. Blood flow from the heart into the aorta is thus reduced, causing, among other urgent problems, congestion in the veins and arteries of the lungs. Aortic stenosis is a serious consequence of 'rheumatic heart disease' and 'rheumatic fever'. See the *rheumatic* entry.

aortic valve

aortic + *valva* Latin, the leaf of a folding door < *volvere* to roll up, to fold up

A valve is a flap or fold of membranous tissue in a tube, canal, or hollow organ of the body that acts to stop what has already passed through the tube from coming back through it. Valves prevent reflux (flowing back of liquids). Artificial valves made of plastic materials may sometimes replace natural structures that are diseased or malformed.

The aortic valve of the heart is between the left ventricle and aorta. This valve prevents blood already pumped through the heart from flowing back into the heart from the aorta.

aperture

apertura Latin, an opening, a hole, an orifice in an anatomical space or canal < *aperire* to open, to uncover

For example, the aperture of the frontal sinus, or in formal anatomical nomenclature, *apertura sinus frontalis*, is the opening of the front sinus, the sinus above the eyebrows, into the nasal cavity. A sinus here is an air cavity in the bones around the nose. These sinuses act as resonators for the human voice. See the *sinus* entry.

apex

apex, apicis Latin, the little wool tuft on the top of the cap of a
Roman chief priest or *flamen* < *apere* to attach; with developed
meanings of attachment, the top of anything, the tip, summit,
the pointed end of a structure
In medicine, an apex is the top or extremity of a body part, for example, the
apex or tip of the tongue. The plural is apices, and the adjective is apical.

apex beat

In examining the sounds and murmurs of the heart with a stethoscope, and with
more complex instruments, a physician can hear, and sometimes see, the apex of
the left ventricle of the heart move against the chest wall. The apex beat can be
felt in the fifth left intercostal space. A weak or displaced apex beat may be
symptomatic of various cardiac diseases and anomalies.

Apgar score

skor Old Norse, a notch cut in a stick for counting, and then
the later, developed meaning of 'a numerical rating'
Named after Virginia Apgar, an American anesthesiologist (1909–1974), it rates a
newborn baby's physical condition based on five factors:

1. heart rate
2. respiration
3. muscle tone
4. color
5. reflexive response

The Apgar score is taken one minute after birth, and then again four minutes
later, and perhaps at further intervals if called for, at which time it is sometimes
called a 'recovery score'. Although this test permits quasi-scientific
quantification of responses, it merely imitates what a mother does naturally
when she first holds her newborn. She checks her baby's general responsiveness.

apo

apo Greek preposition and prefix, away from, off of, derived from
This Greek preposition forms a few words in medicine, and many words in
other sciences and areas of study, including common words like aphorism,
apology, apostle and apostrophe. Apostle derives from the Greek verb
apostellein, 'to send away'. An *apostolos* in New Testament Greek was 'one who
is sent away', that is, sent forth into the world to preach the word of Christ.

ap-her-esis

apo > aph away from + *hair* Greek root form, take, choose + *esis* noun ending here meaning 'process of' so that the Greek word signifies 'removal'

Apheresis, also called pheresis, is a blood-cleaning and blood product-collecting process during which the donor's blood passes into an external machine that removes a portion of it (perhaps some plasma, platelets etc.), and then the blood is returned to the donor's body.

apo-gee

apo away from + *gaia* Greek, the earth

Apogee was first a term in astronomy to denote the point when an orbiting body like the moon is farthest from the earth. It then came to mean 'the highest point of anything, the culmination, the climax'. In medicine, the apogee is the climax of a disease, when symptoms are most severe.

apo-crine

apo away from + *krinein* Greek, to separate

Apocrine denotes certain cells in secretory glands, cells which cast off their ends along with the products they secrete. Examples are the apocrine sweat glands located in the armpit, and in the anal, genital and mammary areas. These sweat glands open into nearby hair follicles instead of opening on the skin surface. Apocrine sweat glands are responsible for the telltale odor of perspiration, when bacteria act on material secreted by these glands. See the *endocrine* entry.

apo-neur-osis

apo away from + *neuron* Greek, nerve, tendon + *osis* condition, state

Aponeurosis was a tricky word in medical Greek and still is in English, because of the double meaning of *neuron*. Neuritis is inflammation of nerves. Neurosis originally was a nervous disorder. But the *neuron* root here means tendon. Tendons are white fibrous bands of tissue that connect muscles to bones. An aponeurosis is a white extension or expansion of a tendon that connects flat muscles to other body parts. One example is the lingual aponeurosis, the connective tissue that supports the inner and outer muscles of the tongue and attaches them. *Lingua* is the Latin word for 'tongue'.

41

apo-physis

apo away from + *physis* Greek, growth, nature, natural quality
Apophysis meant 'offshoot, outgrowth' in Greek, in reference to bone. It is a
bony outgrowth that is not separated from its originating bone, like a process or
a tubercle. See the *epiphysis* entry. But don't try to say apophysis and epiphysis
in the same sentence as pithy apophthegm!

apo-plexy

apo down, away from + *plexia* Greek, a striking
One of the oldest medical terms still used, apoplexy is a striking down – by a
stroke. The term is older than Hippocrates. Today apoplexy has an old-
fashioned sound. Its modern synonyms are more often used, e.g. cerebrovascular
accident (see entry).

apo-thec-ary

apo away + *theca* Greek, storehouse, storage place + *arius*
Latin, agent noun suffix
The original *apothecarius* kept the warehouse where drugs were stored, then the
word came to mean the person who prepared the drugs, hence apothecary, a
druggist or pharmacist. The term is almost obsolete in modern English, but is
still seen in phrases like 'apothecaries' weight' and 'apothercaries' measure', non-
decimal systems of measuring small weights (grains) and small liquid volumes
(minims). Shakespeare has the poisoned Romeo utter these dying words: 'O true
apothecary! Thy drugs are quick. Thus with a kiss I die'.

ap-pend-ix

appendix Latin, *ad* > *ap* Latin, to, on + *pendix* Latin, hanging
part
In Latin *appendix* meant 'addition or appendage'. In anatomy it is any supplementary part of a main structure, like the vermiform appendix. See next entry.

appendic-itis

appendix + *-itis* Greek suffix added to the end of a medical word
that signifies inflammation
The word *appendicitis* was coined in 1886 by Boston surgeon Reginald Fitz, to
refer to acute inflammation of the vermiform appendix, a worm-like process
jutting out 3 to 6 inches from the caecum, the pouch-like first part of the large

intestine. 19th Century scientific Latin *vermiformalis* means 'with a form like a worm' from Latin *vermis*, 'worm'.

arachno-

arachne Greek, spider, spider's web

arachn-oid

arachne spider + *oid* like, similar, a common English suffix from the Greek noun *eides* which means 'form, shape'

Designated by its zoological class, a spider is an arachnid. Poisoning by spider bite is arachnidism or arachnoidism. Fear of spiders is arachnophobia, also the title of a 1990 horror-comedy film produced by Steven Spielberg.

arachnoid membrane or sheath

arachnoid + *membrana* Latin, thin skin

The arachnoid membrane or sheath is the second or middle layer of the three meninges, the membranes of connective tissue that enclose and protect the brain and spinal cord. Early anatomists thought the arachnoid membrane's tissues were very webby or spider-like. Its loose attachment to the dura mater and the pia mater permits space for cerebrospinal fluid, which is the watery shock absorber that flows through the brain and spinal cord tissues, cushioning them against injury. This area is called the subarachnoid space.

arachnoid villi

arachnoid + *villus* Latin, fine hair, fleece, nap of a cloth; plural *villi*

The arachnoid villi are small projections of the arachnoid membrane, part of the protective cushioning of the brain provided by the meninges.

An older name for arachnoid villus is Pacchionian body, but medical eponyms (terms named after persons) should be avoided. Although such a term credits Italian anatomist Antonio Pacchioni (1665–1726), it often turns out that the name attached to a structure is not that of the person who first identified it. This is sometimes true for the names of diseases and syndromes as well. See the subsection entitled *Eponyms* in the introduction to this book.

are-ola

area open space + *ola* noun suffix indicating smallness, a diminutive ending; the Latin plural *areolae* is used in medicine.

An areola can be a small cavity within tissue. It also names the discolored area encircling a pustule or other pimple.

areola mammae

areola + *mammae* Latin, of the breast

The areola mammae is the pigmented area surrounding the nipple of each breast. Under this area are areolar glands, large sebaceous glands (modified sweat glands) around the nipples of female breasts that secrete a fatty fluid that protects and lubricates the nipples.

artery

arteria Greek, airpipe < *aerterion* air duct < *aer* air + *terein* to carry; now in medicine, any of the large vessels that carry blood away from the heart

Some medical word origins show us the mistakes of early anatomists. Ancient Greek doctors thought arteries carried air, instead of blood being circulated away from the heart. They erred because most ancient anatomy lessons had to be learned from corpses. But, after death, arteries are nearly empty, most post mortem blood being found in veins. In arterial bleeding, arterial blood spurts and is bright red. Venous blood, on the other hand, having lost most of its oxygen, is a darker red and flows rather than spurts.

arterial blood gases (ABG)

Laboratory determination of the blood pH (see *pH* entry) and of levels of oxygen and carbon dioxide in arterial blood are important in diagnosis and treatment of diseases like emphysema.

arteri-ola

arteria + *ola* noun suffix indicating smallness

An arteriola or ateriole is the smallest branch of an artery, leading to a network of capillaries.

arterio-gram

arteria + *gramma* letter, something written, something drawn, picture, then with the modern meaning of 'recorded or X-rayed or digitized image'

An arteriogram is an X-ray of an artery that has been injected with a radiopaque contrast medium (dye) so that the possibly clogged lumen of the artery will show up on the X-ray.

arterio-scler-osis

arteria + *skleros* Greek, hardened + *osis* diseased condition

Arteriosclerosis is hardening of the arteries, which may accompany old age or be symptomatic of diseases like hypertension. The arterial walls lose their elastic quality and calcium salts accumulate in arterial tissue so that blood flow to the brain and the arms and legs is severely reduced.

arterio-venous

arteria + *vena* Latin, vein + *ous* common adjectival ending

Arteriovenous means 'pertaining to the arteries and the veins'; for example, arteriovenous, arteriovenous fistula, and arteriovenous shunt all refer to abnormal connnections between arteries and veins that permit blood to flow from an artery to a vein, bypassing the capillaries. Such irregular arteriovenous joinings may be of genetic, pathologic, or surgical origin.

arthro-

arthron Greek, joint

arthr-itis

arthron joint + *itis* inflammation

Arthritis is inflammation of a joint. Rheumatoid arthritis is a severe form involving the membranes and fluids of the joints and possible deformity.

Though rare, there is a Greek plural form of *-itis* words that should be recognized because it is sometimes seen in medical literature. The plural of arthritis can be arthritides, as well as arthritises. Likewise, appendicitides and hepatitides are the rare plural forms for appendicitises and hepatitises.

arthro-cent-esis

arthron joint + *kent* puncture + *esis* Greek noun ending, 'action of'

Arthrocentesis is the surgical puncture of a joint with a needle, either to obtain a diagnostic sample of synovial fluid, or to drain an accumulation of excess fluid from the joint.

arthro-scler-osis

arthron joint + *skleros* Greek, hardened + *osis* noun suffix meaning 'diseased condition'

Arthrosclerosis is any joint-hardening condition, which may be a symptom of arthritis.

arthro-desis

arthron joint + *desis* a fixing, a binding

Arthrodesis is an arthritic joint locking in one position or the subsequent, last-resort surgery to fuse the joint. A rigid joint is not painful, and the patient gains some mobility from the surgery.

arthro-endo-scopy

arthron joint + *endon* Greek, within + *skopein* to look at, to examine + *y* noun ending

Arthroendoscopy may also be seen in its shorter form arthroscopy, in which the interior of a joint, often the knee, is examined by inserting an endoscope (see the *scope* entry) through a tiny incision.

articul-ar

articulus Latin, knuckle or any joint of the body + *ar* adjectival ending

Articulus was the Latin translation of the Greek *arthron*, 'joint'. Articular cartilage is a smooth tissue covering surfaces that rub together in synovial joints.

articul-ate

articulus Latin, knuckle or any joint of the body + *ate* common verb ending

To articulate is to move together like a joint. At the shoulder, the head of the humerus articulates with the scapula. A physiotherapist may articulate the femur gently as part of therapy. Thus the noun, articulation, can be the place bones meet to move together. Articulation can be a synonym for joint. Articulation can also describe the range of motion of a bone.

ascites

askites Greek, abnormal fluid in the abdomen < *askos* leather bag, pouch, sac, used to carry oil, wine and water

Ascites is the abnormal accumulation of a watery fluid in the peritoneal cavity, a possible complication of liver and kidney diseases, of congestive heart failure, certain cancers and of inflammation of the peritoneum or peritonitis. This abnormal escape and accumulation of fluid in a body part is called effusion = *ex* > *ef* out of + *fusio* a pouring forth, a rushing out, a flooding. The procedure of aspirating ascitic fluid from the abdominal cavity is sometimes called paracentesis = *para* beside + *kentesis* puncturing.

a-spir-ate

ad > *a* to, towards + *spiritus* Latin, breath + *ate* verb ending

Aspirare meant 'to breathe' in Latin. In modern medicine, to aspirate is to draw air or fluid out of a cavity. In some poisonings, stomach contents must be aspirated by suction pump as part of the treatment. A pustule may be aspirated by means of a syringe. A dentist may use an aspirating syringe to inject a local anesthetic, drawing up on the syringe to insure that the anesthetic is not being injected into a vein or artery. Certain patients are at high risk for aspiration of vomitus, that is, inhaling vomited stomach contents into their lungs. Aspiration pneumonia may result. Glue-sniffers are engaging in aspiration drug abuse (breathing in noxious chemicals to get high).

asthma

asthma Greek, breathing hard, gasping, panting < *azein* to breathe hard

This breathing difficulty is caused by constrictive spasm of the little muscles that surround the bronchi (see *bronchi* entry) brought on by factors like allergies, air pollution, infection, strenuous exercise, or excessive emotional stress.

athero-

athere Greek, gruel, porridge, gritty meal, with modern medical meaning of hard, fatty plaque deposits

ather-oma

athere gruel + *oma* noun ending meaning 'swelling, tumor, mass'

Atheroma is a fatty plaque or mass in thickened arterial linings or in a sebaceous cyst.

athero-sclerosis

athere gruel + *skleros* Greek, hardened + *osis* noun suffix meaning 'diseased condition'

Atherosclerosis is a disease in which arteries become hard and inflexible, a form of arteriosclerosis due to deposits of hard, fatty plaque in the arterial linings. Atheromatous masses contain cholesterol and other lipids and lipoid debris. The disease may also be called atheromatosis.

atlas

A giant in Greek mythology; in medicine the first cervical vertebra

Atlas or *Atlantos* was a mythical king who became a minor god charged with upholding the pillars of heaven. His name derives from the Greek verb *tlenai* 'to suffer, to endure hardship'.

In anatomy, the atlas is the first cervical vertebra, at the top of the spinal column where the neck meets the skull. Like the legendary giant who holds the world on his shoulders, the atlas may be said to hold the skull. The atlas forms a joint with the base of the skull and permits the head to nod to and fro. The atlas as a 'guidebook' was named after an early book of maps by Mercator who put an engraving of the giant holding up the world on the book's cover. The Atlantic ocean is named after Atlas or the island of Atlantis.

atrium

atrium Latin, hearth-place, with modern medical meaning of the upper chamber of the heart; plural *atria*, combining forms *atri-*, *atria-*, *atrio-*

The atrium is either of the two upper chambers of the heart. The atrium of an ancient Roman house contained an open-fire hearth, and visitors to the home were first greeted there. This metaphor appealed to Victorian doctors who, about 1870, named these heart chambers. For blood is indeed received first into the atria, from all tissues except the lungs. The atria are like the reception rooms of the heart.

inter-atrial septum

inter Latin, between + *atrialis* of the atria + *saeptum* Latin, fence, wall

The interatrial septum is the wall that divides the two atria. In older medical literature, it is sometimes called the interauricular septum, from auricle, an old name for the atrium, because each atrium is roughly ear-shaped, and *auriculum* is the Latin word for 'little ear'.

sino-atrial node

sinus Latin, fold, cavity, hollow channel + *atrialis* of the atria; *nodus* knot, cell cluster

The sinoatrial node is the natural pacemaker of the heart, located in the upper right atrial septum. This node is a clump of modified heart-muscle cells capable of generating bioelectric impulses. The heartbeat starts with electrical impulses from the sinoatrial node, stimulating waves of heart muscle contractions in the atria, which send blood into the ventricles. Sinoatrial node electrical impulses are picked up by another node, the atrioventricular node, and transmitted to the Bundle of His in the interventricular septum that separates the two ventricles of the heart. This bundle branches out to carry impulses to ventricles, causing them to contract.

auris

auris Latin, ear; adjective aural

auris dexter

Latin, the right ear

The chart abbreviation for the right ear is AD, auris dexter.

auris externa (auricula, auricle or pinna)

Latin, the external ear

The auris externa is the part of the ear that sticks out to collect and channel sound waves. It is also called the pinna (Latin, feather). Auricula or auricle, the Latin diminutive form of auris, are also used in medicine to label the outer ear and the ear hole or external auditory meatus.

auris interna

Latin, the internal ear

Auris interna comprises the semicircular canals, the vestibule, and the cochlea of an ear.

auris media

Latin, the middle ear

Auris media labels the middle ear or tympanic cavity, an air-filled space in the temporal bone whose openings include the Eustachian tube, the ear drum and the round window, the last two being covered openings.

auris sinistra

Latin, the left ear

The chart abbreviation in medicine for the left ear is AS, auris sinistra.

auto-

autos Greek adjective which retains its ancient meaning 'self, same' in modern languages

auto-nomic

autos self + *nomos* law + *ikos* adjectival ending

Autonomic means self-regulating. The autonomic nervous system regulates involuntary vital functions like actions of the heart and the smooth muscles. See the *sympathetic* entry.

auto-immune response

The auto-immune response occurs in certain diseases that involve the body producing an immune response that attacks its own tissues. Rheumatoid arthritis and multiple sclerosis are such disorders.

auto-matic

autos self + *matos* acting

In medicine, automatic means 'self-acting, spontaneous, involuntary'.

aut-ism

autos self + *ismos* Greek noun ending indicating disordered condition

Autism is a childhood disorder in which the child does not respond normally to sound and sight stimuli, and seems sealed up inside himself.

axilla

axilla Latin, armpit < *axis* axle, turning point + *illa* diminutive ending signifying 'little'

For ancient Roman medicine, the axilla was the turning point where the arm articulated with the shoulder. The axillary node is one of the lymph glands in the armpit. The axillary temperature of the body is recorded by a thermometer placed in the armpit.

axis

axis Latin, axle, turning point, pivot about which a round object turns

In anatomy, the axis is the second cervical vertebra, the bone under the first neckbone. The axis has a thick knob or process. The first neckbone (the atlas) pivots around this knob on the second neckbone making movement of the head from side to side possible.

axial

axialis scientific Latin, pertaining to an axis

Axial refers to the other common medical meaning of axis, an imaginary line through a body part, around which that body part may be said to rotate. It is part of the scanning technique called computerized axial tomography (CAT). See the *CAT* entry.

axon

axon Greek, axle of a wheel, axis, main stem; in medicine, a long extension of a neuron

The basic cell of the nervous system is a neuron. One of the neuron's extensions or processes is the axon which carries impulses away from an individual neuron.

B

bacillus

bacillum Latin, little iron rod, little stick; plural bacilli
Bacillus is the genus-name for a family of bacteria shaped like little rods, a few of which are pathogenic (disease-producing), including the one that causes anthrax, a virulent bacterial disease of cattle transmittable to humans. *Bacillus anthracis* can be fatal, especially when it invades the lungs.

bacill-em-ia

bacillus rod-shaped bacterium + *em* short for Greek *haim-*, blood + *ia* medical condition
Bacillemia is the presence of bacilli in circulating human blood.

bacill-ur-ia

bacillus rod-shaped bacterium + *ouron* Greek, urine + *ia* medical condition
Bacilluria is the presence of bacilli in urine.

bacteria

baktron Greek, rod, cane, wooden pole + *ion* Greek diminutive ending meaning 'little, small'; a *bakterion* was the small staff of office carried by some officers in ancient Greek armies
Bacteria are unicellular (one-celled) micro-organisms, widespread in air, water, and soil. Some are pathogens (disease-producers). Many bacterial infections can be treated with antibiotics, although overuse of such antibiotics has produced mutated strains of some bacteria that have developed a resistance to older, too widely-used antibiotics. The singular is bacterium. Bacteria are classified by their shapes, among which are:

Spherical	micrococcus	a single ovoid cell (*mikros* small + *kokkos* berry)
	diplococcus	in pairs (*diploos* twofold + *kokkos* berry)
	staphylococcus	in clusters (*staphylos* a bunch of grapes + *kokkos* berry)
	streptococcus	in chains (*streptos* twisted + *kokkos* berry)
	sarcinae	square or cubical groups (*sarcina* bundle)
Rod-shaped	coccobacillus	in oval rods (*kokkos* berry + *bacillus* rod)
	streptobacillus	rods end to end in a chain (*streptos* twisted *bacillus* rod)
Spiral	spirilla	rigid spiral (*spirilla* little spiral)
	spirochetes	flexible spiral (*spira* coil, helix, spiral + *chaite* long hair)
	vibrio (pl. *vibriones*)	curved, comma-shaped, motile (*vibrare* to wiggle, to shake)

bacterial food poisoning

Caused by several species of bacteria like *Salmonella* and *Clostridium botulinum*. See *botulism* entry.

bacteri-cide

bacteria + *caedere* Latin, to kill
Any chemical agent that kills bacteria is a bactericide.

bacterio-logy

bacteria + *logos* Greek, study of + *y* noun ending
Part of the broader science of microbiology, bacteriology is the scientific study of bacteria and their effects, both bad and good, on human tissue.

bacterio-lysis

bacteria + *lysis* Greek, breaking up, breakdown, decomposition, dissolution
Bacteriolysis is the breaking down of a bacterial cell and the consequent release of its cellular contents. Sometimes the bacteriolytic agent is a virus. A chemical substance capable of doing this is called a bacteriolysin.

bacterio-phage

bacteria + *phagos* Greek, eater

A bacteriophage is a virus that infects bacteria and causes bacteriolysis. One often sees used the short form, *phage.*

bacterio-stat

bacteria + *statos* Greek, stopped, brought to a standstill, set, placed
A bacteriostat is an agent that inhibits or retards the growth of bacteria. This process of stopping the reproduction of bacteria is termed bacteriostasis. The adjective is bacteriostatic or bacteristatic.

bar-

baros Greek, heaviness, weight, pressure
The root appears in words and phrases like barometer and baritone voice.

bar-iatrics

baros weight + *iatros* Greek, doctor, physician + *ikos* adjectival ending
Bariatrics is a modish term for the medical treatment and prevention of obesity and related diseases. It is, however, euphemistic gobbledygook invented to obscure the concept of being too fat, to spare its patients embarrassment, and to provide its practitioners with a high-sounding job description. Soon we can expect to see such 'fat' doctors referred to as bariatricians. This pompous and unnecessary addition to the already hefty hoard of medicalese demonstrates that not every new medical word is legitimate.

baro-receptor

baros pressure + *receptor* Latin, receiver
A baroreceptor is a nerve ending sensitive to changes in pressure. Baroreceptors in the atrial walls of the heart, for example, trigger reflex mechanisms that dilate or constrict the blood vessels to permit the heart to adjust to changes in blood pressure.

hyper-baric

hyper Greek, over, above, akin to Latin *super* + *barikos* pertaining to pressure
A hyperbaric chamber is a room or sealed area in which a patient, perhaps a diver suffering decompression illness, can receive pressurized oxygen as part of

therapy. Such hyperbaric oxygenation therapy may be useful in treating carbon monoxide and cyanide poisoning, smoke inhalation, some anemias, and, as mentioned, the bends, when divers resurface too quickly. Such injuries suffered by divers are referred to collectively as barotrauma = *baros* pressure + *trauma* Greek, wound, physical injury.

iso-bar

isos equal + *baros* pressure

An isobar is a line on a weather map or scientific graph that connects points of equal air pressure. In medical procedures that use radioactive elements, an isobar is one of two isotopes that have the same mass but different atomic numbers. In biochemistry, isobaric means 'having equal specific gravity'.

Bartholin-itis

Bartholin, a Danish family with three generations of anatomists (1585–1738) + *-itis* Greek suffix added to the end of a medical word that signifies inflammation or disease

Bartholinitis is inflammation of one or both of Bartholin's glands, small mucus-secreting organs, one on each side of, and whose ducts open into, the vestibule of the vagina, at the base of the labia majora. The mucus protects and lubricates the vaginal entranceway. Chronic inflammation may produce a benign Bartholin's cyst. Acute inflammation may cause Bartholin's abscess.

basal

basis Greek, the ground level, bottom part, foundation, beginning, first cause

Basal pertains to the fundamental, basic, or lowest stage or level of a thing or process. For example, basal body temperature is that measured, and often charted daily, in the morning before exercise or eating. Basal cell carcinoma is a malignant tumor in epithelium, a cancer often caused by over-exposure to sunlight or X-rays.

benign

benignus Latin, mild, favorable; in medicine, not cancerous, the opposite of malignant

A benign tumor or neoplasm (see *plasm-* entry) does not invade other tissues or spread to other parts of the body. Benign prostatic hypertrophy is a common enlargement of the prostate gland seen in men over 50 years old. It is not malignant or inflammatory, but if it progresses it can lead to blockage of the urethra and urinary tract infections. Such symptoms may be alleviated in the short term by balloon dilatation of the prostate, or eliminated by surgical resection of the part of the prostate that presses on the urethra.

beta (β)

The second letter of the Greek alphabet is widely used in science, e.g. in chemical names like beta-carotene and beta-lactamase, and in disease names to indicate a type II or second type of a blood disorder, like hyperbetalipoprotein-emia, which differs slightly from hyperlipoproteinemia.

A beta-blocker is one of several drugs which are therapeutic in some forms of hypertension and cardiac arrhythmia. They block certain receptors in the autonomic nervous system and thus decrease the rate and force of heart contractions.

Beta cells produce insulin from specialized cell clumps called the islets of Langerhans in the pancreas. Beta rays are streams of particles emitted during the decay of some radioactive elements such as tritium. Beta waves are one of the four types of brain waves displayable as oscillations in the output of, for example, an electroencephalogram. This beta rhythm occurs when a human is awake and alert, with both eyes open. High beta activity indicates heightened functioning of the nervous system.

bi-

bis Latin adverb, two times, now a combining form for twice, double, both, two

Bifocal eye glasses have two lens; binoculars let you look with both eyes; a biped has two feet; bisexual pertains to both sexes.

bi-ceps

bi two + *ceps* < *caput* Latin, head

A biceps is a muscle with two heads or divisions. The *biceps brachii* (Latin from Greek, of the arm) is the muscle of the upper arm that flexes the arm, forearm, and elbow.

bi-cuspid

bi two + *cuspis, cuspidis* Latin, point, sharp end

Bicuspid means 'having two points'. A bicuspid tooth has two points. A bicuspid valve in the heart has two valvular leaves and looks a bit like a bishop's hat or miter, and so it was first called the mitral valve.

bi-lateral

bi two, both + *lateralis* Latin, of a side

Bilateral in medicine means 'having two sides, occurring on both sides'. One of the chief arteries carrying blood to the head and neck is the bilateral carotid artery which branches first into left and right divisions and then into internal and external divisions. Bilateral symmetry means that both sides of an organ or structure are quite similar in size and shape. Externally, the human body is bilaterally symmetrical – usually.

bin-ary

bini twofold + *arius* common ending of Latin agent nouns and adjectives

In histology, the branch of medicine that studies cells and tissue, binary fission (Latin, *fissio, fissionis* a splitting) is the simple, asexual reproduction of, for example, a bacterium that grows by splitting into two equal parts.

bi-polar

bi two + *polus* Latin, either end of an axle, the North or South pole + *ar* adjectival ending

In neurology, a bipolar neuron has a process that leads stimuli in and one that leads stimuli out. In psychiatry, bipolar disorders have two phases, one of which sometimes dominates in a patient at one time. An older name for such a disorder is manic–depressive psychosis. There is a hint of euphemism in psychiatry's rush to adopt *bipolar* to replace the now too stark *manic–depressive*.

bis in die (b.i.d.)

bis in die the Latin of prescriptions, (take) twice a day

bili-

bilis Latin, bile, gall

Bile or gall is an important digestive juice secreted in the liver, stored in the gallbladder, and then passed down through the common bile duct into the duodenum. The structures associated with this pathway of bile from the liver to the gallbladder to the duodenum are called the biliary tract. Bile emulsifies fat, a major digestive process in the intestines. Certain salts in the bile form compounds with fatty acids, a necessary step in fat being absorbed into the body to provide fuel for life processes.

bili-ous-ness

bilis bile + *osus* Latin adjectival suffix meaning 'full of' + *ness* English noun suffix here indicating 'condition'
Various liver disorders cause the symptoms labeled with this general term. Symptoms may include headache, appetite loss, constipation and vomiting of bile.

bili-rub-in

bilis bile + *rubus* Latin, red + *in* common noun ending for organic chemical compounds
Bilirubin is an orange–yellow pigment in bile, a product of the breakdown of hemoglobin in old red blood cells. Bilirubin normally passes in the bile into the duodenum and is excreted in the feces, to which it contributes part of the characteristic fecal color.

hyper-bilirubin-emia

hyper Greek, over, above, akin to Latin *super* + *bilirubin* + *em* short for Greek *haim-*, blood + *ia* medical condition
Hyperbilirubinemia is abnormal and excessive amounts of bilirubin in the blood. When this pathologic excess of bilirubin reaches the skin, it displays as jaundice (*jaunisse* Old French, yellowness from *jaune,* yellow).

bio-

bios Greek, life
The root appears in words like autobiography, microbe, aerobics and symbiosis.

anti-bio-tic

anti against, counter to + *biotikos* pertaining to life
An antibiotic is a chemical naturally made by micro-organisms or synthetically made, that suppresses the growth of or kills other disease-producing micro-organisms like bacteria.

bio-ethics

bios life + *ethikos* Greek, pertaining to or possessing moral habits

The adjective is derived from *ethos*, Greek for 'custom, habit, moral character'. *Ethics* entered the major languages of the West early because it was the title of a famous treatise by the ancient Greek philosopher, Aristotle.

Medical bioethics is the study of what is morally correct in the actions of those who practice the health professions, often with a focus on biological research, scientific advances, and their moral implications, but touching also on controversial actions such as abortion and euthanasia (see *eu-* entry).

bio-nics

bios life + *nics* an ending borrowed from the term *mechanics*
Bionics is the study of how electronic and mechanical devices like computers may solve certain medical problems. Bionics encompasses the design and application of machines like cardiac pacemakers and artificial arms. It is a branch of biophysics.

bio-logy

bios life + *logos* Greek, word, writing, science, study of + *y* noun ending
Biology is the scientific study of life and living organisms. Microbiology (*mikros* Greek, small) is concerned with micro-organisms like bacteria, fungi, protozoa and viruses.

bi-opsy

bios life + *opsis* Greek, vision, seeing, looking at
Biopsy is the removal of a minute sample of tissue from a living body for analysis. Biopsy specimens are often taken by suction through a needle, but surgical means are sometimes necessary.

blasto-, -blast

blastos Greek, young growth, bud, sprout; in medicine a prefix and a suffix denoting pre-embryonic, or an immature stage
Note that in medicine, the developing fertilized ovum is not called an embryo until after the long axis appears. From the end of the second week after fertilization until the end of the eighth week, it is termed an embryo.

blasto-cyst

blastos bud + *kystis* Greek, little bag

The blastocyst is a stage of pre-embryonic growth in which there are two layers of cells surrounding the fluid-filled cavity of the blastula.

blast-oma

blastos young growth, bud, sprout + *oma* common medical noun suffix that means 'tumor, swelling'
A blastoma is a tumor or neoplasm composed of immature cells from the undifferentiated cell mass out of which a particular organ or tissue develops.

blasto-mere

blastos young growth, bud + *meros* Greek, part
The blastomere is one of the first two cells that result from the first division of the fertilized ovum.

blast-ula

blastos young growth, bud, sprout + *ula* Latin diminutive ending meaning 'small'
The blastula is an early stage of development of the pre-embryonic ovum in which it is a hollow sphere one-cell thick. The single-celled layer is called the blastoderm (*derma* Greek, skin). The cavity of the blastula is the blastocele or blastocoele (*koilos* Greek, hollow) which is filled with fluid. This fluid is called the blastochyle (*chylos* Greek, juice). The cavity increases the amount of surface area through which the developing blastula can absorb oxygen and nutrients.

endo-blast

endon Greek, within + *blastos* young growth, bud, sprout
An endoblast is the immature cell that is the precursor of an endoderm cell (*derma* Greek, skin). Endoderm makes up the innner layer of cells in an embryo.

epi-blast

epi Greek prefix and preposition, on, upon, over + *blastos* young growth, bud, sprout
The epiblast is the outer layer of cells in a plate-like group of cells in a mammalian pre-embryo. The embryo proper develops from this cell group, which is called the blastoderm (*derma* Greek, skin).

erythro-blast

erythros Greek, red + *blastos* young growth, bud, sprout
An erythroblast is an immature precursor of a red blood cell or erythrocyte
(*kytos* Greek, cell).

erythro-blast-oma

erythros Greek, red + *blastos* young growth, bud + *oma* tumor
An erythroblastoma is a cancer of bone marrow in which the malignant cells
look like erythroblasts.

leuko-blast

leukos Greek, white + *blastos* young growth, bud, sprout
A leukoblast is an immature precursor of a white blood cell or leukocyte. It is
also called a leukocytoblast.

megalo-blast

megas, megalos Greek, big + *blastos* young growth, bud, sprout
A megaloblast is a big, abnormal red blood cell found in the circulating blood of
patients with certain severe anemias (see *anemia* entry).

odonto-blast

odous, odontis Greek, tooth + *blastos* young growth, bud, sprout
Odontoblasts are cells inside the pulp chamber of a tooth that produce dentin
(*dens, dentis* Latin, tooth + *in* suffix denoting organic chemical compounds).
Dentin is the calcium-rich part of the tooth covered by the much harder enamel
on the crown of the tooth and by cementum in the root area.

bleb

English, variant of the earlier word *blob*
A bleb is any large, flaccid blister or vesicle filled with serous fluid. It may be as
small as 1 cm, or as large as a golf ball.

blephar(o)

blepharos Greek, eyelid

blephar-ectomy

blepharos eyelid + *ex* out + *caesio, caesionis* Latin, a cutting
Blepharectomy means excision of all or part of an eyelid. It can be because of disease, or be part of cosmetic facial surgery.

blephar-ism

blepharos eyelid + *ism* disordered condition
Blepharism is continuous blinking and twitching of the eyelids.

blephar-itis

blepharos eyelid + *itis* inflammation of
Blepharitis is inflammation of the eyelids, sometimes caused by allergens. Eyelids are red, swollen, painful and encrusted with dried mucus. The eyelash follicles may be affected, and also inflamed may be the tiny meibomian glands on the posterior margin of each eyelid, which secrete an antibacterial and antifungal sebum that also protects the eyelid skin from drying out.

blepharo-ptosis

blepharos eyelid + *ptosis* Greek, drooping
Blepharoptosis is drooping of the upper eyelid.

-bol-

bole Greek, a throwing < *ballein* to throw; developed meaning of 'throw together, build, develop'

ana-bol-ic

ana up + *bole* Greek, the act of building + *ikos* adjective ending
Anabolic substances help the process of changing nutrients into chemicals that build body cells. In anabolism, simple chemicals are converted into the more complex chemicals found in living cells. For example, controversial anabolic steroids (see *stereo* entry) help athletes build muscle, but at the cost to their future health of deleterious side-effects.

cata-bol-ism

kata Greek, down + *bole* Greek, throwing + *ism* noun suffix denoting 'process of'

Catabolism is the breaking down of complex cells and biochemicals by living cells into simpler chemicals which body systems use to make heat and energy. The combined processes of anabolism and catabolism are called metabolism.

em-bol-ism

embolos Greek, plug, stopper; *en > em* in + *bolos* anything thrown + *ism* a disordered condition

Embolism is the blockage of a blood vessel by a foreign clump of material, often a blood clot travelling through the bloodstream that becomes stuck in a vessel and obstructs normal flow. Pulmonary embolism occurs when either or both of the two main arteries of the lungs is obstructed by such clumps. *Pulmo, pulmonis,* Latin for lung.

em-bol-us

embolus, scientific Latin from *embolos* Greek, plug, stopper; *en > em* in, into + *bolos* something thrown or put in, a ball

An *embolos* was something put into an opening, like a wedge in a door or a cork in a wine bottle.

An embolus is a mass of matter that may clog a blood or lymph vessel. Emboli may consist of solid, liquid or gaseous substances.

meta-bol-ism

meta Greek, across, with developed meaning of 'change' + *bole* throwing + *ism* 'process of'

Metabolism comprises all the physical and chemical processes the body uses to maintain itself, including the conversion of food into energy.

botul-ism

botulus Latin, little sausage + *ism* noun suffix indicating disordered condition

Botulism is a severe food poisoning, first observed in early 19th Century Germany in carelessly prepared sausages. The botulinus neurotoxins in the poisoned food can be fatal if ingested in great quantity. The culprit is excessive growth of a bacterium called *Clostridium botulinum.*

bowel

botellus Latin, little sausage > *boel* Old French > *bouel* Middle English > *bowel* modern English

The plain English word for intestine goes all the way back to a Roman battlefield, where soldiers first saw disembowelled cohorts. Exposed coils of intestines extruding from the gutted corpses of slain soldiers looked like sausages.

brachi-, brachio-

brachion Greek, upper arm; it came into English from its Latin form *bracchium*

brachi-al

brachialis scientific Latin adjective, pertaining to the upper arm

The *brachialis* is an upper-arm muscle lying directly under each biceps. The *brachioradialis* is a muscle on the lateral side of the forearm. The brachial artery is the main vessel that brings oxygenated blood to the upper arm.

brachial plexus

brachialis + *plexus* Latin, a braid, an interwoven rope

The brachial plexus is a network of cervical and spinal nerves that innervate the upper arm, forearm, and hand.

    An interesting word derived from *bracchium* is pretzel. A Latin diminutive form was *bracchiolum* meaning 'little arm'. Medieval German monks who read Latin would have pronounced the word *bretziolum*. Take off the Latin noun ending *-um* and you've got the dialect German *Bretzel*, with the High German pronunciation of *pretzl*, and the modern German *Brezel*, a biscuit of baked dough strips folded into 'little arms'. The form with *p*, pretzel, is an American spelling. German priests originally gave pretzels to children as rewards for saying their prayers, the little arms of the pretzel reminding the children of their own arms folded in prayer.

brachy-

brachys Greek, short

brachy-cephal-ic

brachys short + *kephale* Greek, head + *ikos* adjective ending

A brachycephalic cranium has a smaller than usual capacity. However, this short-headedness need not be abnormal, since the cephalic index has a range of normal cranial volumes. The noun is brachycephaly. On the other hand, certain congenital malformations of the skull do accompany retardation.

brachy-dactyl-ous

brachys short + *daktylos* finger or toe + *ous* English adjective ending

A brachydactylous individual has fingers and/or toes shorter than normal. The noun is brachydactylia or brachydactyly.

brady-

bradys Greek, slow

brady-cardia

bradys slow + *kardia* Greek, heart

Bradycardia is an abnormally slow heartbeat, that is, under sixty beats per minute. The opposite is tachycardia (*tachys* fast, speedy, swift), an abnormally elevated rate of the heartbeat, more than one hundred beats per minute in an adult. Bradytachycardia is a heartbeat that alternates between abnormally slow and fast rates.

brady-lalia

bradys slow + *lalia* Greek, talking, speaking

Bradylalia is abnormal slowness of speech. Bradyglossia (*glossa* Greek, tongue) is a synonym.

brady-phrasia

bradys slow + *phrasis* thing spoken, utterance, speech

Bradyphrasia is abnormal slowness of speech seen in certain types of mental disease.

bronch-

brogchos Greek, windpipe

bronch-itis

brogchos windpipe + *itis* inflammation of

Bronchitis is an inflammation of the mucous membranes lining the bronchi, bronchioles, and trachea. It may follow the common cold. Bronchitic agents include dust, fumes, allergens, the influenza virus, and streptococcal and staphylococcal bacteria, as in 'strep or staph throat'.

bronchi-ole

brogchos windpipe + *ole* diminutive suffix denoting 'small'

Bronchioles are smaller subdivisions of the bronchi that lead inspired and warmed air into the alveoli of the lungs where oxygen is transferred into the blood.

broncho-dilator

brogchos windpipe + *dilatare* Latin, to widen, to stretch + *or* agent noun suffix = -er in English

A bronchodilator is a chemical agent that acts to widen the air-carrying lumen of bronchioles, by reducing smooth-muscle contractions of the tubes. Patients suffering from asthma, bronchitis and emphysema then find breathing less strenuous.

broncho-pneumon-ia

brogchos windpipe + *pneumon* Greek, lung + *ia* medical condition

Bronchopneumonia is inflammation of the bronchioles and alveoli of the lungs, often caused by bacteria known as pneumococci. Elderly, bedridden patients are most at risk of contracting bronchopneumonia.

broncho-scopy

brogchos windpipe + *skopein* to look at, to examine + *y* noun ending

Bronchoscopy is visual examination of the bronchi through the insertion of an instrument called a bronchoscope. Optic fibers carry light down the scope and images of what is seen inside back to an external cathode ray tube monitor for viewing. This particular endoscope also may permit suctioning of bronchial secretions, biopsies, fluid and sputum samples for analysis, and removal of foreign matter from the bronchi. A patient to be 'bronchoscoped' is usually given a sedative and a topical anesthetic.

bucca

bucca Latin, cheek

buccal fat pad

buccalis scientific Latin, pertaining to the cheek

A buccal fat pad gives human babies that plump-cheeked look. It is a disc-shaped lipid deposit under the subcutaneous layer of the skin directly over the buccinator muscle. It is sometimes called the sucking pad, and generally loses prominence by the time the infant is weaned.

buccal glands

buccalis scientific Latin, pertaining to the cheek + *glans, glandis* acorn, small organ

The buccal glands are minor glands that secrete saliva, located between the buccinator muscle and the vestibule of the mouth.

buccal smear

A buccal smear, obtained on a swab from the mucus lining the interior cheek, can be used to determine the genetic sex of a person.

buccina-tor

buccinator, Latin, trumpet-player < *buccina*, trumpet + *tor* Latin agent noun suffix

To play the trumpet, one uses, among other body parts, the cheeks or *buccae*. The buccinator muscle is one of the facial muscles that horn-players refer to when they speak of 'getting their chops in shape'. The buccinator is the chief muscle of the cheek, acting to compress the cheek and hold food under the teeth during chewing.

bu-limia

bous ox + *limia* hunger

Ancient Greek medicine recognized and named this disorder in which they thought human patients ate like oxen. Cycles of eating binges followed by self-induced vomiting and then depressive fasting are symptomatic of this appetite disorder.

bulla

bulla Latin, bubble; plural bullae

Bulla is the technical term for a large blister or vesicle, raised from the surface of the skin, containing serous fluid. It is more than 5 mm in diameter. But note emphysematous bullae, air-filled sacs in the lung caused by destruction of elastic tissue of the lung. This stage of emphysema may lead to pulmonary failure.

bursa

bursa Greek, a leather wine-skin, an ox-hide pouch; in medicine, a sac of fluid near joints; plural, bursae

A bursa is a small pouch or sac associated with a joint and filled with synovial fluid. A bursa reduces friction by permitting body parts to glide smoothly over one another. Typical bursal sites are under muscles, under skin, under tendons and under fascia.

burs-itis

bursa leather pouch + *itis* inflammation of

Bursitis is inflammation of bursae, commonly of subdeltoid bursae located under the deltoid muscles that cover each shoulder.

The Romans used *bursa* in Latin, whence it gave rise to many words in European languages, like English *purse* and *bursary*, French *la Bourse* and Spanish *la Bolsa*, 'stock exchange', with the sense of the nation's purse. One disbursed funds originally by taking money out of a purse. If one puts money back into someone's purse, one reimburses them.

C

caduceus

caduceus Latin, the wand carried by a professional Roman messenger; as a medical symbol, a winged stick encircled by a snake or two snakes. Compare *kerukeion*, Greek, herald's wand < *kerux*, herald, messenger.

When the Greeks created their messenger of the gods, Hermes – and later the Romans created their equivalent, Mercury – they depicted them both wearing winged sandals and a winged hat to show their speed, and holding the caduceus, traditional sign of a herald who comes in peace to bring news.

However, the stick encircled by the snake had been a symbol of magic healing in the ancient Near East for millennia. Long before Hermes was ever depicted carrying the messenger's rod, the same caduceus – with one snake – was the magic wand of pre-Hellenic healers from whom the cult of Asklepios arose. Among the ancient Greeks, Asklepios was revered as the founder of medicine and achieved divine status as the god of healing. So popular was he in ancient Greece that shrines were devoted to his worship, where the sick or their relatives came, made an offering, and hoped for a specific cure to be revealed magically in dreams. Part of the ceremony in the chief temple of Asklepios at Epidaurus involved snakes kept by the attending priests.

In Greek mythology, the god Hermes is associated with the myth of Asklepios. Apollo sent Hermes to take the unborn Asklepios from his dying mother's womb. Hermes also conveyed the infant Asklepios to the centaur Cheiron who taught him the arts of healing and hunting. It was probably to remind their audience of this association that Greek artists began to show Hermes carrying Asklepios' caduceus. The Romans borrowed Asklepios as Aesculapius, and much of the mumbo-jumbo, even the magic snake wand.

The first systematic collection of practical medical knowledge is attributed by tradition to Hippocrates (460–377 BC), a real physician who travelled throughout ancient Greece and may have operated a school for doctors on the Aegean island of Kos.

The snake has been a worldwide symbol of healing, probably since the dawn of *homo sapiens sapiens*. The snake symbolizes fertility, rejuvenation (shedding its skin annually), keen sight, wisdom, and finally active health. The

US Army Medical Corps uses a two-snaked caduceus as its symbol. Their British equivalent, the Royal Army Medical Corps, uses a caduceus with one snake.

caecum

caecum Latin, blind thing; in medicine the first part of the large intestine; plural caeca

An old name for the caecum is the blindgut or blind intestine, namely, the first part of the large intestine, which comprises a large pouch. The ileum, the colon and the vermiform appendix open into the caecum. The combining form modifies the root to *cec-*, giving cecal, cecocolon, cecostomy, cecotomy, etc.

ceco-pexy

caecum blindgut + *pexis* Greek, a fastening to, a fixation

Cecopexy is a surgical procedure to correct a disorder called mobile caecum, in which the opening pouch of the large intestine moves around too much, due to a congenital malformation or later mechanical injury. Such cecofixation involves suturing small areas of this pouch to the abdominal wall.

calc-

calx, calcis Latin, chalk, limestone, stone, heel; acquired scientific meaning 'calcium' and 'heel'

calc-aneus

calx, calcis heel + *aneus* Latin adjectival and noun suffix 'pertaining to, characteristic of'

The calcaneus is the heelbone, the largest of the seven tarsal bones that facilitate articulation of the foot with the leg. A still-seen, older name for the same bone is *os calcis*, bone of the heel, first used in *De Medicina* (AD 30) by the Roman medical writer Celsus.

calcar

calcar spur, Roman army term for a rider's spur, named because spurs were first affixed to the heel of military footwear

In anatomy, a calcar is a spur-like projection of a bone, for example, the *calcar femorale* is a bony process that gives extra rigidity to the neck of the femur. An older anatomical name for the heel, still seen in some European and British medical literature is *calcar pedis*, the spur of the foot. But note that calcareous goes back to the prime root and means 'chalky, made of limestone'.

calci-fer-ol

calx, calcis calcium + *ferre* Latin, to carry + *ol* biochemical suffix indicating an alcohol

Calciferol or vitamin D_2 is an unsaturated alcohol that occurs in milk and fish-liver oils. A synthetic version is part of the treatment of bone deficiency disorders like rickets.

calci-tonin

calx, calcis calcium + *tonos* Greek, quality of being stretched, like a musical note (tone) or a muscle, from *teinein*, to stretch + *in* common noun ending for organic chemical compounds

Calcitonin is a thyroid hormone that helps regulate calcium levels in blood and hence muscle contraction and the depositing of calcium in bone building.

calc-ium

calx, calcis limestone + *ium* Latin noun suffix 'thing containing or related to', hence its modern adoption as the general suffix to indicate the chemical elements: helium, magnesium, potassium, radium, sodium, uranium, etc.

Calcium (chemical symbol Ca) is the fifth most common chemical element in the human body, found in bones, blood and other tissues, because the body needs calcium ions to transmit nerve impulses and perform muscle contraction, blood clotting, heart actions and various other body functions.

calc-ulus

calx, calcis limestone + *ulus* Latin, diminutive suffix indicating smallness, therefore *calculus* = limestone pebble; in medicine pathologic accretion or stone

A calculus is an abnormal stone that forms in body organs from the concretion of urinary mineral salts, and therefore the organs usually affected are the gallbladder, kidneys, ureter and urethra. Consequent inflammation and obstruction may impede the natural flow of fluids through these organs.

   In ancient Rome, round limestone pebbles were used as gambling tokens and voting ballots. Roman children used limestone pebbles to learn counting on a device much like an abacus, hence the origin of English words like calculate, calculation, and the branch of mathematics, calculus.

calor

calor Latin, heat

Calor can be the moderate heat of normal human metabolism, or the heat of fever, but is most frequently used in medicine as follows. The four classic signs of inflammation, the reaction of tissue to injury, are stated as Latin nouns:

calor heat;
dolor pain;
rubor redness;
tumor swelling.

Inflamed tissue is red, swollen, warm to touch, and painful because of increased blood supply whose white cells fight infection and remove dead tissue. Blood also flows to injured tissue to bring extra cell food for the generation of new cells.

calor-ie

calor heat + *ie* French noun suffix

A calorie is a unit of heat measurement, namely, the total heat needed to raise the temperature of one gram of water by one degree Celsius. Calorimetry is the act of scientific heat measurement. The device used is a calorimeter, e.g. respiration calorimeter.

cancer

cancer Latin, crab, a disease of malignant tumors

Both early Greek and Roman physicians used their nouns for *crab* to refer to the disease. The English words *canker* and *chancre* derive from *cancer*, crab, Latin. Cancer as a crab is one of the signs of the zodiac. The Roman doctor Galen (AD 131–201), like many of the best physicians of the Roman empire, was a Greek who wrote in Greek. His writings summarize ancient anatomy and medical procedure, adding new observations based on his own practice. For 1400 years Galen's writings were *the* authority on medicine in the Christian world. Galen wrote that 'cancerous veins' extend out from the disease site like the claws of a crab. Another early medical writer claimed that, like a crab, cancer reaches out when it metastasizes and seizes many different parts of the body.

Much earlier than Galen, in the Hippocratic school of ancient medicine, *karkinos* meant 'a non-healing ulcer', and *karkinoma* was 'a malignant tumor' (a cancer). The Greek word for crab is *karkinos*. Carcinoma is *karkinos* plus the common suffix *-oma*, which has the medical meaning of benign or malignant tumor or swelling.

A note on medical euphemism and cancer jargon

Suppose a bedridden person has just been told he has cancer. In the initial days of his adjustment to this fact, his attending physician may have to refer to the cancer and may judge the blunt word too unbearable to repeat in front of his patient. Years ago, a doctor could have used the word *carcinoma* and been reasonably sure most patients would not have known this synonym for cancer. That is not always true today, when public awareness of the major diseases and the vocabulary used to describe them has grown. But medical jargon provides a long list of euphemistic alternatives. Doctors can and do refer to cancer as 'the mitotic figure', 'a neoplasm', or 'a neoplastic figure'. If a cancer has spread to form new foci of disease distant from the original site, they might say 'the mitotic incident has metastasized'. But plenty of patients know and fear the word 'metastasis'. So more obscure levels of technical language and circumlocution may have to be plumbed, as when a physician might refer to one specific cancer site as a 'melanosarcomatous excrescence'. In general, however, obscure technical jargon is not necessary during doctor–patient interchanges. Even in medical literature, one seldom *needs* to call a black eye 'a circumorbital hematoma'. Naturally, that is not said to deny the legitimacy of specialized medical vocabulary items like cholecystostomy, the *raison d'être*, after all, of this book. On the other hand, yes, there are compassionate reasons for employing euphemism now and then in the practice of medicine.

candid-

candidus, shining white; a Roman candidate for office wore a symbolically white toga

Candida is a yeastlike fungus normally found in mucous membranes of the mouth, intestines and vagina. *Candida albicans,* with a *double* white name (see *alb* entry), is the usual microbial culprit in so-called yeast infections. Its proliferation causes white patches in the mouth called thrush. The body's natural bacteria usually keep *Candida* within bounds, but powerful antibiotic drugs can control it until natural bacterial suppression returns.

candid-iasis

candidus white + *iasis* < *osis* diseased condition

Candidiasis is infection by *Candida* fungi. A former name is moniliasis, itself from the former name of the fungi genus *Candida*.

cannula

canna Latin, hollow reed + *ula* diminutive suffix indicating smallness; now a medical device: a hollow tube that guides a sharp-pointed puncturing instrument

A cannula is a hollow tube inserted into any body cavity to act as a guide for another instrument, or to draw off any abnormal volume of fluid, or to introduce a solution of drugs. A trocar can be inserted through the lumen of a cannula. The trocar is a sharp, three-pointed instrument for piercing the wall of a body cavity. After it pierces the wall, the trocar may be withdrawn, leaving the cannula in place. An example is trocar cystostomy, placing a catheter in the urinary bladder. Cannulation is the process of inserting a cannula into a duct or cavity.

capillary

capilla Latin, hair + *arius* adjectival ending

Capillaries are the tiny blood vessels that connect arterioles and venules. The very thin walls of a capillary are permeable. They permit the diffusion of arterial oxygen from the blood into individual cells. From the cell into the capillary, products of cell metabolism enter the bloodstream for eventual filtering and excretion.

capillary nail refill test

The time taken for capillaries to refill after pressure has been exerted upon them can provide a gross estimate of the force of the blood pressure. A capillary nail refill test or nail blanch test involves pressing on a finger nail briefly until it turns pale, then measuring the time required for the nail to turn pink again. Normal time is two seconds or less (from pale to pink). Three to five seconds shows a sluggish circulation, at least in the fingers. More than five seconds is abnormal.

caput

caput, capitis Latin, head, adjective *capitalis*, of the head

caput costae

caput head + *costae* Latin, of the rib

The caput costae is the head of a rib which articulates directly with a vertebra.

caput femoris

femur, femoris Latin, of the big leg bone
The head of the femur articulates with the acetabulum (see entry).

caput humeri

humerus, humeri Latin, of the humerus
Caput humeri is the formal anatomical name of the head of the humerus bone, which articulates in the glenoid cavity of the scapula (shoulder blade). Glenoid = *glene* Greek, joint socket + *oid* like, similar.

oc-ciput

ob > *oc* Latin, behind, at the back of + *ciput* < *caput* head
Occiput is a general term for the back of the head or skull. Two occipital arteries branch from each of the external carotids and together form six branches that supply blood to parts of the head and scalp. The occipital bone forms the saucer-shaped back of the skull and part of the skull base. It has a large opening, the *foramen magnum* (see entry) where the occipital bone articulates with the atlas, the first vertebra of the spinal column. The occipital lobe is one of the five lobes of each cerebral hemisphere. It is the posterior lobe and is shaped like a small pyramid.

sin-ciput

sin < *semi* half + *ciput* < *caput* head
The sinciput is the upper part of the head, the anterior part of the head, a term sometimes seen in anatomy texts.

capitate

capitatus with a head
In anatomy, the capitate bone is one of the bones of the wrist, one of the carpal bones, having a rounded extremity or head.

capit-ulum

caput, capitis head + *ulum* Latin, diminutive suffix indicating smallness

A capitulum is a small process on a bone where it articulates with another bone. For example, the *capitulum humeri* is the round process at the distal end of the humerus where it articulates with the radius.

cardi-

kardia Greek, heart

Cardiac arrest is the sudden stopping of the heart function of pumping out blood, with the consequent cessation of circulation.

cardio-pulmon-ary

kardia heart + *pulmo, pulmonis* Latin, the lung + *arius* adjectival ending

Cardiopulmonary resuscitation (CPR) is an easily learned method of restoring heart function and normal breathing to some victims of cardiac arrest. CPR involves artificial respiration and massage of the heart by external hand pressure on the chest.

electro-cardio-gram (ECG)

elektron Greek, amber, then modern meaning 'electric' + *kardia* heart + *gram* something written or recorded

An electrocardiogram is a graphic record of the heart's electrical impulses and changes due to disorders. Frequently in science, the word ending in *-gram* is the actual record, while the machine that makes the record is a word ending in *-graph*, in this instance, an electrocardiograph.

myo-card-

mys, myos Greek, muscle + *kardia* heart

Myocardium is heart muscle, cardiac muscle that surrounds the heart in a tough, thick layer.

myocardial infarction

myocardialis scientific Latin, of the heart muscle + *infarctio, infarctionis* Latin, stuffing a sausage until it is full

A myocardial infarction is a heart attack due to the closing off of a coronary artery that causes an infarct of the heart muscle. In an infarct, part of the heart muscle dies from lack of oxygen because blood supply via the coronary artery has been interrupted. Infarction is a 17th Century coinage belonging to the discredited theory of humors, and so the word is not truly appropriate to modern cardiology – but some old words die slowly. Originally, infarction referred to a 'stuffing together' of bodily humors.

cardio-myo-pathy

kardia heart + *mys, myos* Greek, muscle + *pathos* Greek, disease + *y* noun ending
A myopathy is any muscle disease. A cardiomyopathy is any disease of heart muscle.

idio-pathic cardiomyopathy

idios Greek, peculiar to one person + *pathikos* of a disease
'Idiopathic' first described a disease unique and particular to one patient, and then developed its current meaning 'pertaining to a disease of unknown cause'. Therefore, an idiopathic cardiomyopathy is any heart-muscle disease of unknown cause. Although the cause may be unknown, an idiopathic disease may exhibit known symptoms and be curable.

carotid

karotides Greek, the arteries of the neck < *karos* heavy sleep < *karoun* to choke, to stupefy
Ancient Greek physicians named the principal arteries of the neck as the carotid arteries with that adjective because they thought pressing hard on these arteries made mammals and humans become sleepy or lose consciousness.

The two carotid arteries are the main blood supply to the head and neck from the heart. If they are obstructed, brain tissue loses oxygen with a damaging, sometimes fatal result. In martial arts, there are two places on the neck where, if sufficient pressure is applied on a carotid artery, the victim may lose consciousness.

carpus

carpus Latin, wrist; *carpalis* adjective, of the wrist
The carpus is the anatomical name for the wrist, the joint between an arm and a hand that consists of eight wrist bones called carpals. The carpals are arranged in two rows.
The proximal row of carpals includes:

1.	The scaphoid bone, *os scaphoideum*	the boat-shaped carpal with a little hollow; *skaphe* Greek, boat, skiff + *oid* similar to *os* Latin, bone

2. The lunate bone, *os lunatum* — the vaguely moon-shaped carpal lying between the scaphoid and the triquetral carpals; *lunatus* moon-shaped

3. The triangular or triquetral bone *os triquetrum* — the carpal that roughly resembles a little pyramid; *triquetrus* three-cornered, triangular

4. The pisiform bone, *os pisiformis* — the smallest carpal, an oval, pea-shaped nodule of bone located in a wrist tendon. It is one of the sesamoid ('tiny as a sesame seed') bones of the human body which protect certain tendons subject to repeated compression and tension by adding extra internal support; *pisum* Latin, pea + *formis* shaped like

The distal row of carpals includes:

5. The trapezium bone, *os trapezium* — the most lateral bone of the distal row of carpals; *trapeza* Greek, table + *ion* diminutive suffix, 'little'

6. The trapezoid bone, *os trapezoideum* — the carpal between the trapezium and capitate bones; *trapezion* little table + *oid* similar to

7. The capitate bone, *os capitatum* — the large carpal bone at the center of the wrist with a rounded head that fits the hollow part of the adjacent scaphoid and lunate carpals; *capitatus* with a round prominence or *caput*, head

8. The hamate bone, *os hamatum* — the little wrist bone that rests on the fourth and fifth metacarpals was named because of its tiny, hook-like, bony process, the hamulus (little hook); *hamatus* having a hook, hooked

meta-carpals

meta Greek, after + *carpalis* pertaining to the wrist
The metacarpals are the five bones of the middle part of the hand that come after the carpals; they form the palm of the hand.

carpal tunnel syndrome (CTS)

The flexing tendons of the fingers and the median nerve of the hand pass through a very small tunnel near the wrist bones. Numbness and great pain may result if the tendons press on the nerve due to repetitive wrist actions from, for example, certain keyboarding movements in computerized word processing, or from wrist stress in carpentry and sports such as rowing and tennis. Pregnancy and menopause may aggravate CTS. The aching, tingling pain and/or numbness may radiate to the forearm and shoulder.

carpo-ptosis

carpus wrist + *ptosis* Greek, a falling down, a drooping, a dropping

Ptosis is displacement of a body part from its normal position, also called prolapse. Therefore, carpoptosis is wrist drop. Wrist drop is a condition in which the hand is bent at the wrist and cannot be straightened or extended. Wrist drop is a symptom of muscular paralysis of the extensors of the hand and fingers, or of other injury to the radial nerve which innervates these extensor muscles.

computerized axial tomography (CAT)

One example of a CAT scan might involve hundreds of X-ray pictures taken as a machine revolves around the head. The X-rays of these sectional brain views, compared in a computer to previous X-ray series, help the physician, with other scanner data files, assess the size and spread of a brain tumor. Axial refers to an axis, an imaginary line drawn through the center of a body part, around which the body part could be said to revolve. By minutely altering the axis of the part being scanned, many different axial views are made.

tomo-graphy

tome Greek, cutting, slicing + *graphe* writing, recording

A tomograph is a machine that moves an X-ray tube through an arc, so that the X-ray shows one plane of tissue clearly. Tomography is the process of recording such multiple planes for later study.

cata-

cata- Greek, down, under, against; combining forms: *kata, kat, cat, cath*

cathar-sis

katharos pure, clean + *(o)sis* Greek noun ending here indicating process of = *katharsis* a cleansing

In physiology, catharsis is purging the bowels. In Freudian psychiatry, catharsis is cleansing the mind of repressed incidents that may have caused neuroses by bringing feelings and ideas into consciousness through free association, sometimes while the patient is under hypnosis.

cathartic

kathartikos Greek adjective, purgative
A cathartic is an agent that induces evacuation of the bowel.

cath-eter

kath < *kata* down + *hienai* to send, to cause to go, so *katheter* Greek, thing put in, thing let down into, inserted, lowered
A catheter is a flexible tube put into a body part, either to drain liquid from that part, or add liquid to it. The word is first found in Hippocratic Greek, referring to a metallic instrument used for emptying the bladder. Ancient Roman catheters were found in the ruins of Pompeii.

Some of the modern types of catheter are:

Balloon catheter	an inflated balloon is filled with water, air, saline or a contrast medium after the catheter is inserted. The balloon holds the catheter in place until the bladder is empty
Double-channel catheter	has two passageways so that liquids can pass in and out of a body cavity
Elbowed or prostatic catheter	an acute bend near the tip is designed to allow this catheter to pass a prostatic enlargement
Foley catheter	invented by American urologist Frederick Foley (1891–1966), this self-retaining urinary tract catheter has a balloon that is filled with air or a sterile liquid after insertion, to prevent the catheter from leaving
Indwelling catheter	a catheter permitted to remain in a body tube for a period of time
Triple-lumen catheter	contains three separate passageways

cata-lysis

kata Greek, down + *lysis* a breaking, so that *katalysis* = a dissolving, a breakdown

cata-lyst

kata Greek, down + *lystes* loosener, separator

The Greek agent noun suffix *-istes* is equivalent to *-or, -tor* in Latin words like actor, donor and senator; and *er* in English words like baker, maker and singer. Words borrowed by English with this Greek agent noun suffix include antagonist, evangelist and protagonist. English and many European languages use this ending as a prolific source of agent nouns, e.g. alarmist, biologist, chemist, dentist, pianist, sociologist and terrorist.

A catalyst is a substance that speeds up a chemical reaction, or is necessary for that reaction to occur, but is not itself altered in the reaction it assists. Such a catalytic process is catalysis.

cata-rrh

kata Greek, down + *rrhoia* Greek, a flowing (see *-rrhea* entry)

Catarrh is any discharge due to inflammation of a mucous membrane, e.g. from a runny nose. In medicine, catarrh usually refers to inflammatory discharge from the airways of the nose and trachea.

cata-ract

kata Greek, down + *rrhaktes* something that rushes, drops quickly; in medicine, a loss of transparency in the lens of the eye

Modern medical dictionaries state that this term comes from the Greek word for waterfall. A cataract is a loss of transparency in the lens of the eye. In what way might this progressive opacity of the lens be related to a waterfall? In no way whatsoever. Cataract in fact derives from a Greek noun whose prime meaning is sluice gate, portcullis, or dense iron grating over a window, that is, something that obstructed a view – as a cataract may be said to do.

cata-tonia

kata Greek, down + *tonos* Greek, stretching + *ia* medical condition

Although Hippocrates used the verb *katatenein* to mean 'to stretch for the purpose of setting a bone', the noun was coined by the German psychologist Karl Kahlbaum (1828–1899) in his journal article 'Die Katatonie' (1874), where it means, as it still does, 'lack of muscle tone or tension symptomatic of a schizophrenic phase characterized by motor disturbance, often rigidity and stupor'.

cauda

cauda Latin, tail, tail-like anatomical structure
The Latin word for tail, *cauda*, has reflexes (modern linguistic derivatives) in several common words. The tail-end of a piece of music, the finale of a classical ballet, a part added at the end of a sonnet, each is a coda. *Cauda* transformed into Old French as *cue* and *queue*, which English then borrowed to give us words and phrases like billiard cue, cue ball, to queue up in a line for tickets, a queue of cars at the gas station.

cauda equina

cauda Latin, tail + *equinus* of a horse
At the first lumbar vertebra a bundle of nerves goes through the spinal canal of the sacrum and coccyx (see entries). To early anatomists, this nerve bundle looked like a little horse's tail.

cauda pancreatis

cauda Latin, tail + *pancreatis* of the pancreas
The cauda pancreatis is the formal anatomical name for the left tail of the pancreas that touches the spleen and the area where the transverse and descending colon join.

caudal an-esthesia

caudalis of the tail + *an* not + *esthesia* feeling, sensation
Caudal anesthesia is the injection of a local anesthetic into the lower end of the spinal canal through the sacrum, sometimes indicated in childbirth and for surgery of the anus, rectum and urogenital area.

cavity

cavitas Latin, an empty space, a hollow place, a hole; compare the English word cave

A cavity is the site of dental caries, or a body space that often contains internal organs, for example:

Abdominal cavity	contains stomach and intestines;
Buccal cavity	the space between the cheeks for food; *bucca* Latin, cheek;
Cranial cavity	contains the brain;
Orbital cavity	contains an eyeball;
Pelvic cavity	contains organs of reproduction and excretion;
Spinal cavity	contains the spinal cord;
Thoracic cavity	contains the lungs.

-cele

kele Greek, hernia, swelling

cysto-cele

kystis Greek, sac, bladder; usually in medicine, the urinary bladder + *kele* Greek, hernia
A cystocele is the hernial protrusion of the urinary bladder through the wall of the vagina. One surgical procedure to correct cystocele is cystopexy, the suturing of the bladder to the abdominal wall (*pexis* Greek, a fastening).

hydro-cele

hydros Greek, of water + *kele* Greek, hernia
Hydrocele was so named because the Roman medical writer Celsus mistakenly thought it was a hernia. Hydrocele is a contained accumulation of fluid in the serous membrane that surrounds the testes, caused by inflammation of a testis or the epididymus. Hydrocele can also occur along the spermatic cord if adjacent veins or lymphatic vessels become blocked. One operation to relieve it is hydrocelectomy, draining and excising the accumulation.

celio-

koilia Greek, belly, abdomen

celiac artery

coeliacus Latin, abdominal
The celiac artery is a stout branch of the abdominal aorta that typically divides into three smaller arteries: the left gastric, the common hepatic and the splenic.

celiac disease

Celiac disease is an inherited defect of metabolism, in which the body cannot properly digest gluten, a protein in grains like wheat. Symptoms are swollen abdomen, vomiting, diarrhea, wasting and lethargy. An older plain-English term for celiac disease was sprue. A medical name much more accurate and descriptive is gluten-induced enteropathy, which is gaining acceptance. Enteropathy = *enteron* Greek, intestines + *pathos* disease.

celiac plexus = solar plexus

plexus Latin, a braid, a plait

In medicine, a plexus is a tangled intermingling of blood vessels, nerves or lymph vessels. We have all heard of a boxer getting a hard back slam, or getting punched in the solar plexus. It is also called the *celiac* plexus, a network of nerve fibers and ganglia at the upper back of the abdomen. It is named solar from the Latin word *solaris* 'of the sun', because sympathetic and parasympathetic nerves radiate out from this plexus like rays from the shining sun.

cell

cella Latin, a small room, from *celare* to hide, to conceal

The cell is the basic structural unit of body tissue. A cell membrane encloses the protoplasm, all the material inside a cell. A cell nucleus controls cell activities and carries genetic information. The study of cells is cytology (*kytos* Greek, cell). Cytoplasm is all the material inside the cell except the nucleus. Protoplasm = *protos* Greek, first, basic + *plasma* Greek, thing formed.

sickle cell anemia, an-em-ia

an not + *em* short for *haima*, Greek, blood + *ia* medical condition

Sickle cell anemia is a serious and painful genetic disorder, mostly of negroid peoples, in which faulty hemoglobin formation produces severe damage to the blood system. The fragile red blood cells characteristic of the disorder look wizened and sickle-shaped.

cent-esis

kent Greek verbal root, puncture + *esis* Greek noun ending, action of = *kentesis*, a surgical puncturing

Centesis is the surgical puncture of a cavity or hollow structure often to aspirate accumulated fluid, both to drain the fluid and obtain a sample of the fluid for testing.

amnio-centesis

amnion Greek, inner sac enclosing fetus + *kentesis* Greek, a puncturing

Amniocentesis is a diagnostic procedure in which, early in a pregnancy, about the 16th week, a small sample of amniotic fluid is aspirated through a hollow needle put through the uterine wall. If done late in the pregnancy, the procedure can be performed through the cervix. Chemical analyses of the fluid and genetic analysis of the fetal cellular debris in the fluid may help determine the health of the fetus and the presence of some congenital defects like Down's syndrome or Tay–Sachs disease.

arthro-centesis

arthron Greek, joint + *kentesis* Greek, a puncturing

Arthrocentesis is puncturing the cavity of a joint and drawing off a small volume of synovial fluid for analysis.

-ceps

-ceps < *caput* Latin, head, as medical suffix: with head(s), part(s), end(s), etc.

bi-ceps

bis Latin, twice + *ceps* head

The biceps is an arm muscle with two heads, that is, two points of origin or two divisions, a long head and a short head. The biceps helps flex the forearm and turn it up or down.

tri-ceps

tris thrice < *tres* three + *ceps* head

The triceps is a muscle of the upper arm with three points of origin called the long head, lateral head, and medial head. The triceps helps extend the arm and forearm.

quadri-ceps femoris

quadri of four + *ceps* head + *femoris* of the femur

The quadriceps is the large front thigh muscle, made up of four smaller muscles, all of which work together to extend the leg.

cephal-

kephale Greek, head

cephal-ic

kephalikos of the head

Cephalic means pertaining to the head, or, as an anatomical direction, located toward the head, but the better anatomical descriptive is cephalad.

cephalic vein

The cephalic vein carries used blood anteriorly up the arm and then empties into the axillary vein. So why is a vein of the arm labeled with an adjective meaning 'of the head?'

The cephalic vein is an example of a badly named body part, and a thus confusing medical word, all based on a translator's mistake. Some important early medical texts were in Arabic, for example, the Canon of Avicenna. This was written by a Persian physician named Ibn Sina (AD 980–1037), known in European languages as Avicenna, who wrote books collecting the medical knowledge of his times. The Canon of Avicenna was an important textbook in medieval medical schools, with more than 14 editions in the 15th Century alone. In Avicenna's Arabic, this vein of the arm was named *al-kifal,* 'the outer (vein of the arm)'. When the Canon was translated into Latin in AD 1564, the translator thought *al-kifal* was related to Greek *kephalikos* 'pertaining to the head' and its Latin form *cephalicus.* He was wrong, but the naming error stuck, and became sanctified by tradition. This happens too often in the conservative realms of medical nomenclature.

en-cephal-on

en > eg in + *kephale* head + *on* common ending of Greek neuter nouns, therefore *egkephalon* is the brain, literally 'the part in the head'

en-cephal-itis

egkephalos brain + *itis* inflammation of

Encephalitis is any one of many inflammatory diseases of the brain, e.g. vernal encephalitis of Russia, acquired from tick bites in the spring, also passed on in infected milk and flesh.

electro-encephalo-gram (EEG)

elektro modern meaning 'electric' + *egkephalos* brain + *gram* something written or recorded

An electroencephalogram is a graphic record of the brain's electrical activity, captured by electrodes placed on the scalp. The recorded brain waves are categorized by their frequencies as alpha, beta, delta, or theta waves. The machine that makes such recordings is an electroencephalograph.

hydro-cephalus

hydros of water + *kephale* head

Hydrocephalus is a disease characterized by excess cerebrospinal fluid in the brain. The popular name for the disorder is apt: water on the brain.

micro-cephal-y

micros Greek, small + *kephale* head + *y* noun ending

Microcephaly is a congenital irregularity in which the head is abnormally small in relation to the rest of the body. The brain of microcephalic individuals is underdeveloped, causing some mental retardation.

cer-

cera Latin, wax; akin to *keros* Greek, wax, beeswax; in medicine the combining form means 'wax' or 'waxy'

cer-oma

keros wax + *oma* common medical noun suffix that means 'tumor, swelling'

A ceroma is a benign tumor of waxy composition.

cerumen

cerumen scientific Latin, earwax

Cerumen or earwax is secreted by tiny, modified sweat glands (ceruminous glands) in the external ear canal which produce a waxy substance instead of sweat.

cerumin-osis

cerumen earwax + *osis* diseased or abnormal condition
Ceruminosis is a buildup of earwax that may lead to discomfort, infection, and mild temporary hearing loss. Relief is provided by ceruminolytic medications that loosen earwax and permit its removal. Cerumino-lysis = *cerumen* earwax + *lysis* Greek, 'a breaking up of'.

cereb-ellum

cerebrum Latin, brain + *ellum* diminutive suffix meaning 'small, little'
The Latin word for 'little brain' denotes a part of the brain located behind and under the cerebrum. The cerebellum regulates voluntary muscular activity like walking, getting dressed, scratching an itch, etc.

cerebra-, cerebri-, cerebro-

combining forms denoting cerebrum, the largest, uppermost part of the brain; see *cerebrum* entry

cerebral cortex

cerebralis of the brain + *cortex* Latin, bark, outer covering
The cerebral cortex is the thin layer of gray matter on the outer surface of the cerebral hemispheres, where many higher mental functions are integrated.

cerebral edema

cerebralis of the brain + *oidema* Greek, fluid-filled swelling
Cerebral edema is an abnormal accumulation of fluid in brain tissues, due to infection, tumor, or trauma. As mounting pressure injures nearby brain tissues, symptoms include involuntary muscle contractions, dilation of pupils, and a slow loss of consciousness that may lead to fatality.

cerebral hemo-rrhage

cerebralis of the brain + *haima* Greek, blood + *rrhagia* Greek, bursting, gushing forth
A hemorrhage is a bleeding, an escape of blood from its vessels. Cerebral hemorrhage is a flow of blood from a ruptured vessel in the brain. One frequent instance occurs when high blood pressure causes the rupture of a sclerotic artery

near the basal ganglia. Cerebral hemorrhage may also be due to injury to the head or the bursting of an aneurysm (see entry). Symptoms may include dizziness, numbness, loss of certain mental functions, coma, or even death.

cerebral palsy

cerebralis of the brain + *palsy* Medieval French contraction of *paralysie* < paralysis < *para* Greek, beside + *lysis* Greek, a breaking up of function, a loosening; ancient Greek medical writers referred to any disabling of the limbs as *paralysis*

Cerebral palsy is permanent impaired control of muscles due to brain damage at or just before birth. Symptoms may include spastic paralysis of the arms and legs, mental retardation and seizures.

cerebrum

cerebrum Latin, brain

The cerebrum comprises the largest mass of brain tissue. Its two cerebral hemispheres at the top of the cranial cavity control conscious activities like speech, writing and emotional responses, as well as other sensory, motor and integrative functions including memory.

cerebrospinal fluid (CSF)

Normally a clear, colorless, watery liquid, CSF flows through and fills the cavities of the brain and spinal cord. It is a shock absorber, acting to cushion brain and spinal tissue from physical impacts when the body moves or suffers accidents. Chemical analyses of CSF provide diagnostic clues in the detection of certain diseases like some forms of meningitis, brain abscesses, polio and syphilis. Cerebrospinal fluid is often sampled by means of a lumbar puncture, in which an aspirating needle draws a small volume from a space in the lumbar portion of the spinal canal. A popular name for this procedure is spinal tap.

cerebro-vascular

cerebralis of the brain + *vasculum* < *vas* vessel + *culum* diminutive suffix meaning 'little'

cerebrovascular accident (CVA)

A cerebrovascular accident is a stroke. Brain hemorrhage or blockage of cerebral blood vessels causes brain tissue to become starved of oxygen. Symptoms may include sudden loss of movement of an arm or leg, and impaired speech. Often only one side of the body is affected. Physiotherapy may help recover some use of affected body parts.

cervix

cervix, cervicis Latin, neck, any neck-like structure, combining forms: *cervica-, cervico-*
The cervix is the lower, narrower, neck-like part of the uterus that extends into the vagina. Among other functions, the cervix is a conduit for spermatozoa on their way to fertilize an egg. Menstrual blood also passes out of the uterus through the cervix during menstruation (see entry).

It is sometimes specified as the uterine cervix or *cervix uteri* in *Nomina Anatomica*, Latin for 'anatomical names'. The anatomical names are a set of Latin terms for parts of the body, agreed upon by the International Congress of Anatomists who meet regularly to revise and update medical nomenclature.

cervical cap

The cervical cap is a barrier method of contraception not common in North America. Women who do not retain a diaphragm easily may be fitted for the cap, which looks like a big thimble. It fits over the cervix and is held in place by suction. A spermicide must be used with the cap.

cervical vertebra

cervicalis of the neck + *vertebra* Latin, a turning place, a joint, a bone of the spine that turned < *vertere* to turn
The first seven segments at the top of the spinal column are the neck bones or cervical vertebrae.

cheilo-

cheilos Greek, lip, combining form meaning 'lip of the mouth'

cheil-itis

cheilos Greek, lip + *itis* inflammation of
Cheilitis is inflammation of the lips due to sunburn, vitamin lack or allergy. For example, *cheilitis actinica* (*aktis, aktinos* Greek, ray of sunlight) is lip inflammation from too much sun exposure; *cheilitis venenata* (*venenatus* Latin,

poisoned) is lip inflammation from chemical irritants in lipsticks, lip creams and other cosmetics.

cheilo-gnatho-palato-schisis

cheilos Greek, lip + *gnathos* Greek, jaw + *palatum* palate + *schizein* to split + *osis* diseased condition

Cheilognathopalatoschisis is a congenital irregularity in which there is a cleft or split in the lips, in the upper jaw, and in the hard and soft palates.

cheil-osis

cheilos Greek, lip + *osis* diseased condition

Cheilosis or perliche is a riboflavin deficiency that causes the lips and mouth to crack and scale.

cheilo-plasty

cheilos Greek, lip + *plastia* new scientific Greek, a shaping, a forming, with later implication of 'forming by means of surgery'

Cheiloplasty is the surgical correction of any congenital defect of the lips.

cheilo-rrhaphy

cheilos Greek, lip + *rrhaphe* Greek, seam, surgical suture + *y* noun ending

Cheilorrhaphy is surgical suturing to repair a cleft lip.

cheilo-schisis

cheilos Greek, lip + *schizein* to split + *(o)sis* diseased condition

Cheiloschisis is split lip, harelip, or any congenital palatal fissure of varying severity.

chlor-

chloros Greek, green; combining form in chemical names: with a chlorine-containing radical; in medicine: pertaining to chlorides

chlor-ine

chloros green + *ine* common ending for the elements of the halogen family that comprises astatine, bromine, chlorine, fluorine and iodine

Chlorine is a chemical element whose pure form is a greenish, toxic gas. Common salt, an important constituent of body fluids including blood, is sodium chloride, the sodium salt of hydrochloric acid.

hyper-chlor-em-ia

hyper Greek, over, above, akin to Latin *super* + *chlor* chlorine + *em* short for *haima*, Greek, blood + *ia* medical condition

Hyperchloremia is too much salt and other chlorides in the blood.

hypo-chlor-em-ia

hypo Greek, under, below, beneath, less than, akin to Latin *sub* + *chlor* chlorine + *em* blood + *ia* medical condition

Hypochloremia is too little salt and other chlorides in the blood, often due to the frequent urination that accompanies the use of diuretics, or to prolonged gastric suctioning. A saline IV, a solution of salt in water delivered intravenously, corrects the deficiency.

chole-

chole Greek, bile, gall; combining form meaning 'bile, gall'

chole-cyst-ec-tomy

chole Greek, bile, gall + *kystis* Greek, sac, bladder + *ek* out + *tome* Greek, a surgical cutting

Cholecystectomy is surgical excision of the gallbladder. The standard procedure now is laparoscopic cholecystectomy. See *laparoscopy* entry. A popular name is 'keyhole' surgery.

chole-cyst-itis

chole gall + *kystis* bladder + *itis* inflammation of

Cholecystitis is acute or chronic inflammation of the gallbladder, as cystitis is inflammation of the urinary bladder.

chole-cysto-stom-y

chole gall + *kystis* bladder + *stoma* Greek, mouth, opening + *y*
noun ending
Cholecystostomy is the surgical making of a mouth-like opening in the
gallbladder through the abdominal wall, often for the purpose of inserting a
catheter to drain excess fluid accumulation from the gallbladder.

chole-ster-ol

chole Greek, bile, gall + *stereos* Greek, solid, firm + *ol*
biochemical suffix indicating an alcohol
Cholesterol is a solid alcohol of animal fats first isolated in gall stones. Early
doctors thought it was solidified bile, hence the name. But cholesterol, while it is
one of the many chemicals in bile, is not solid bile – so how apt is this name?

melan-chol-y

melas, melanos Greek, black + *chole* bile + *y* noun ending
Melancholy and melancholia mean sadness and brooding because early Greek
physicians, believing in the now discredited theory of humors, thought black
bile made one sad. The word *choler* also means bile or anger, because later
medieval doctors still believed excess bile made a person of angry temperament.

chondro-

chondros Greek, gristle, cartilage; combining form meaning
'cartilage'

chondro-blast

chondros cartilage + *blastos* Greek, a sprout, a bud
A chondroblast is a precursor cell that eventually forms cartilage.

chondro-blast-oma

chondros cartilage + *blastos* a bud + *oma* tumor
A chondroblastoma is any benign tumor of cartilage-forming cells in the
epiphysis of a bone, most commonly of a femur or humerus.

chondro-muc-in

chondros cartilage + *mucus* Latin, slime, goo + *in* ending for organic chemical compounds
Chondromucin is the gluey substance between cartilage cells.

chondro-sarc-oma

chondros cartilage + *sarx, sarkos* Greek, flesh + *oma* tumor
A sarcoma is a cancer that begins in connective tissue such as muscle and bone. A chondrosarcoma is a bone cancer, a malignant tumor arising in cartilaginous cells.

chondro-malacia patellae, or runner's knee

chondros cartilage + *malakia* Greek, softening + *patellae* Latin, of the kneecap
Athletes who strain a knee by the constant pounding shocks of running may suffer chondromalacia patellae, in which articular cartilage degenerates.

Patella means 'saucer' or 'small pan' in Latin. The human kneecap, whose anatomical name is patella, does *not* look like a small pan, but the Latin name is 600 years old. The kneecap bone is actually an irregular rectangle in shape.

hypo-chondria

hypo below + *chondros* cartilage + *ia* medical condition
The ancient Greeks used this word to refer to the area of the upper abdomen below and behind the cartilages of the lower ribs. It is still sometimes called the hypochondriac region. Ancient Greek physicians also believed that feelings of distress, depression, and general anxiety about one's health came from the hypochondriac region, and this is the origin of the term *hypochondriac* for a person with chronic, unrealistic concerns about his or her health.

hypochondriasis

Hypochondriasis is the preferred medical term for the older word *hypochondria*
Hypochondriasis is used by some clinicians for extreme patients who plunge into dangerous depression, convinced that they have diseases that rational medical evidence says they do not have.

chrom-

chroma chromatos Greek, color of the skin, then any color; combining form signifying 'color'

a-chromat-ic lens

a not + *chromatikos* Greek, suited for color

An achromatic lens does not disperse light into its components, although the lens permits light to pass through itself. Such achromatism is one symptom of the color blindnesses. See the next entry for another meaning of achromatic.

chromatic

chromatikos Greek, suited for color

In medicine – particularly in histology, the microscopic study of body cells and tissues – chromatic is said of a substance or tissue able to be stained by a dye. Achromatic is said of a substance that does not stain well. Tissue samples are stained with various agents to facilitate their inspection under a microscope or other instrument of histological analysis.

chromat-in

chromata colors + *in* noun ending for organic chemical compounds

Chromatin is the gene-carrying part of a cell nucleus (DNA and nucleic proteins) that takes color (stains) easily and deeply. Achromatin is the part of a cell nucleus that does not take a stain well and so appears fainter under a microscope.

chromato-phil

chroma chromatos color + *philos* Greek, loving

A chromatophil is any substance, a cell or tissue, that stains easily. An achromatophil is any substance that does not stain easily.

chromo-some

chroma color + *soma* Greek, body

Formed from chromatin – hence the name – a chromosome is a little, threadlike line of DNA in the nucleus of a cell. DNA is the chemical structure that transmits genetic information.

chronic

chronikos Greek, of time, persisting through time

A chronic disorder persists, lasts for a long time. Chronic disease is the opposite of acute disease. An acute (*acutus* Latin, sharp) disease comes to a crisis point quickly, has rapid onset, severe symptoms, and a short duration.

chyle

chylos Greek, digestive juice

Chyle is the white digestive fluid in which emulsified fats enter the bloodstream. Produced in the small intestines, chyle is absorbed, through tiny lymph channels that line the small intestines, into the thoracic duct, the main lymph-transporter tube of the body. The thoracic duct empties chyle into the left subclavian vein in the neck.

chylo-derma

chylos juice + *derma* skin

Fluids can become trapped in lymphatic vessels of the thick skin of the scrotum, due to tropical parasites, local infection, or cancer. A synonym for chyloderma is scrotal elephantiasis, named because the scrotal sac may become extremely swollen.

chylo-rrhea

chylos Greek, juice + *rrhoia* Greek, a flowing through, a discharge

Chylorrhea is escape of chyle from a ruptured thoracic duct, often into the peritoneal cavity, to produce a condition called chyloperitoneum.

chylo-peri-card-ium

chylos juice + *peri* around + *kardia* heart + *ium* Latin suffix 'thing containing or related to'

Chylopericardium is escaped chyle in the membranous sac that encloses the heart and the first parts of the great blood vessels.

chylo-pneumo-thorax

chylos Greek, juice + *pneuma* air + *thorax* chest

Chylopneumothorax is escaped chyle and air trapped in the pleural space, which is the space between the two layers of the protective membrane that enfold the lungs.

chyme

chymos Greek, fluid, juice
Chyme is the thick liquid mixture of partly digested food and digestive juices in the stomach.

chymos-in

chymos Greek, juice + *in* common ending for organic chemical compounds
Chymosin is an enzyme in the stomach of infants that curdles milk. Its old name *rennin* is being dropped because of confusion with renin.

chymo-tryps-in

chymos Greek, juice + *tripsis* Greek, rubbing, friction + *in* ending for organic chemical
Chymotrypsin is a pancreatic enzyme that assists in the digestive breakdown of proteins.

ec-chym-osis

ek, ex out + *chymos* juice + *osis* diseased condition
Ecchymosis is discoloration of the skin, in which large blue-black areas appear due to blood escaping from its vessels into surrounding mucous membranes and other tissues. The hemorrhagic blood eventually changes from blue-black to a greenish brown or yellow.

-cide

caedere Latin, to slay, to cut down with a sword; in medicine the suffix means 'killing, or causing a reduction in pathogenic quantity of'
The suffix is common in scientific terms. An amebicide is a chemical agent that kills amebas, a bactericide kills bacteria, a fungicide kills fungi, and a spermicide kills sperm. A suicide kills himself or herself (*sui* Latin, of one's own).

cilia

cilium Latin, eyelash, small hair; in medicine the plural, *cilia*, refers to hair-like projections on cells, or the eyelashes

Cilia project from the epithelial lining of the respiratory tract where their waving motion helps move particles of mucus and debris out of the tract.

ciliary body

ciliarius new scientific Latin, pertaining to an eyelid or a hairlike cilium

The ciliary body is behind the iris where it secretes the aqueous humor, the clear fluid that fills and circulates through the chambers of the eyeball. Here also is the ciliary muscle, the eye muscle chiefly involved in adjusting the eye to see nearby objects.

circum

circum Latin, around, circling, about

Medical words with *circum* include circumcorneal (around the cornea of the eye), circumlental (around the lens of the eye), and circumrenal (around the kidney); *renalis* Latin, of the kidney.

circum-cision

circum around + *cisio, cisionis* Latin combining form, a cutting < *caedere* to cut

A few days after birth in many cultures the foreskin of a baby's penis is cut off by surgery.

Aside from religious ritual, there is usually no medical reason for circumcision in a newborn male. However, if the father has been circumcized, he wants his son's penis to look exactly like his. The foreskin evolved to protect the head of the penis from injury and to maintain its sensitivity. Indications for circumcision may include a foreskin that is so tight that retraction is painful or often impossible. This condition is called phimosis, from *phimos*, the ancient Greek word for a leather device used to muzzle a dog or horse. The phimotic foreskin looked to ancient physicians somewhat like a muzzled dog.

Female circumcision is partial or complete removal of the clitoris. This useless mutilation of pre-pubertal girls is a tribal abomination of no medical legitimacy whatsoever. It should be made illegal in any country wishing to call itself civilized. It arises from a dread of female sexuality by primitive males and their wish to blame the female for the instigation of all sexual activity not condoned by a particular society.

cirrh-osis

kirrhos Greek color adjective, orange-yellow + *osis* diseased condition

The French physician René Laennec, inventor of the stethoscope, was also first to report orange-yellow deposits in the livers of alcoholics. Cirrhosis is a complex, chronic, degenerative disease of the liver, made worse as the cells and structures of the body's largest organ and main blood-filter lose function. Nutritional deficits, previous inflammations, and poisons other than alcohol may also cause cirrhosis.

clav-

clavis Latin, key, bolt, stick

clav-icle

clavicula Latin, twig, little stick, hoopstick, human collarbone
clavis stick + *-cula* Latin diminutive ending, small

Clavicula meant literally 'little key', but in Latin it also denoted a long hoop-stick, the water-bent wooden branch that Roman children used to trundle a hoop. This hoopstick was *f*-shaped like a human collarbone.

The clavicle is the long, slender, *f*-shaped collarbone that connects the breastbone (sternum) with the shoulder blade (scapula). The clavicle is the most frequently broken bone in the human body.

auto-clave

autos Greek, self + *clavis* Latin, key

An autoclave is a self-locking device for sterilizing medical instruments by steam pressure.

cleft

cleft Middle English past form of cleave, a variant of cleaved and cloven; in medicine a cleft is a split or fissure in a body structure

cleft palate

The palate is the roof of the mouth, a horizontal structure made of muscles and membranes, and supported by bones. The palate separates the mouth from the nasal cavity. Cleft palate or palatoschisis (*schisis* Greek, abnormal splitting) is a congenital defect. The two halves of the palate fail to fuse properly. Results range from a tiny groove at the edge of the lip, to total midline separation of the palate. Plastic surgery corrects this. Often palatoplasty (*plastia* forming by means of surgery) is an operation in two parts, each years apart. In severe cases, where the baby cannot suck milk easily, an early palatorrhaphy (*rrhaphe* surgical suturing) permits palate and lip function. Later, further plastic surgery of a cosmetic nature improves appearance.

clinic

kline Greek, a bed

In Latin, *clinicus* was a bedside lecture by a teaching physician to medical students. Later it also meant examining patients in front of a medical class. Then, in French, *clinique* meant a group of patients with similar diseases attending at one location to see a doctor. A dry clinic is a lecture with case histories of patients who are not present. Clinical diagnosis is the identification of a disease based on signs and symptoms, as opposed to diagnosing by using procedures like blood tests, X-rays, or invasive means such as surgery.

clitoris

kleitoris, kleitoridis Greek, clitoris < *kleis, kleidos* Greek, key + *oris* Greek agent noun suffix

The clitoris is a quarter-inch bud of sexually responsive tissue located just above the vaginal entrance, where the labia minora join. The seat of much sexual pleasure in the female, the clitoris may be hidden under a hood of flesh called the clitoral prepuce. The clitoris is analogous to the penis. *Kleitoris* in ancient Greek means literally 'the man with the key' or 'the gatekeeper'. A playful origin of names for this organ is repeated in many languages. Compare a British folk term, 'the little man in the boat'.

clitorid-itis

kleitoris, kleitoridis Greek, clitoris + *itis* inflammation of

Inflammation of the clitoris, also termed clitoritis.

clitoro-megaly

kleitoris + *megale* enlargement, from *megas* large

Clitoromegaly is abnormal enlargement of the clitoris, due to endocrine diseases, and seen in female athletes overdosing with anabolic steroids.

clone

klon ancient Greek botanical term, twig, slip, plant cutting used to propagate similar plants

A clone is an individual organism or group of cells grown from a single somatic cell of its parent and thus genetically identical to it, for example a plant propagated vegetatively rather than sexually, from a cutting instead of seed. In histology, a clone is a group of cells grown from a single mother cell by mitosis so that all the daughter cells are genetically identical.

clonus

klonos Greek, tumult, convulsion

Clonus is involuntary, rapid contraction and relaxation of skeletal muscle, seen principally in abnormal reflex actions of the ankle, toe and wrist. Clonic spasm is thus different from tonic spasm. Tonic spasm is continuous contraction; clonic spasm is alternating contraction and relaxation of muscle.

myo-clonus

myo of muscle + *klonos* convulsion

Myoclonus is also called clonospasm (*spasmos* Greek, convulsion, tension), clonism, and myoclonia: quick, jittery spasms of muscles. Myoclonic spasm is seen in some forms of epilepsy. Palatal myoclonus displays as quick, up-and-down spasm of the palate and muscles of the face, tongue, pharynx and diaphragm.

co-, con-, cum

cum Latin preposition and prefix, with, together

The Latin preposition *cum* produces thousands of words in plain and scientific English. It is seen unaltered in Latin phrases used in English, like *magna cum laude*, 'with great praise', on diplomas. In informal speech, it appears as a slangy connective, as in 'a house *cum* law office'. But most often *cum* shows up in its combining form *con-*, in words like connect, conjoined, conjunctiva. The final *n* assimilates with or alters owing to the first letter of the root, in words like collaborate (to labor together with), combine, communicate, complex, corrugate and incompatible. The *n* is dropped if the root begins with a vowel or *h*, as in medical words like coagulate, coenzyme, cohesive, coincidence and coition (*cum* together with + *itio, itionis* a going = sexual intercourse). A few other medical words containing this prefix are given below.

co-arct-ation of the aorta

cum together + *arcere* to box in, to enclose + *ation* noun suffix
Coarctation of the aorta is a congenital heart defect in which localized portions of the walls of the aorta are too narrow. The surgical repair of this defect is commonly successful.

co-factor

cum with + *fact-* Latin root, do + *or* agent noun suffix
A substance that acts with another substance to produce certain effects, e.g. a coenzyme.

col-lateral

cum with + *lateralis* pertaining to the side of something
In medicine, collateral means 'side by side, accompanying, nearby, subordinate', as in collateral ligaments which provide side stability to joints.

con-ceptus

conceptus Latin past participle used as a noun, something that has been conceived
Conceptus is a general term for the products of human conception. It might refer to a fertilized egg and its protective membranes, or to an embryo or a fetus, at any intrauterine (within the uterus) stage from conception to birth.

con-genital

cum with + *genitalis* Late Latin, pertaining to birth
A congenital defect or anomaly is one present at birth. These structural abnormalities may be due to genetic inheritance flaws, problems during the pregnancy, or damage inflicted during the process of birth.

in-con-tin-ence

in Latin, not + *con, cum* with + *tenere* to hold + *entia* noun ending
Incontinence is the inability to hold and control urine and/or feces. Urinary stress incontinence occurs in female more often than male patients, and may be brought on by coughing and any kind of straining. There are many causes – mechanical, chemical and physiotherapeutic – and just as many effective treatments.

coccyx

kokkyx, kokkygos Greek, the cuckoo bird, and by analogy its beak; in medicine, the human tailbone

At the base of the human spinal column, three to five rudimentary vertebrae fuse to make up the human tailbone, named after the cuckoo because these bones together vaguely resemble a cuckoo's bill. The rudimentary bones are called the coccygeal vertebrae.

cochlea

cochlea Latin, snail shell, a bony tunnel structure in the inner ear < *kochlias* Greek, spiral snail shell < *kochlos* land snail

The cochlea is a spiral tunnel along the base of which are tiny holes through which stick fibers of the acoustic nerve, the receptor for hearing. A cochlear implant is one form of electronic hearing aid that receives sound and transmits it to electrodes placed surgically in the cochlea, to permit awareness of sounds in certain deaf patients, and possibly the eventual ability to understand speech. It is in an experimental stage at present.

coll-, -col

kolla Greek, glue

colla-gen

kolla Greek, glue + *gen* making

Collagen is a fibrous protein in skin, bone and connective tissue; its tiny fibrils combine to form the shiny, white fibers of tendons, ligaments and fascia.

coll-oid

kolla Greek, glue + *oid* similar to, from Greek *eides* 'form, shape'

A colloid is a thick substance that consists of particles dispersed throughout another substance. Smoke is a colloid of incombustible particulates suspended in air. Colloidal solutions and suspensions in water are used in medicine and sometimes found in disorders like colloid goiter, in which the follicles of the thyroid gland are swollen with colloid. To relieve some forms of dermatitic irritation and skin inflammations, a patient is sometimes given a colloid bath in water in which gelatin, bran and starch are suspended.

proto-col

protos Greek, first + *kolla* glue

In medicine, a protocol is a detailed plan of treatment. In ancient times the first sheet of a papyrus was glued to the scroll. This *protokollon* or first glued sheet displayed the title and summary of the scroll contents. All other meanings, like diplomatic procedure and the use in computerese, arise from this original sense of the first glued sheet.

colon

kolon Greek, Aristotle's word for part of the large intestine

The colon is the large intestine, the last part of the alimentary canal. The colon has three parts, the ascending, transverse, and descending colon, which gives a rough idea of its bodily course. The colon goes up, across, and down, to its last five inches which comprise the rectum.

colic

kolikos Greek, a pain in the intestines

Colic is a vague word for any gas-distension pain in the intestines. The root shows up too in the English dialect word for stomach-ache, the collywobbles.

colo-stomy

kolon large intestine + *stoma* mouth, small opening + *y* noun ending

A stoma is a mouth-like opening of an internal organ to the surface of the body. A stoma may be natural, depending on the structure, but is often surgically cut and kept open for drainage. A colostomy is making a mouth-like opening between the colon and the body surface for the discharge of fecal matter when, for example, the rectum has been removed because it was cancerous.

colpo-

kolpos Greek, vagina

colpo-rrhaphy

kolpos vagina + *rrhaphe* surgical suture + *y* noun ending

Colporrhaphy is suturing the vagina to mend tearing, or in some cases to narrow the vaginal lumen which may have become distended by muscular laxity, various diseases, or childbirth.

colpo-scopy

kolpos vagina + *skopein* to look at, to examine + *y* noun ending

Colposcopy permits a magnified view of interior vaginal and cervical tissues. A colposcope is basically a microscope with a light for direct gynecological examination. If a Pap smear test has shown any unusual tissue change, the colposcope may be able to pinpoint the exact site. A camera or recording device attached to a colposcope keeps a record of any tissue changes.

A vaginal speculum (see *speculum* entry) gently holds open the walls to get a clear view of the cervix. A colpostat (*statikos* Greek, standing in place) is a device for holding an instrument in place in the vagina. Other instruments permit dilation or dilatation of the vagina and cervix. Barnes' dilator is a rubber bag filled with fluid to dilate the cervix.

condyle

kondylos Greek, Aristotle's word for knuckle; in medicine, a spheroid bump on a bone where it articulates with another bone

condyl-oid process

kondylòs knuckle + *-oid,* formed like > *eides* Greek, form, process, a bony knob or projection on a bone

The condyloid process occurs where the lower jawbone articulates with the temporal bone of the skull.

condyl-oma

kondylos knuckle + *oma* tumor

A condyloma is a wart on the surface of the genital or anal skin. It is a tumor vaguely shaped like a knuckle, not a tumor of the condyle of a bone. This confusing medical word ought to be replaced. *Condyloma acuminatum* is the common genital wart. Acuminate is a learned adjective meaning 'tapering to a point'. Compare the word *acumen,* 'sharpness'.

conjunctiva

con, cum with + *iunctivus* Latin, joining

The conjunctiva is a transparent mucous membrane lining the eyelids and part of the eyeball.

conjunctiv-itis

conjunctiva + *itis* inflammation of

Conjunctivitis is commonly termed 'pinkeye', and is inflammation of the conjunctiva whose origin is viral, bacterial, allergic, traumatic or chemical. Eyelids may stick together upon awakening and a thick discharge is present. Conjunctivitis of the newborn presents as pus in the infant's eyes during the first three weeks of life. Gonococcal bacteria can cause conjunctivitis of the newborn which, if untreated, may lead to blindness. A conjunctival test involves dilute solutions of allergens instilled in the eyes to identify possible allergenic causes of conjunctivitis.

corona

corona Latin, crown, wreath, garland

corona dentis

corona dentis Latin, literally, the crown of a tooth

The crown is the upper portion of a human tooth that is covered in enamel.

coronary arteries

coronarius Medieval Latin, like a wreath, crowning

The coronary arteries are so named because they encircle the heart like a garland or wreath. Here is the source of the lay term *coronary* for a kind of heart attack, namely a myocardial infarction or occlusion (see the *cardi-* entry).

coronal suture

coronalis crown-like + *sutura* Latin, a stitch, a seam, a sewing

The coronal suture is the crown-like line of juncture of the frontal bone and the two parietal bones of the skull. A suture is a type of joint found only in bones of the skull. The cranial bones of a newborn baby are not completely joined. This allows compression of the skull during birth, and later permits the brain to grow, before its protective cranium becomes virtually solid bone. In the adult, the two bones united by suture joint are not movable.

corona radiata

corona crown + *radiata* Latin, spread out in rays, like sunbeams < *radius* ray

The corona radiata in the brain is a crown of fibers radiating through the cerebral cortex and mingling with fibers of the corpus callosum.

coroner

coroner Middle English, an officer of the Crown, literally a 'crowner'

Coroner equalled crowner, because in England where the office began, he was always an officer of the British Crown who at first led petitions to the king, and then inquests into suspicious deaths. Nowadays a coroner is often a medical doctor with expert knowledge of pathology.

corpus

corpus, corporis Latin, body; plural corpora

In medicine, a corpus is the main part of an organ, or some specialized tissue or mass. Examples include:

Corpus callosum	a band of nerve fibers that divides the brain's cerebral hemispheres; *callosum* Latin adjective, full of hard parts
Corpus cavernosum	erectile tissue in the penis and clitoris that becomes distended with blood during sexual arousal; *cavernosum* Latin adjective, full of hollow spaces
Corpus luteum	a tiny yellow body of cells in the follicle of an ovary after it ruptures. A corpus luteum secretes the hormone progesterone (see *progesterone* entry); *luteum* Latin adjective, yellow
Corpus spongiosum	a column of spongy, erectile tissue that, with the corpora cavernosa, forms the penis; *spongiosum* new scientific Latin, with sponge-like spaces

cortex

cortex, corticis Latin, bark, rind, any outer covering; plural cortices; in medicine, the outer layer of an organ or structure

The adrenal glands, kidneys, ovaries, lymph nodes, thymi, cerebrum and cerebellum all have an outer layer called a cortex and an inner layer called a medulla (*medulla* Latin, little middle part).

cortico-afferent

cortex, corticis outer layer + *ad > af* to, towards + *ferens, ferentis* carrying, bearing

Corticoafferent nerves carry impulses toward sensory areas of the cerebral cortex.

cortico-efferent

cortex, corticis + *ex > ef* out of, away from + *ferens, ferentis* carrying, bearing

Corticoefferent nerves carry impulses away from sensory areas of the cerebral cortex.

cortico-steroid

Corticosteroids are hormones like androgen secreted by the cortex of the adrenal glands. They help metabolic reactions occur at optimal speed. See the *steroid* entry.

costa

costa Latin, rib; plural *costae*

Costal cartilage connects the end of a true rib to the sternum. Costectomy is the surgical cutting out or resectioning of a rib. A costotome (*tome* Greek, a cutting) is a pair of surgical shears or a knife used to cut through ribs and their cartilage, during, of course, a costotomy.

crani-

cranium Latin, skull < *kranion* Greek, skull

The cranium is the skeleton of the head, the skull, but not including the lower jawbone.

Craniad is an anatomical direction: toward the cranium, toward the superior end of the body. The opposite anatomical direction is caudad, toward the tail (*cauda* Latin, tail), toward the end of the body, away from the head. Cranial nerves along with the spinal nerves make up the peripheral nervous system. Twelve pairs of cranial nerves, all connected to the brain, have a unique safety feature: they come in identical pairs, both nerves of a pair identical in form and function. If one is damaged, the other takes over its function.

cranio-clasis

cranium skull + *klasis* Greek, a fracturing, a breaking into pieces

Cranioclasis or cranioclasty is crushing the head of a dead fetus to permit delivery of the stillborn. The instrument used to crush the fetal skull is a cranioclast (*klastes* new scientific Greek, fracturer). A craniotome is a similar instrument used to divide the stillborn's skull to facilitate delivery.

crepit-

crepitare Latin, to rattle, creak, rumble < *crepitus* a pop, a rattle, a rumble

crepitant rale

crepitans Latin present participle, creaking, rattling + *rale* French, bubbling noise in the lungs

Crepitant rale is heard with a stethoscope (see *stethoscope* entry) after one draws in breath, as an abnormal bubbling sound. Higher-pitched crackling rale is produced as air enters alveoli or bronchioles that have collapsed or are plugged with mucus, or serous or fibrous exudate, in diseased conditions like pulmonary edema, pneumonia, congestive heart failure or early tuberculosis. Lower-pitched, bass-note rale happens in the larger bronchi or trachea under similar pathological conditions.

crepitation and crepitus (synonyms)

crepitatio, crepitationis scientific Latin, crackling, rumbling, and *crepitus* a crackle, a rumble

Crepitation and crepitus may both mean farting or flatulence, and may both mean the grating sound in a joint when bones have suffered arthritic damage. Both words also refer to the dry, crackling sound when fractured bone splinters grate together.

Decrepit, meaning 'worn out, run-down' is said of people and buildings, but originally it meant 'so old that one's bones creak'. Decrepitation is the explosive crackling of certain substances when heated, e.g. salt and other crystals. The Latin prefix *de* intensifies the meaning of a root. Thus decrepitation means a really noisy crackling. Originally in Latin, discrepancy was a metaphor referring to people who did not (*dis*) rumble or crackle together when speaking, and so discrepancy was a disagreement. Later in English a discrepancy was not only lack of agreement, but an instance of this, an inconsistency or variance.

crin-

krinein Greek, to secrete, to separate

apo-crine

apo Greek, from + *krinein* Greek, to secrete

Apocrine cells secrete and contribute part of their protoplasm to their secretion. The apocrine sweat glands located in the armpit and pubic area open into hair follicles.

ec-crine

ek, ex Greek, out + *krinein* Greek, to secrete

Eccrine sweat glands open directly onto the skin's surface.

endo-crine

endon Greek, within, inside + *krinein* Greek, to secrete

Endocrine glands are groups of specialized cells that secrete hormones inside the body and empty them directly into the bloodstream, e.g. the thyroid glands and the pancreas.

endo-crin-ology

endon inside + *krinein* Greek, to secrete + *logos* Greek, study of

Endocrinology is the study of diseases of the endocrine glands and their treatment.

exo-crine

exo Greek, outside + *krinein* Greek, to secrete

Exocrine glands pour out their secretions through ducts on to a surface or to other organs, e.g. the sweat glands whose ducts open on the skin.

holo-crine

holos Greek, entire, whole + *krinein* Greek, to secrete

Holocrine glands are those whose secretions consist of their own altered cells. The oil glands of the skin secrete sebum to lubricate and protect the skin. The product of these sebaceous glands, sebum, consists of fat and epithelial cell debris from the deepest layer of the epidermis.

mero-crine

meros Greek, a part of + *krinein* Greek, to secrete

Merocrine glands are those whose secretions come from cells that remain unaltered during their process of secretion. The salivary and pancreatic glands are merocrine.

crisis

krisis Greek, separation, moment of separation, judgment point

A crisis is (1) a turning point of a disease after which it gets better or worse, (2) a sudden change for the better in an acute disease, or (3) a sudden intense spasm of painful symptoms during the course of a disease. A *psychological* crisis in life may be the death of a loved one, a divorce, or the loss of a job.

critical

criticalis Latin < *kritikos* Greek, pertaining to a crisis point

A critical time may be a time dangerous or vulnerable to a patient. A critical period is a biological time-span in which to acquire specific traits or responses. In children there is a critical period, a span of years, for the acquisition of primary language skills.

crista

crista Latin, ridge, crest, comb of a rooster; plural *cristae*

cristae cutis

Anatomical Latin, ridges of the skin

Cristae cutis are dermal ridges on the palm of the hand and the sole of the foot that give humans individual fingerprints and footprints.

crista galli

Anatomical Latin, the comb of a rooster

The crista galli is a little process on the ethmoid bone of the nose that resembles a cock's comb.

inter-cristal diameter

inter Latin, between + *cristalis* Latin, pertaining to a crest

Intercristal means between two crests of a bone, organ, or bony process. In measuring the pelvis to determine possible problems in childbirth, one measurement is of the distance between the iliac crests. This is called the intercristal diameter.

cryo-

kryos Greek, very cold

cryo-bank

kryos Greek, very cold

The machine or the act of storage to freeze and preserve semen at very cold temperatures. Cryobank is a synonym for 'sperm bank'.

cryo-gen

kryos Greek, very cold + *gen* Greek, making, producing

A cryogen is any substance that produces very cold temperatures. Cryogenics is the science of producing cold temperatures.

cryonics

Fraudulent word formed on the analogy of bionics, to make it sound scientific. It is not.

Cryonics is the pseudo-medical scam of freezing diseased corpses. These dead cannot be restored to life, because freezing and thawing inflict obliterative tissue damage on the major organs of the body needed for life. Only a very few cellular entities, like human semen, are capable of being returned to useful function after deep freezing.

cryo-probe

kryos Greek, very cold + *probare* Latin, to test

A cryoprobe is an instrument that applies extreme cold to tissue. Often the cryogen is liquid nitrogen.

cryo-surgery

kryos Greek, very cold + *chirurgia* Latin < *cheir* Greek, hand + *ergos* Greek, work

Surgery in Classical Greek was *cheirourgia*, 'a working with the hands', as it originally applied to non-invasive, external manipulation of the patient's body by the hands of a physician. Only later in medieval France, and then in England, did surgery attain its present meaning of invasive procedures to correct and to cure.

Cryosurgery is destroying tissue, usually malignant, by the application of extreme cold through a cryoprobe that uses liquid nitrogen. This therapeutic injury or destruction of tissue may be termed cryolesion.

curette

curette French, scraper, cleaner < *curer*, to clean

A curette is an instrument with a sharp-edged blade formed in a loop, to scrape uterine walls, often in a procedure called a 'dilatation and curettage'. This is a common surgical procedure under local or general anesthetic. Dilatation derives from *dilatatio*, Latin, a widening. A vaginal speculum holds open the vaginal walls, while other rods may help dilate the cervix. Then the curette carefully scrapes the uterine lining. This procedure may be carried out to treat certain menstrual disorders, to terminate some pregnancies, to clean adhesions, or to diagnose uterine cancers, among other reasons.

cutis

cutis Latin, skin

The cutis, or skin, is the outer covering of the body, made up of the dermis and the epidermis (*epi* Greek, on + *dermis* Greek, skin). The epidermis is on the surface, its cells rich in a tough, horny protein, keratin (*keras, keratos* Greek, horn), that helps the skin be an efficient protector. The dermis beneath is the true, living skin tissue, full of nerves, blood vessels and glands. Occasionally one meets this word in anatomical names for simple phenomena like gooseflesh, which is *cutis anserina*, from Latin *anserinus* 'pertaining to geese'.

cut-icle

cutis Latin, skin + *icula* Latin diminutive suffix, meaning 'little, small'

The epidermis of the skin is sometimes called the cuticle. The more frequent use in medicine sees cuticle meaning the enamel cuticle of the tooth. The capsule of the lens of the eye is also termed a cuticle.

per-cut-aneous

per Latin, through + *cutis* skin + *anius* common Latin adjectival suffix

Percutaneous means done through the skin, e.g. percutaneous rubbing on of ointment or salve. Percutaneous also refers to injecting or removing fluid by a needle through the skin. It is a favorite adjective of certain modern procedures, as follows:

percutaneous balloon valvuloplasty, in which uninflated small balloons are inserted through the skin to widen a narrowed heart valve;

percutaneous endoscopic gastrostomy (PEG), in which feeding tubes are inserted through a hole in the skin over the stomach by means of an endoscope. Gastrostomy = *gastron* Greek, stomach + *stoma* mouth + *y* noun ending = making a mouth-like hole in the stomach. A PEG may be performed to feed a patient with cancer of the esophagus, or one expected to be unconscious for an extended time;

percutaneous transhepatic cholangiography (PTC), in which, to determine the cause of jaundice, a needle is inserted through the skin over a space between the ribs. The needle punctures a bile duct of the liver and injects a radiopaque dye to make a picture of the bile duct to more clearly show any pathological condition. Transhepatic = *trans* Latin, through + *hepar, hepatos* Greek, liver. The procedure is transhepatic because it seeks to trace the course of bile flow through the biliary tract, from little channels in the liver to the opening of the bile duct into the duodenum. Cholangiography = *chole* bile + *angeion* duct, vessel + *grapheia* making a picture or recording;

percutaneous ultrasonic lithotripsy, in which high frequency sound waves, above 20 000 cycles per second and thus inaudible to human ears, are applied from outside on the skin to travel inside and break up gallstones and kidney stones. Lithotripsy = *lithos* Greek, stone + *tripsis* Greek, a fracturing by rubbing together.

sub-cut-aneous

sub Latin, below + *cutis* skin + *anius* common Latin adjectival suffix

Subcutaneous means beneath or under the skin. Injections may be given subcutaneously (s.c., sub-cu).

cyan-

kyanos Greek, dark blue

This Greek color adjective is widely used in scientific naming. Blue-green algae belong to a species of cyanobacteria. Cyanide was first obtained from a chemical process one of whose reagents was a blue dye called Berlin blue or Prussian blue.

cyan-osis

kyanos dark blue + *osis* diseased condition
Cyanosis is reduced blood oxygen, a pathological condition that gives a bluish color to skin, lips and mucous membranes. The cyanotic victim needs immediate medical attention, as cyanosis may be symptomatic of poisoning, choking, or severe internal disorders, including faulty oxygenation of the blood in tissues of the lung. An extreme state of this condition is labeled hypercyanosis (*hyper* Greek, over, above, akin to Latin *super*).

cyano-philous

kyanos Greek, dark blue + *philos* Greek, loving, fond of + *ous* adjective ending
Any tissue or cell is cyanophilous that is stainable with a blue dye.

cyan-ops-ia

kyanos Greek, dark blue + *opsis* Greek, vision + *ia* medical condition
Cyanopsia is a defect of vision in which eveything appears of blue hue.

cyst, cysti-, cysto-

kystis Greek, sac, urinary bladder, bag

cyst

kystis Greek, sac, urinary bladder, bag
Cyst can refer to a natural anatomical structure like a dacryocyst whose better, clearer, less confusing name is lacrimal sac. But, far more often in medicine, a cyst is pathological. A cyst is an abnormal sac or pouch, with a wall lined with epithelial cells, and usually distended by liquid or semi-solid material. There are dozens of named cysts. A blue dome cyst is one close to the surface of the skin on the breast, whose blueness indicates that venous blood fills the sac of the cyst. An ovarian cyst is an abnormal sac of serous fluid in an ovary. A sebaceous cyst is a wen in ordinary English, a cyst found in the epidermis whose sac is filled with keratin and fatty, sebum-like material. Note, however, and see below, that in its combining forms, this confusing root almost always refers to natural structures like the urinary bladder.

cystic duct

kystis Greek, in this case the bladder referred to is the gallbladder + *ductus* Latin, canal, channel, any hollow tube which conveys liquids < *ducere* to carry, to lead

The cystic duct of the gallbladder joins the hepatic duct from the liver to form the common bile duct which empties bile into the duodenum.

cystic fibrosis

kystikos Greek, pertaining to sacs + *fibra* Latin, fiber + *osis* diseased condition

Cystic fibrosis is an hereditary disease that is the most common cause of severe chronic lung disorders in children. It is a genetic defect producing dysfunction of the exocrine glands, and thus affecting particularly the pancreas, the mucous glands of the bronchi, and the digestive glands. Fibrosis is the abnormal formation of fibrous tissue, often full of cysts. In cystic fibrosis, these fibrotic cysts may clog the ducts of the pancreas.

cyst-itis

kystis urinary bladder + *itis* inflammation of

Cystitis is inflammation of the urinary bladder by micro-organisms, often associated with urinary tract infections.

chole-cyst-itis

chole gall + *kystis* bladder + *itis* inflammation of

Cholecystitis is inflammation of the gallbladder.

cysto-pexy

kystis urinary bladder + *pexis* Greek, an attaching of, a fastening to

Cystopexy is a surgical procedure to suture a urinary bladder to the wall of the abdomen, usually after the bladder has protruded in a hernia-like manner through a weakened wall of the vagina. This herniation of the urinary bladder through the wall of the vagina is termed cystocele (*kele* Greek, hernia).

cysto-scope

kystis urinary bladder + *skopos* Greek, viewer, spy

A cystoscope is an instrument for viewing the urinary bladder, the ureter and the kidneys. The word was formed on the analogy of telescope. Cystoscopy is performed through the urethra while the patient is in the lithotomy position (see *lithotomy* entry) under sedation or anesthesia. The urinary bladder is distended with air or water to reveal as much of the interior lining as possible. The cystoscope also contains a light source usually of fiber-optic wire, and a tube to carry catheters and other surgical instruments.

cysto-stomy

kystis Greek, urinary bladder + *skopein* to look at, to examine + *y* noun ending
Cystostomy is making a mouth-like opening in the urinary bladder for drainage.

en-cyst-ed

en Greek, in + *kystis* sac
The adjective encysted means enclosed by a membrane, encapsulated, or, to use the synonym from Latin, saccate (*saccatus*, having a pouch or sac).

endo-cyst

endon Greek, inside + *kystis* sac
The endocyst is the innermost tissue of an hydatid cyst.

hydatid cyst

hydatis Greek adjective, water-filled + *kystis* sac, pouch
This cyst is formed usually in a human liver infested with dog tapeworms. It can be surgically removed.

poly-cystic ovary

polys Greek, many + *kystis* sac + *ovarium* Latin, ovary < *ovum* egg
An ovary with many ovarian cysts may be labeled polycystic.

cyto-, -cyte

kytos Greek, hollow vessel, hence a cell

cyto-toxic

kytos cell + *toxicon* Greek, a poison

Cytotoxic drugs destroy cancerous body cells, ideally without damage to normal cells.

leuco-cyte

leukos Greek, white + *kytos* cell

A leucocyte is a white blood cell. Many cell names end in *-cyte*: phagocyte, granulocyte, monocyte, thrombocyte; all are studied in cytology, the scientific study of cells. A lymphocyte is a white blood cell involved in immunity, a cell produced by lymphoid tissue.

D&C or dilatation and curettage

see *curette* entry.

dacryo-

dakryon Greek, tear, akin to Latin *lacrima*

dacryo-cyst

dakryon Greek, tear + *kystis* Greek, sac

Dacryocyst is an alternative name for the lacrimal sac, a reservoir for tears which are secreted by the lacrimal glands. Tears are stored in each of two dacryocysts, one for each eye. A dacryocyst is the enlarged end of a nasolacrimal duct. The word is used in compound nouns denoting pathology of the lacrimal sac, as shown below.

dacryo-cyst-itis

dakryon tear + *kystis* sac + *itis* inflammation of

Dacryocystitis is inflammation of the tear sac with involvement of mucosa and submucosa, and surrounding tissue, often due to a blocked tear duct.

dacryo-cysto-blenno-rrhea

dakryon tear + *kystis* sac + *blenna* Greek, mucus + *rrhoia* Greek, a flowing through, a discharge

Dacryocystoblennorrhea is chronic inflammation of the tear sac with discharge of mucus.

dacryo-cysto-cele

dakryon tear + *kystis* sac + *kele* Greek, tumor, swelling

Dacryocystocele is a hernia-like protrusion of the tear sac.

dactyl-

daktylos Greek, digit, finger, toe

sickle cell dactyl-itis

daktylos finger, toe + *itis* inflammation of

Sickle cell dactylitis is a painful inflammation of the hands and feet of infants afflicted with sickle cell anemia.

dactylo-megaly

daktylos finger, toe + *megale* enlargement < *megas* big

Dactylomegaly is abnormal size in the fingers and toes, often seen in acromegaly, a post-maturity growth defect in which the pituitary gland secretes extra growth hormone, causing gross enlargement of the skeletal extremities: fingers, toes, nose and jaw.

de

de Latin, down, away from, not, opposite of, thoroughly

The Latin preposition and prefix *de* has a basic meaning of 'down, away from', with a negative force indicating removal, as in decay, deciduous tooth, decongestant, deform, degenerate, dehydration, demented, deviant. In English and the Romance languages, *de* is added to the front of words to produce their antonym, as in deactivate, the opposite of activate; debility, almost an opposite of ability; delouse, deplane, devitalize, de-emphasize, and devalue. *De* can also be a merely intensive prefix, that boosts the force of a verb's basic meaning, as in words like declare, dedicate, delay, denominate, depend, independent, depict, deprive and devastate.

débride-ment

débrider French, to unbridle, then in medicine, to remove adhesions + *-ment* French < *mentum* Latin noun suffix

To débride a wound is to remove foreign material and cut away dead or damaged tissue. Débridement was originally borrowed by English from French (1880) to refer to treating gunshot wounds by enlarging them through surgical removal of nearby tissue damaged by a bullet.

de-cubitus ulcer

de down + *cubitus* Latin, lying in bed + *ulcus* Latin, a sore, an ulcer, akin to *elkos* Greek, a sore

An ulcer is a limited lesion of the skin or mucous membranes that line many organs and body parts, an open sore with dead tissue due to infection, inflammation, or malignancy.

A decubitus ulcer is a bedsore, an ulceration of tissue lacking blood supply because blood vessels are pressed against bones, common in immobile, elderly, bed-ridden patients. Bedsore sites include elbow, hip, buttocks and shoulder.

de-fec-ate

de away from + *faex, faecis* Latin, dregs, dung, shit (plural *faeces, feces*) + *ate* verb ending

To defecate is to excrete waste matter from the digestive tract through the rectum.

de-fibrill-ate

de not (to stop an action) + *fibrilla* Latin, little thread, little fiber, fibril + *ate* verb ending

Fibrillation is the abnormal, involuntary contraction of muscle and nerve fibers. When this happens in the atria and ventricles of the heart during sudden cardiac arrest, blood flow to the brain will decrease or cease, causing severe damage. Hence the heart muscles and nerves must be defibrillated immediately. Drugs or physical means may be effective. Various devices called defibrillators deliver variable electric shocks to the heart muscle through the chest wall. Such resuscitators may be used when the heart is fibrillating or has stopped beating completely.

de-myelin-ation

de not (removal of) + *myelos* Greek, of myelin + *ation* noun ending

Confusingly, in medicine *myelo-* also denotes 'bone marrow' (see *myelo* entry).

The myelin sheath is a white, greasy cover that protects most nerve cells and fibers. Myelin also covers parts of the spinal cord and the white matter of the brain. Neural tissue that is not myelinated, or not covered with myelin, is gray, hence the term 'gray matter' of the brain and spinal cord. Demyelination occurs in certain diseases of the nervous system, when the myelin sheath disintegrates and nerve cells fail to transmit impulses well. Multiple sclerosis is an example.

de-squam-ation

de off of (removal) + *squama* Latin, scale of a fish or snake + *ation* noun ending

Desquamation is the scaling off of skin. Usually epithelial tissue comes off in sheets or scales. This is also sometimes called desquamative exfoliation (*ex* out of + *folium* leaf, sheet).

Squamous means consisting of thin, plate-like structures, for example squamous epithelial cells that make up the outer layer of the skin. They are flat, scaly, and arranged in many layers. They are one of the reasons our skin peels after a sunburn or scratch. One type of skin cancer is squamous cell carcinoma.

delirium

de away from + *lira* Latin, furrow in a field + *ium* common noun ending in Latin; hence *delirium* Latin, a going off the ploughed track, a madness

Delirium, often a learned word in English, has its origin in a homey Latin metaphor. If an ancient Roman farmer was driving an ox before a plough, made a mistake, and went off the line of the furrow or *lira*, he committed a *delirium*. He got off the track. It's a small jump in meaning to: he went out of his mind, he became delirious. The same root resides in the English verb *learn*, whose root *lir-en* goes back to a stem meaning 'track, rut, furrow'. To learn is to keep on the track of wisdom. Delirium as a technical term in psychiatry is an acute organic mental disorder.

delirium tremens (the 'd.t.'s')

delirium madness + *tremens* Latin, trembling

Delirium tremens is an acute and sometimes fatal brain disorder affecting alcoholics, sometimes called alcohol withdrawal delirium, which happens a few days after one stops booze intake of many years. Symptoms may include raving, hallucinations, trembling and rapid heartbeat, among others. There is also alcohol hallucinosis which is associated with years of constant alcohol abuse. Now, in slang use, it's the d.t.'s, the heebie-jeebies, the shakes, the blue devils, and 'when those pink elephants turn nasty'. Delirium also accompanies abuse of drugs like amphetamines. It may be of slow or rapid onset.

delta

Delta is a Greek *d*, the fourth letter of the Greek alphabet. Because the capital delta written in Greek looks like a triangle (Δ), any structure or area that is roughly triangular may be referred to as a delta, such as the delta of a river where it empties into a larger body of water. In medicine, the slowest of the four brain wave patterns is called the delta rhythm, seen in deep, dreamless sleep.

delt-oid

delta the letter *d* + *eides* Greek, form, shape; hence *-oid* means 'formed like, similar to'
Deltoid means triangular. The deltoid muscle is a thick, triangular muscle that covers the shoulder joint and helps move the arm. Bodybuilders work on their 'delts'. In the ankle joint, the middle ligament is the deltoid ligament.

-dem-

demos Greek, town, populace, then: people, whole population
The root appears in many common English words, like democracy, demographics, demagogue.

en-demic

en Greek, in + *demos* population
Endemic is said of a disease that lasts a long time in any particular group or area. Chronic lung disorders are often endemic to miners.

epi-demic

epi Greek, upon + *demos* population
An epidemic is a rapid outbreak of disease affecting many persons in one area. Sudden multiple cases of influenza may be an epidemic. Epidemiology is the scientific study of the outbreaks, distribution, causes and control of disease in human beings.

pan-demic

pan Greek, neuter form of the adjective *pas* 'all' + *demos* population
A pandemic disease spreads over a very large area, even the whole world. AIDS is now pandemic.

dendrite

dendrites Greek adjective, branching like a tree < *dendron* tree

A dendrite is one of several branching extensions of a neuron that receive impulses. For example, dendrites in a sensory neuron will transmit impulses from nerve endings in the skin back to the main cell body of the neuron. Dendritic is tree-like.

dendritic keratitis

dendritic tree-like + *keras, keratos* Greek, horn, cornea of the eye + *itis* inflammation of
Keratitis is any inflammation of the cornea. Dendritic keratitis presents as branching ulcers on the surface of the cornea.

dent-

dens, dentis Latin, tooth; akin to *odous, odontos* Greek, tooth
The root appears in common English words like indent, literally 'toothed in'; dentifrice, a synonyn for toothpaste (*fricare* Latin, to rub, to brush); and trident, a spear with three prongs or teeth. The root is hidden in dandelion, from French *dent de lion* 'lion's tooth', from the shape of the leaf or the yellow petals. The Greek word for tooth appears in some names in dental pathology, like odontia (see entry) and odontoma.

dens in dente

Latin, a tooth inside a tooth
A dental genetic anomaly, *dens in dente* appears in X-rays as the outline of a second dental structure inside a tooth.

dentia

new scientific Latin, teething
Dentia is the normal process of the eruption of teeth.

dent-in

dens, dentis tooth + *in* noun ending for organic chemical compounds
Dentin is bony tissue that comprises the major portion of a tooth. Dentin covers the soft interior pulp. Dentin is covered by the enamel.

e-dentia

ex, e Latin, out of, without + *dens, dentis* tooth

Edentia is absence of teeth, congenital or acquired. Dentulous means having one's natural teeth, and edentulous means having no teeth.

derm-, derma, dermat-, dermato-

derma, dermatos Greek, skin

derma

derma Greek, skin

Derma, sometimes called dermis in medicine, is the true skin, also known by its Latin name, cutis vera (true skin).

dermat-itis

derma, dermatos skin + *itis* inflammation of

Dermatitis is inflammation of the skin. There are many dermatitides (note formal plural of words ending in *-itis*). Symptoms include itching, redness, and a variety of skin lesions.

dermato-glyphics

derma, dermatos skin + *glyphikos* Greek, pertaining to carving or marking a surface

Dermatoglyphics is the scientific study of markings on the surface of the skin of the hands and the feet. This includes fingerprint comparison in identification and also finding markers for various genetic events and disorders.

derma-tome

derma, dermatos skin + *tome* a cutting

Dermatome is a particular area of skin innervated by a specific spinal cord segment. The location of these skin areas is important in procedures such as skin grafting. Another meaning of dermatome is an instrument for cutting thin slices of skin to be used in transplantation surgery.

ecto-derm

ektos Greek, outside + *derma* skin

A human embryo has three primary cell layers. The outermost is the ectoderm, from which arise the nervous system, eyes, ears, skin and associated glands.

endo-derm

endon Greek, inside + *derma* skin

The endoderm is the innermost layer of the three primary cell layers of the human embryo; from it arise linings of body cavities, passages through the body, and covering tissues for organs of the body.

meso-derm

mesos Greek, middle + *derma* skin

The middle layer of the three primary cell layers of a human embryo is the mesoderm, from which arise bone, muscle, blood, connective and vascular tissues.

-desis

desis Greek, fusion, a binding together

arthro-desis

arthron Greek, joint + *desis* Greek, fusion, a binding together

Arthrodesis is an arthritic joint locking in one position or the subsequent, last-resort surgery to fuse the joint. A rigid joint is not painful, and the patient gains some mobility after joint fusion. The immobility of a joint can be called ankylosis, from *ankyle* stiff joint + *osis* diseased condition. Thus artificial ankylosis, the surgical fixation or fusion of a joint, is a synonym for arthrodesis.

spondylo-syn-desis

spondylos Greek, vertebra + *syn* together + *desis* fusion

Spondylosyndesis is spinal fusion, the surgical joining together of two or more spinal vertebrae.

di-

dis Greek, two, twice, double; akin to Latin *bis, bi-*

dicentric	having two centers
dicoria	congenital anomaly in which there are two pupils in each eye
dicyclic	having two cycles
diencephalon	the second part of the brain (*enkephalos* Greek, brain)
diglossia	congenital anomaly in which there are two tongues
dimorphic	having two forms
diphasic	having two phases
diplegia	paralysis of similar parts on both sides of the body

diplo-

diploos Greek, double, twin

dipl-oid

diploos double + *eides* Greek, form, hence *-oid* means 'formed like'

A body cell is diploid if it contains two sets of chromosomes, that is, twice the number of chromosomes in the egg or sperm.

dipl-opia

diploos double + *ope* Greek, sight + *ia* medical condition

Diplopia is double vision, of which there are several varieties. A diplopiometer is a device to measure the extent and kind of double vision present.

dia

dia Greek, through, throughout, among, apart, between, across, very

dia-betes

dia through + *betes* Greek, passing

The word itself refers to a chief symptom of some of the many forms of diabetes, the 'passing through' of excessive urination. The most common form is diabetes mellitus, a disorder of carbohydrate metabolism resulting from too little or inefficiently used insulin. *Mellitus* means 'honey-sweet' from the early observation that some diabetics had excessive amounts of sugar in their urine.

dia-gnosis

dia among + *gnosis* Greek, knowledge

Diagnosis is finding the cause of a disease, so the sense of diagnosis is distinguishing among many causes. Diagnostics is the science and practice of diagnosis, as conducted by an expert called a diagnostician. A differential diagnosis tries to pinpoint which precise disease of several is causing the symptoms. Plural, diagnoses.

dia-lysis

dia through + *lysis* Greek, loosening, dissolving, breaking up

Dialysis is filtering waste materials in the blood through a semi-permeable membrane as a replacement for natural kidney function. Hemodialysis filters blood using an artificial kidney machine.

dia-phragm

dia through + *phragma* Greek, wall, fence; *diaphragma* partition, dividing sheet

The diaphragm is a tough wall of muscle that divides the chest from the abdomen, and functions by moving up and down when breathing out and in. Diaphragm also refers to a barrier contraceptive device, a rubber cap that fits over the cervix. It is used with spermicidal jelly. It is not 100% effective.

dia-rrhea

dia through + *rrhoia* Greek, a flowing, a discharge

Diarrhea is too-frequent bowel movements of watery stools, a flowing through of waste material.

dia-stole

dia apart + *stole* Greek, a drawing, a pulling

Diastole is a drawing apart, the relaxing and expanding of the ventricles, when blood flows into the heart. Its complementary action is systole (*sys* < *syn* together), a drawing together, the contraction of the ventricles of the heart, when blood is pumped out.

diastolic and systolic

Blood pressure measures the pressure against the vessel walls. When the ventricles contract, the highest pressure is produced, the systolic. When the ventricles relax, the lowest, the diastolic pressure, is produced.

didym-

hoi didymoi Greek, 'the twins', i.e. the two testicles

epi-didym-is

epi Greek, on + *didymoi* testicles + *is* Greek noun suffix
The epididymis, resting on and beside each testis, is part of the excretory duct of each testis, a long tube through which sperm begin their journey out of the male body.

dis-

dis Latin, apart; as a prefix: negated, reversed, removed, excluded, separated, moved apart
Verbs and nouns with this prefix are common in English: discover, disease, disgrace, disgust, dismiss, dispose, disrespect, dissect, dissolve, distend, distort.

dis-soci-ation

dis Latin, apart + *socius* friend + *ation* noun ending
In psychiatry, dissociation is the interruption of normal thought processes in a patient who is not aware or conscious that this breaking off has occurred.

distal

A scientific coinage of the 19th Century, from *dist*-ance + *al*, which is a common adjectival ending
In anatomy, distal means remote from the point of attachment, or away from the center of the body. For example, each finger and toe except for the thumb and big toe has three end bones called phalanges. The distal phalanx of a finger is the bone farthest away from the center of the body, so it's the very last, outermost bone at the tip of the finger.

The opposite of distal is proximal (*proximus* Latin, the nearest). Proximal as an anatomical position means nearest the center of the body, or at the beginning of a structure. The proximal part of the ureter is near the kidney. The distal part of the ureter is nearest the bladder.

Bones are said to articulate proximally and distally with other bones. The proximal end of the thigh bone, the femur, forms a joint with the socket of the hip bone. The distal end of the femur articulates with the tibia and the knee-cap.

dolor

dolor Latin, pain. See the *inflammation* entry.

donor

donor Latin, one who gives – blood, organs, etc.

dorsum

dorsum Latin, the back; *dorsalis* adjective, of the back
Dorsum is the back surface of a body or body part, e.g. the dorsum of the hand. Dorsal is an anatomical direction: to, on, or near the back side of the body; the opposite of ventral. Dorsad means toward the back. Dorsocephalad means toward the back of the head (*kephale* Greek, head). Tabes dorsalis is the late stage of syphilis, a painful wasting away (*tabes*) of the dorsal column of the spinal cord.

drom-

dromos Greek, a run, a course
A hippodrome was originally a place in which horse races were run. A dromedary camel runs well. A palindrome is a word that is spelled the same backward as forward.

dromo-mania

dromos a course, a travelling + *mania* Greek, madness
In psychiatry, dromomania is one of the many manias, and is an obsessive desire to travel, to get away from daily concerns and problems with the self. It is seldom a useful ploy. Travel is a 360-degree mirror. Who do you travel with? Yourself.

pro-drome

pro Greek, in front of + *dromos* a running
A prodrome is a symptom near the onset of a disease, announcing a disorder.

syn-drome

syn together + *dromos* a running
A syndrome is a running together of symptoms that predict one particular disease.

duct

ductus Latin, canal for conduction of fluids
A duct is a tubular passage for secretions and excretions. The cystic duct (*kystikos*, of the gallbladder) connects the neck of the gallbladder to the common bile duct which unites the cystic duct and hepatic duct (*hepatikos*, of the liver). The common bile duct then carries its bile to empty into the duodenum, the first portion of the small intestine, where it helps digest food. All three are thus called biliary ducts.

ductus deferens

ductus; *de* away from + *ferens* carrying
In the testicle, the ductus deferens carries sperm away from the epididymis and to the ejaculatory duct.

-duct

ductum Latin, past participle of *ducere* to carry, to lead, to draw
To adduct is to draw a body part toward the midline of the body. The adductor longus is a long muscle that lies along a ridge on the back of the femur. This muscle helps adduct, rotate and flex the thigh.

To abduct is to draw a body part away from the body midline. The abductor muscle of the thumb is used when one raises a hand with the thumb stuck up to indicate success; this muscle abducts the thumb.

dupp

In the common heart sounds, 'lubb dupp'
Among the most prominent regular heart noises heard through a stethoscope are lubb and dupp. The heart and its major vessels have valves to insure that blood flows one way, that no backflow occurs. The slamming shut of the tricuspid and mitral valves makes a *lubb* sound. The semilunar valves of the aorta and pulmonary artery then close with a shorter, higher *dupp*.

dura mater

dura mater Latin, tough mother

Three meninges or membranes wrap around and protect the brain and spinal cord. The tough outer meninx, singular of meninges, is the dura mater, the 'tough mother'. *Mater* is a translation into Late Latin from the Arabic term *oum al-dimagh,* 'tough mother'. Arabic uses *oum* 'mother' to mean 'the greatest of, the most important of'. Compare this with the dictator Saddam Hussein's phrase 'the mother of all wars'.

epi-dural

epi on + *dura,* short for *dura mater* + *alis* common adjectival suffix

Epidural means located on or outside the dura mater. Epidural space surrounds the dura mater of the brain and of the spinal cord. Epidural anesthesia is the injection of local anesthetics into the epidural space of the spinal column to obtain anesthesia of specific body regions, such as the pelvic or the genital area. In clinical abbreviation, the injection itself is sometimes simply called 'an epidural'.

dys-

dys Greek, bad, difficult, painful, abnormal; indicates difficult or disordered function

dys-entery

dys painful + *enteron* Greek, gut; in medicine refers to the small intestine

Dysentery is an inflammation of the intestine, particularly the colon, caused by bacteria, protozoa, parasites, or chemical irritants; for example amebic dysentery. The symptoms are pain in the abdomen, frequent bloody stools and spasms of the rectum. Treatment includes rehydration (replacement of lost fluids orally or intravenously) and antibiotics.

dys-meno-rrhea

dys painful + *men, menos* Greek, month + *rrhoia* Greek, a discharge

Dysmenorrhea is a monthly period that is painful due to various inflammations or mechanical obstructions.

dys-plasia

dys abnormal + *plasis* Greek, a forming; so in medicine the development and growth of tissue and cells
Dysplasia is abnormal cell growth, usually pre-malignant.

dys-pnea

dys abnormal + *pnoe* Greek, breathing
Dyspnea is breathing that is labored or difficult.

dys-tocia

dys difficult + *tokos* Greek, childbirth + *ia* medical condition
Dystocia is prolonged or difficult labor, due to a large fetus, its abnormal position, or an obstruction or constriction of the birth canal. Eutocia is normal labor in childbirth (*eu* Greek, well, good, normal).

dys-tonia

dys abnormal + *tonos* Greek, tone + *ia* medical condition
Dystonia is abnormal muscle tone in a muscle or a muscular sac like a bladder. It might be a spasm due to a drug reaction or to a rare genetic disorder like dystonia musculorum deformans.

dys-trophy

dys bad + *trophe* Greek, nourishment
Dystrophy is any disease due to faulty nutrition in a body part. Note the many muscular dystrophies which are serious degenerative diseases.

E

ec-

ek, ex Greek, out, out of

The prefix appears in many common words. Something eccentric was originally outside the center of what was usual or normal. Ecstasy, in Greek *ecstasis*, first meant a trance, a feeling of standing outside oneself. Some people get ecstatic at the sight of an eclipse, in Greek *ekleipsis*, a leaving out, an abandonment, an omitting where one celestial body obscures and thus leaves out part of another celestial body, as in a lunar eclipse, that is, a lunar leaving out, when part of the normal view of the moon is left out as the moon passes through the dark umbra of the earth's shadow. Eclectic means 'picking out, selecting' from various options, what seems best for the patient.

ec-crine

See under *crin-* entry

ec-lampsia

ek out + *lampsis* Greek, a sudden flashing, a bright shining

The term eclampsia was coined by François-Boissier de Sauvages, an 18th Century French pathologist, to describe toxic convulsions during pregnancy, one of whose most remarked but not most severe symptoms was flashes of light seen before the eyes of the pregnant woman. Eclampsia, of unknown cause, often occurs between the 20th week of pregnancy and the end of the first postpartum week. Convulsive seizures, edema, elevated blood pressure and coma leading to death may result. This is best prevented by careful monitoring for pre-eclampsia: symptoms like elevated blood pressure, headaches, albuminuria and edema of the legs.

-ec-tomy

ek, ex Greek, out, out of + *tome* Greek, a surgical cutting
This common suffix in words of medical procedure indicates a surgical excision.

append-ec-tomy

appendix + *ectomy* surgical cutting out of
Appendectomy is surgical excision of the vermiform appendix (*vermiformis* scientific Latin, shaped like a worm).

chole-cyst-ec-tomy

chole Greek, bile, gall + *kystis* Greek, sac, bladder + *ek* out + *tome* Greek, a surgical cutting
Cholecystectomy is surgical excision of the gallbladder. The standard procedure now is laparoscopic cholecystectomy. See *laparoscope* entry. A popular name is 'keyhole' surgery.

mast-ec-tomy

mastos breast + *ek* out + *tome* a surgical cutting + *y* noun ending
Mastectomy is partial or complete removal of a breast or the breasts usually as treatment for breast cancer. A radical mastectomy involves excision of not only the breast but also pectoral muscles, skin, lymph nodes of the armpit, and some subcutaneous fat. Simple mastectomy is sometimes termed lumpectomy, in which only the tumorous mass is removed and other tissues and structures are left intact.

splen-ectomy

splen Greek, spleen + *ectomy* surgical cutting out of
Splenectomy is the surgical cutting out of the spleen. Because most spleen functions can be carried out by other organs, in an otherwise healthy adult splenectomy has few bad effects.

ec-topic

ek out + *topos* Greek, place + *ikos* adjective ending
Ectopic means 'out of its normal place'. The noun is ectopia. This abnormal position, often congenital, may refer to any organ or structure or to the

products of conception, as in an ectopic pregnancy; for example, a tubal pregnancy where the fertilized ovum has implanted outside the uterine cavity in one of the Fallopian tubes.

ec-zema

ek out of + *zeein* Greek, to boil, gives a noun form *eczema*, literally, a boiling out of bad humor to form an eruption of the skin

In modern medicine, eczema is any superficial dermatitis, either a contact dermatitis or one of unknown cause.

edema

oidema, *oidematos* Greek, a swelling

Edema results when salt retention causes excess fluid build-up in the intercellular spaces and thus puffy swelling. Ultimate etiology (see entry) is manifold and complex, including trauma, heart disease, kidney failure, cirrhosis and allergens. The adjective is edematous. The older English word was dropsy. Pitting edema is present when one presses a finger on edematous skin tissue and a temporary pit or depression results. Non-pitting edema may be severe, e.g. myxedema.

myx-edema

myxos Greek, of mucus + *oidema*, swelling

Myxedema is a non-pitting edema seen in cretinism and also associated with severe thyroid disorders. It is edema with mucin deposits and many other symptoms including fatigue, weight gain and thick skin.

ef-ferent

ex > *ef* Latin, away from + *ferens, ferentis* Latin adjective, leading

A nerve is a bundle of fibers that conduct impulses. A neuron is a nerve cell, the basic cell of the nervous system. There are three kinds of neurons. Motor or efferent neurons conduct impulses away from the brain and spinal cord. Sensory or afferent (*ad* > *af* to + *ferens* leading) neurons lead impulses to the brain or spinal cord. Connecting or associative neurons conduct impulses from one neuron to another.

elbow

eln-boga Old English, literally the forearm bend, the place where one can make an L-shaped bend; compare Old English *ell*, the letter *l*

Three arm bones interact at the elbow in two joints: a hinge joint between the humerus and the ulna, and a ball-and-socket joint between the humerus and the radius.

tennis elbow

A common cause of tennis elbow is tendonitis of the forearm muscles which are attached to a bony bump on the outer side of the elbow. The backhand movement in tennis strains this tendon. A tendon is a fibrous cord of connective tissue at the end of muscles where they attach to bones. Inflamed tendons need rest, physiotherapy, or injection of anti-inflammatory drugs.

embolus

embolos Greek, a plug, an insert < *en* in + *bolos* thing thrown or stuffed

An embolus is anything that plugs up a tube or blood vessel. An embolus may be a blood clot, a gob of fat, a bubble of air, a tumor, or a little ball of cellular debris. Embolism is the condition of having emboli plugging up an artery or vein. One speaks of an air embolism, fat embolism, or a pulmonary embolism plugging up vessels in the lungs. An anti-embolism hose is an elastic stocking worn to prevent the formation of emboli or thrombi (see entry) by post-operative patients or the bed-ridden. The stocking promotes the venous circulation and prevents dilated veins, both of which help stop embolism.

embol-ec-tomy

embolos a plug + *ek* out + *tome* cutting

Embolectomy is the surgical cutting out of emboli from blood vessels.

embryo

en > *em* Greek, in + *bryon* something that grows in another body < *bryein* to grow

An embryo is the product of human conception from its second to its eighth week, that is, the stage of growth between the ovum and the fetus. Embryology is the science that studies the origin, growth, function and development of an organism from fertilization to birth.

embry-oma

embryon + *oma* tumor
An embryoma is a tumor arising from embryonic tissues or cells.

emetic

emetikos Greek adjective, pertaining to vomiting
An emetic is any substance that induces vomiting, such as ipecac syrup. Emesis is the noun. An emesis basin is a bowl shaped to fit against a patient's neck to collect vomitus, a medical word for the material expelled from the stomach during vomiting.

hyper-emesis gravidarum

hyper Greek, above, abnormal, excessive + *emesis* Greek, vomiting; *gravidarum* Latin genitive plural, of pregnant women; compare English adjectival synonym of pregnant, gravid
Hyperemesis gravidarum is severe and excessive vomiting, of far longer duration than the simple vomiting of early pregnancy popularly called 'morning sickness'. Untreated hyperemetic pregnant women suffer salt depletion, dehydration, weight loss and possible liver damage. Hyperemesis gravidarum can be fatal, but early treatment saves both mother and fetus.

em-phys-ema

emphysema, emphysematos Greek, inflation < *en* in + *physan* to blow + *ema* noun ending
Emphysema is over-inflation of the pulmonary system. The walls of emphysematous alveoli lose elasticity and rupture during the efforts of difficult breathing. Acute emphysema may accompany bronchopneumonia, whooping cough, or suffocation. Chronic emphysema is seen with the chronic bronchitis caused by smoking, and sometimes subsequent to asthma or tuberculosis.

emphysematous bullae

bulla Latin, a bubble; plural *bullae*
Bulla is a technical term for a large blister or vesicle more than 5 mm in diameter, raised from the surface of the skin, containing serous fluid. But emphysematous bullae are air-filled sacs in the lung caused by destruction of

elastic tissue of the lung. This stage of emphysema may lead to pulmonary failure.

em-py-ema

en in + *pyon* Greek, pus + *ema* Greek noun ending meaning 'the act or action of'
Empyema was originally a Greek word meaning the formation of pus. It was Hippocrates' word for suppuration. Now empyema is pus in any body cavity but especially in the pleural cavity. It is usually a symptom of a primary infection of the lungs. Antibiotics and aspiration of the pyothorax, and sometimes surgical drainage, are indicated.

en-cephal-on

en > *eg* in + *kephale* Greek, head = *egkephalos*, the brain, that is, what's in the head
The encephalon is the brain.

en-cephal-itis

enkephalos brain + *itis* inflammation of
Encephalitis is one of many inflammatory diseases of the brain, e.g.vernal encephalitis of Russia, acquired from tick bites in the spring, also passed on in infected milk and flesh. Equine encephalitis affects horses bitten by a virus-carrying mosquito. It can be passed to humans by mosquito bite.

encephalo-myel-itis

enkephalos the brain + *myelos* spinal cord + *itis* inflammation of
Encephalomyelitis is an acute inflammation of the brain and spinal cord.

encephalo-myelo-pathy

enkephalos the brain + *myelos* spinal cord + *pathos* disease
An encephalomyelopathy is any disease of the brain and spinal cord.

encephalo-scler-osis

enkephalos the brain + *skleros* hard + *osis* diseased condition
Encephalosclerosis is hardening of the brain tissues.

endo-

endon Greek, within, inside

endocrine

See under *crin-* entry

endo-metrium

endon inside + *metra* Greek, literally, mother thing, hence womb or uterus = *endometrium*, scientific Latin, tissue inside the womb

The endometrium is the inner lining of the uterus consisting of epithelial mucosa. The superficial layers, called decidua, are shed during menstruation if pregnancy does not occur.

end-orphin

endon inside + *morphine* < *Morpheus* the Greek god of dreams + *in* ending for organic chemical compounds

Endorphins are proteins called neuropeptides that reduce the sensation of pain by acting on the central and peripheral nervous systems. Their pharmacologic effects are similar to those of morphine, hence the name. Acupuncture may activate the production of some endorphins.

endo-scope

endon inside + *skopia* Greek, a watching

An endoscope is a tube with room for a fiber-optic instrument and a source of illumination, for viewing the interior of a body cavity or organ. It may be introduced through a natural body opening or a small incision. Endoscopy is the act of examining the inside of a body cavity with any of various instruments called endoscopes.

end-osteum

endon inside + *osteon* Greek, bone

Endosteum is the tissue that lines the bone marrow or medullary cavity of a bone.

endo-thelium

endon inside + *thele* Greek, nipple

Endothelium is epithelial tissue, composed of flat and scale-like cells that line the internal organs of the body like the heart, as well as the veins and arteries. The name was conceived on the analogy of epithelium, itself first coined in 1700 to refer to the cells just surrounding the nipple. Later, when the use of the narrow term was broadened, the inappropriate Greek root for 'nipple' stayed in the word.

endo-tracheal

endon inside + *tracheia* Greek, rough. It is the feminine form of the adjective *trachys*.

The Greeks called the windpipe *arteria tracheia,* 'rough air vessel'. By AD 1500, in medical books, artery had another meaning, so artery was dropped and the windpipe was termed, for clarity, trachea.

An endotracheal tube is a large-diameter, rubber or plastic catheter inserted through the mouth into the trachea to deliver pressurized oxygen from a ventilator. An inflated cuff keeps the system closed. It is often used when a face mask proves ineffective. Endotracheal intubation is common too in some procedures to induce general anesthesia. Anesthetic gases are introduced into the respiratory system through the endotracheal tube. Such an airway catheter is also used to keep passages open, to prevent aspiration of vomitus in unconscious or paralyzed patients, and to allow suctioning off of tracheal and bronchial secretions.

enteron

enteron Greek, gut < *entos* inside, hence literally 'the part inside'; in medicine it refers to the small intestine

The enteron is the small intestine, the first twenty feet of gut after the stomach, comprising the duodenum, jejunum and ileum. The adjective is enteric. An enteric coating may be applied to certain tablets to prevent drug release until the tablet reaches the small intestine.

dys-entery

dys painful + *enteron* small intestine

Dysentery is an inflammation of the intestine, particularly the colon, caused by bacteria, protozoa, parasites, or chemical irritants; for example amebic dysentery. The symptoms are pain in the abdomen, frequent bloody stools and spasms of the rectum. Treatment includes rehydration (replacement of lost fluids orally or intravenously) and antibiotics.

enter-itis

enteron small intestine + *itis* inflammation of
Enteritis is inflammation of the small intestine; some enteritides are severe and life-threatening.

gastro-enteritis

gaster Greek, stomach + *enteron* small intestine + *itis* inflammation of
In gastroenteritis, the inflammation involves the stomach as well as the small intestine.

Entero-virus

enteron Greek, gut + *virus*
Enterovirus is a large category of very small, parasitic micro-organisms (viruses) that replicate chiefly in the intestinal tract. Enteric viruses cause, among other diseases, the common cold and polio. Enteroviruses have been recently reclassified as a genus of picornaviruses, that is, pico-RNA-viruses (*pico* Italian, small + RNA ribonucleic acid).

ento-

entos Greek, within, inside. This is a Greek variant of *endos*, within.

ent-optic

entos within + *optikos* Greek, seeing
Entoptic means 'pertaining to or happening in the interior of the eye'. Entoptic phenomena are visual irregularities due to causes within the eye. Most humans have seen little specks floating across their field of vision. Many are utterly benign, due to cellular debris floating in the vitreous humor of the eyeball. Some are the viewer's own blood cells flowing through retinal arteries and veins. One delightful medical name for these floaters or benign black floating specks is muscae volitantes, which is Latin for 'flitting houseflies' which seem to flit about as the eyeball is moved. Another benign entoptic phenomenon is called Moore's lightning streaks in which older patients think they see little zigzag flashes of

light in their peripheral fields of vision in the dark. These are due to little vitreous polyps or growths on the retina. Sometimes the Latin word for flashing is used to label this phenomenon: coruscation.

Less benign and indicative of retinal irritation or possible cerebral lesions is photopsia (*photos* light + *opsis* vision): seeing sparks or flashes of light in one's field of vision when no outer light source is producing such effects.

epi-

epi Greek, on, on top of, above, upper, upon
This prefix is widespread in English words like epoxy glue, epicenter, epigram, episode, epitaph, epitome and the Christian festival of Epiphany.

epi-dermis

epi on top of + *derma* Greek, skin
The epidermis is the outermost layer of the skin, itself made up of five layers of squamous epithelium.

epi-dural

See under *dura mater* entry

epi-glottis

epi on top of + *glottis* Greek, the back of the tongue. It is related to *glotta* and *glossa*, Greek words for the tongue
The epiglottis is the lid of cartilage that flaps shut over the larynx and the trachea when one swallows, to prevent food entering the lungs.

epi-lepsy

epi on + *lepsis* a seizing = *epilepsis* a seizure. Aristotle used the form *epilepsia* for any convulsive seizure.
Epilepsy, known of old as the falling sickness, is uncontrolled electrical discharges in the neurons, producing recurring episodes of seizure, convulsions, impaired consciousness and other symptoms. Anticonvulsant drugs provide some relief of symptoms. The French names for two common types of epilepsy, *grand mal* and *petit mal* (powerful disease and small disease), go back to a time in French medical history when the disorder was known as 'the disease of Hercules' because some epileptic patients seemed to have superhuman strength

when in the throes of a *grand mal* seizure, but no strength at all when experiencing a *petit mal* seizure.

epi-nephrine

epi on top of + *nephros* kidney + *ine* common ending for organic chemicals

Epinephrine is a synonym for adrenaline, a hormone produced by the adrenal medulla when stimulated by the sympathetic nervous system. It helps prepare the body for 'flight or fight' when fear and anxiety reactions occur. It narrows the blood vessels. Synthetic epinephrine is administered to treat shock, bronchial spasm, nasal congestion, and to make certain local anesthetics more effective.

epi-physis

epi on top of + *physis* Greek, growth

Epiphysis is an anatomical term for the wide end of a long bone, like the femur or the humerus, that is cartilaginous until the bone stops growing, at which time the epiphyseal plate of cartilage disappears and the head and the shaft are solid, united bone.

episio-tomy

epision Greek, Hippocrates' word for the pubic area + *tome* a surgical incision

An episiotomy is an incision made to enlarge the vaginal opening during a difficult birth, for example during a forceps delivery, when the baby's head is too large to pass out of the birth canal without severely stretching and tearing the muscles and tissues of the vagina. An episiotomy can hasten delivery and make the birth easier for mother and child. Afterwards, the fine suturing of the cut perineum is an episiorrhaphy (*rrhaphe,* a suture).

epi-thel-ium

epi on + *thele* Greek, nipple

Epithelium is the varied, external tissue that covers the body, the outer layer of the skin. Epithelium also forms the surface layer of mucous and serous membranes, and thus it lines hollow organs such as the bladder, and the passages of the respiratory, digestive and urinary tracts. Epithelium as a word was first coined in 1700 to refer only to the cells surrounding the nipple. Later, the meaning was expanded but the specific root was not changed. Related words containing the 'nipple' root are thelitis, meaning sore nipples due to inflammation, and the rarer term thelalgia, or pain in the nipples.

epitheli-oma

epithelio + *oma* tumor
Epithelioma is a malignant tumor, a carcinoma, made up of epithelial cells. The tumor originates in the skin or in a mucous membrane. One form is basal cell epithelioma, in which the tumor derives from cells in the basal layer of the epidermis, also called the stratum germinativum.

erythro-

erythros Greek, red

erythro-cyte

erythros red + *kytos* cell
An erythrocyte is a red blood cell or red corpuscle. They hold hemoglobin, the protein in blood that carries oxygen molecules to most body cells. Erythrocytes are manufactured in the red marrow of bones.

erythro-mycin

erythros red + *mykes* fungus, mushroom + *in* common ending for organic chemical compounds
Erythromycin is an antibiotic of wide application, named because it is produced by a red bacterium called *Streptomyces erythreus* that was originally isolated in a mushroom.

erythrism

erythrismos Greek, redness
Erythrism is red-hairedness, of normal occurrence, with red hair or beard, and a ruddy complexion.

-escent, -escence

This common suffix to nouns and adjectives derives from the present infinitive form, *-escere*, of what are called inchoate verbs in Latin (*inchoare*, to begin). The basic meaning of the suffixes *-escent* and *-escence* is 'just beginning to, starting the initial stage of'. For example, someone who is senescent displays some initial signs of senility or old age. An adolescent is beginning to be an adult. A phosphorescence is the initial glow of a phosphorus-like light. Obsolescent techniques are just beginning to become obsolete. A convalescent is just beginning to heal, to get his or her strength back. A patient with a chronic disease who is tabescent is beginning to suffer a progressive wasting and withering away, as in tabes.

eso-phagus

oiso- Greek dialectic variant of *es* or *eis* which means 'to, toward, into' + *phagos* Greek, eater, so the sense of the Greek word is the 'in-eater'

The esophagus is the muscular gullet tube, about 9 inches long in a North American adult. The esophagus connects the pharynx to the stomach. Peristaltic (see entry) contractions of muscles that encircle it pass food through the esophagus.

essential

essentialis Latin, of the essence of a thing, from *esse* to be

A special medical use of this adjective makes *essential* a synonym for idiopathic (see entry), that is, having no obvious cause. For example, essential hypertension is high blood pressure for which no specific cause or set of causes can be found. The sense of the adjective is 'of essence'. It has being, it exists, but the cause is unknown or of obscure origin. Humility in the face of not knowing is at times required of all health professionals. Not to admit that medical knowledge has limits is arrogant, and is certainly not productive of the impulse to discover something new beyond current limits of knowledge.

etio-logy

aitia Greek, cause + *logos* Greek, study of

Etiology is the study of the causes of diseases. In everyday medical parlance, etiology is used as a synonym for cause.

etio-tropic

aitia cause + *tropikos* Greek, turning toward

An etiotropic drug or treatment destroys the agent that causes a disease. A nosotropic (*nosos* Greek, sickness, ailment) drug treats the symptoms or effects of a disease.

eu-

eu Greek, good, well, normal

eu-phoria

eu well + *phoros* Greek, bearing, carrying oneself + *ia* noun
ending indicating condition
Euphoria is a general sense of well-being, feeling good. But inappropriate feelings
of euphoria may also accompany certain manic states in some mental disorders.

eu-rhythmia

eu well + *rrhythmos* Greek, timed beat in music + *ia* medical
condition
Eurhythmia is sometimes used in its ancient Greek sense, to mean 'harmony' or
'harmonious development of organs or structures in the body'. Eurhythmia is
also having a good, regular rhythm in the pulse. Often the opposite of a benign
condition has a Greek-derived name with *a-* or *dys-* as a prefix, thus, arrhythmia,
irregular pulse and heart-beat.

eu-pepsia

eu well + *pepsis* Greek, digestion
Eupepsia is good digestion, often indicating a sufficient amount of the chief
enzyme, pepsin, among the stomach juices. So lack of good digestion is
dyspepsia, and in daily language, a grumpy, out-of-sorts person, possibly with
stomach troubles, may be said to be dyspeptic.

eu-pnea

eu well + *pnoe* Greek, breath
Eupnea is normal breathing, regular respiratory activity. Abnormal breathing
then is dyspnea.

eu-thanas-ia

eu good + *thanatos* Greek, death
Euthanasia is making death painless. Active euthanasia involves administering a
lethal drug to an incurable and terminally ill patient. Passive euthanasia permits
death by withholding treatment that might extend life even for brain-dead
patients. A common synonym to be avoided is mercy killing.

eutocia

See under *dystocia* entry

ex

ex Latin preposition and prefix, out of, away from, outside

ex-cise

ex out of + *cisio* Latin, a surgical cutting
To excise is to cut out a body part. The noun is excision.

ex-pector-ate

ex out + *pectus, pectoris* Latin, chest + *ate* common verb ending
To expectorate is to spit mucus, phlegm, or other secretions out of the chest
through the mouth. A chemical substance that promotes this spitting up by
making a patient's sputum more liquid and less sticky is called an expectorant.

ex-sanguin-ate

ex out + *sanguis, sanguinis* Latin, blood + *ate* common verb
ending
To exsanguinate is to bleed to death, to suffer massive and fatal hemorrhage.

ex-udate

ex out + *sudatus* sweated out
An exudate is a fluid with protein and cell debris that has escaped, exuded, from
blood vessels to surrounding tissue. Exudation is part of inflammation.

extra

extra Latin adverb, on the outside, beyond, or additionally

extra-corporeal

extra outside + *corpus, corporis* Latin, the human
body > *corporealis* scientific Latin, of the body

Extracorporeal means 'outside the human body'. For example, extracorporeal shock-wave lithotripsy (*lithos* stone + *thrypsis* Greek, a breaking into small pieces, a crushing), hence the popular name: the stone-crushing machine. The medical name for the machine is a lithotriptor. In this procedure, sound waves conducted through water disintegrate kidney stones, and the debris is washed out of the system. The shock wave generated is similar to that produced by a 'depth charge'.

extra-ocular

extra outside + *ocularis* scientific Latin, of the eye
Extraocular muscles (EOM) are muscles attached externally to each eyeball to control movement and the co-ordination necessary for depth vision.

extra-vasate

extra outside + *vas* Latin, vessel + *ate* common verb ending
Blood, lymph, or serum may extravasate, that is, escape from the carrying vessel into surrounding tissues and spaces. The word can be used as a noun too. The fluid so escaped can be called the extravasate. The suffusion (see *sub* entry) of such fluids into nearby tissue is extravasation.

facies

facies Latin, face, external appearance

In formal anatomical nomenclature expressed in scientific Latin, facies is the face or surface of a body structure, for example, the facies gastrica splenis is the surface of the spleen in contact with the stomach.

Facies also refers to the pathological appearance of the human face, as an informal aid to diagnosis, for example, in facies abdominalis, the patient's face is anxious, pinched up, furrowed in pain, characteristic of one suffering abdominal pain. Parkinsonian facies is mask-like, expressionless, with unblinking eyes, characteristic of parkinsonism.

factitious / factitial

factitiosus Latin, full of artifice and pretense

Patients with factitious disorders make up their diseases in order to remain patients. This severe personality disturbance is seen in chronic hypochondriasis and in Munchausen's syndrome, where patients feign pains, vomit, faint, and develop fevers, seemingly at will. Deliberate misinterpretation of normal body sounds and functions is common. In Munchausen's syndrome, patients may even mutilate themselves in order to retain constant medical attention, sometimes moving from emergercy ward to emergency ward in larger cities. As soon as they are detected, these patients require psychiatric diagnosis and therapy.

Fallopian tube

Named after Gabriele Fallopio (AD 1523–1563), an Italian anatomist who first described the tubes accurately

One of two ducts between the uterus and the peritoneal cavity over the ovary. The Fallopian tubes are passages where ova are carried from the ovary to the uterus, and spermatozoa move out from the uterus toward the ovary.

fascia

fascis Latin, a bundle of sticks, firewood tied up to take back to the fire

A fascia (plural *fasciae*) is a band of fibrous connective tissue that wraps protectively around muscles and some organs. Fasciae cover the body under the skin in two layers. The superficial fascia is a layer of fat with fiber strands. The deep fascia is a tough shield, but not so thick over the chest and abdomen, to permit them to expand during breathing, food intake and pregnancy.

fasci-culus or fascicle

fascia + *culus* little = a small fascia

A fasciculus is a little bundle of nerve, tendon, or muscle fibers. Fasciculation is a localized, uncontrollable twitching of a single muscle group.

fasci-itis

fascia + *itis* inflammation of

Inflammation of connective tissue may be due to infection, trauma, or autoimmune responses. In pseudosarcomatous fasciitis (*pseudos* Greek, false, fake + *sarx, sarkos* flesh + *-oma* tumor), connective tissue in the cheek develops a benign growth that only resembles a cancer.

feces

faex, faecis Latin, dung, dregs, stool

Synonyms include excreta, excrement, stools, and the vulgar word shit. All label body waste discharged from the bowels through the anus.

defecation

de away + *faex, faecis* stool + *-atio, ationis* noun ending 'action of', so that *defaecatio* meant originally 'passing stools away from the body'

Defecation is the act of evacuating the bowels, or 'having a bowel movement' in common speech.

fecal impaction

impactus Latin, pressed together + *io, ionis* noun ending indicating process or condition

In fecal impaction, large, hardened fecal masses lodge in the distal colon or rectum, too large to be passed. A hard, rounded mass of fecal matter may be called a scybalum or scybalous feces, from *skybalon,* a Greek word for stool or dung, although this term is somewhat rare. A hard mass of feces in the colon is sometimes referred to as a fecalith (*lithos* Greek, stone). A large mass of impacted feces in the rectum which resembles a tumor is called by some a fecaloma (*faecalis* Latin, pertaining to stool + *-oma* tumor). However, this is not a useful or an appropriate coinage, because it labels with an ending that means 'tumor' something that is not a tumor.

femur

femur, femoris Latin, the thigh; plural *femora* or femurs

The longest and strongest bone in the human body, the femur is the thigh bone, extending from the pelvis to the knee. The uppermost end of the femur forms a ball-and-socket joint with a cup-shaped pelvic indentation called the acetabulum, permitting great freedom of movement of the legs.

femoral condyle

femoralis Latin, of the thigh bone; *kondylos* Greek, Aristotle's word for knuckle

The femoral condyle is one of two spheroidal projections on the distal end of the thigh bone where it articulates with adjacent bones and where ligaments and tendons are anchored.

fetus

fetus Latin noun, offspring, spawn, brood

This word is not, as many medical dictionaries state, from the Latin adjective *fetus* that meant 'fruitful, pregnant'. The Latin words are related, but not the same.

In medicine, the fetus is the product of human conception from its 8th week until birth.

fetal alcohol syndrome (FAS)

FAS is a group of birth defects and abnormalities seen in infants whose mothers consumed alcohol during pregnancy. The severity of the infant's physical defects and retardations increases in direct proportion to the amount of alcohol drunk by the mother.

fetal distress

During labor, abnormal fetal heart rate and rhythm, abnormal fetal blood, or abnormalities in the amniotic fluid may indicate this clinical diagnosis of fetal pathology.

feto-metry

fetus + *metria* new scientific Greek, measurement

Fetometry is measurement of the fetus *in utero* to anticipate birth problems, hence the size of the fetal head and the circumference of the trunk are important.

fibro-

fibra Latin, thread, fibrous tissue

The prefix denotes fibers or fibrous tissues.

fibril

fibrilla Latin, little thread

A fibril is a very small fiber found inside a cell or as a component of a fiber. Fibrillation is quivering, abnormal contractions of muscle and nerve fibers, particularly in the heart, in atrial or ventricular fibrillation. Ventricular fibrillation is seen widely in cases of sudden cardiac arrest. Hence the heart muscles and nerves must be defibrillated immediately. Drugs or physical means may be effective. Various devices called defibrillators deliver variable electric shocks to the heart muscle through the chest wall. Such resuscitators may be used when the heart is fibrillating or has stopped beating completely.

fibula

fibula Latin, the needle or pin of a brooch; plural *fibulae*

The fibula is the smaller bone of the lower leg. The fibula articulates proximally with the tibia, much as a pin clicks into a brooch. There is distal articulation of the fibula with the tibia again, and with the ankle bone. The Greek word for fibula is *perone*. One muscle attached to the fibula is the peroneus longus.

in-fibul-ation

in + *fibula* pin + *atio, ationis* noun ending

Infibulation was and is a barbarous and woman-hating sewing together of the labia to stop copulation in tribal women. It often followed a clitoridectomy, and was done by closing the labia with little pins or fibulae.

fimbria

fimbria Latin, lacy fringe; plural fimbriae

A fimbria is a body structure that forms a fringe-like edge or border. For example, the fimbriae at the distal ends of Fallopian tubes are little finger-like projections which assist in the movement of ova and spermatozoa.

fissure

fissura Latin, groove, cleft

There are two meanings for fissure in medicine, one physiologic, the other pathologic. In the anatomy of the brain, natural clefts or grooves occur in the cerebral hemispheres. They are deep folds in the cerebral cortex, the outer covering of the brain. They are named after early anatomists, e.g. the fissure of Rolando, the fissure of Sylvius. Certain areas of the brain are named after them, e.g. the perisylvian slope. An example of a pathological fissure is an anal fissure, a painful groove-like ulcer at the margin of the anus, often caused by straining at stool while constipated. A minor surgical operation repairs anal fissure.

fistula

fistula Latin, waterpipe, tube

A fistula is an abnormal passage between two internal organs or surfaces lined with epithelium, or between an organ and the surface of the body. Anal fistula or fistula *in ano* is a pathological opening from the rectum to the skin near the anus. It begins with a localized infection of the mucous membranes of the rectum or anus that does not heal but grows and ulcerates. Surgical correction is effective. A vesicovaginal fistula (*vesica* Latin, bladder) is an abnormal passage from the urinary bladder to the vagina, reparable by surgery.

flamm-

flamma Latin, flame

inflammation

inflammatio, inflammationis Latin, a burning, a flaming

Inflammation is the reaction of tissue to injury. The four classic signs are easy to remember as Latin nouns: *rubor* redness, *tumor* swelling, *calor* heat and *dolor* pain. Inflamed tissue is red, swollen, warm to touch, and painful because of increased blood supply whose white cells fight infection and remove dead tissue. Blood also flows to injured tissue to bring extra cell food for repair and healing.

flatus

flatus Latin, a blowing, a wind, flatulence

Flatus is air or gas in the stomach and intestines, or air or gas expelled through the anus. The activity is subject to a flurry of nervous euphemisms in English: break wind, carminate, flatulate, make a rude noise, pass intestinal gas – all to avoid use of the common, useful word: fart. The same Latin root is the basis of such English words as conflate, deflate, inflate, inflationary. Flatulence is the condition of having air or gas in the stomach or intestines. Speaking of euphemisms, a delightful medical word for the rumbling of intestinal gas inside the body is borborygmus, which in ancient Greek meant 'to make a low sound like bor-bor'.

flavi-

flavus Latin color adjective, straw-yellow

Flavedo is yellowness of the skin, seen in jaundice. The flavivirus is the virus that causes yellow fever. There is also a genus called Flavobacterium which produces a yellow pigment when cultured. Flavone is a biochemical responsible for the orange-red-yellow colors in many vegetables.

ribo-flavin

ribo- combining form indicating ribonic acid or ribose + *flavus* yellow + *in* ending for organic chemical compounds

Flavins are yellow pigments in many animals and plants. Riboflavin is also called vitamin B_2 and is required during the oxidation of other body chemicals.

flavo-proteins

flavus yellow + *proteios* Greek, primary, of basic importance

Flavoproteins are also called yellow enzymes, proteins chemically linked with flavins that take part in intracellular chemical processes like oxidation and reduction.

flex-

flexus Latin, a bending

hepatic flexure

hepatikos Greek, of the liver, *flexura* Latin, a bending, a folding

The hepatic flexure or right colic flexure is a bend in the large intestine where the ascending colon flexs just under the liver to go across the body as the transverse colon.

splenic flexure

splenikos Greek, of the spleen

The splenic flexure or left colic flexure is where the transverse colon bends near the spleen to begin its downward descent as the descending colon.

flexor

flexor Latin, thing that bends

A flexor is any muscle that bends a limb at a joint.

follicle

folliculus Latin, little bag < *follis* bag + *iculus* diminutive ending meaning 'small'

A follicle is a small secretory cavity or sac, like a hair follicle: a pit in the epidermis from which the hair develops. Most hair follicles have sebaceous glands associated with them, whose sebum coats and protects the skin and each strand of hair. Lymph follicles are the dense layers of lymphocytes and lympho-blasts that comprise the outer part or cortex of a lymph gland. In follicular tonsillitis, the follicles on the surface of the tonsil become filled with pus.

foramen

foramen Latin, hole, aperture; plural *foramina*

A foramen is an opening into or through a bone for passage of veins, arteries, nerves, or ligaments.

foramen magnum

Latin, the big hole

The foramen magnum is the great aperture in the occipital bone at the back of the skull. The spinal cord goes through this hole to connect to the brain.

mental foramen

mentalis Latin, of the chin, from *mentum* chin; not to be
confused with a different root that is spelled the same, *mentalis*,
of the mind, from *mens, mentis*

The mental foramina are two small holes in the lower jawbone that permit
passage through the jawbone of the nerves and blood vessels of the chin.

for-ceps

forceps Latin, tongs, pincers < *formu-ceps* literally, taker of
something hot (*formus* Latin, warm + *capire* to take)

The first use of Roman forceps was by blacksmiths, then by teeth-extractors. But
an alternative origin may lie in *ferrum* Latin, iron + *-ceps* < *caput* Latin, head,
giving an early, unattested form like *ferriceps*, 'iron-head' tongs or pincers.

Forceps originated as flattened blades with a handle in ancient ironmongery.
Some ancient blacksmith thought of joining the blades by crossing them at their
centers and fastening them with a bolt that permitted their movement. There
are many kinds of medical forceps used to grasp, handle, compress and join body
tissues or medical equipment. Clamp forceps have an automatic locking device.
Mosquito forceps are very tiny hemostats (see entry) with fine points, used to
clamp off blood vessels. Towel forceps clip towels to the site of a surgical
incision or operative wound. Chamberlen forceps are the classic set of obstetric
forceps: high, mid and low, used in forceps delivery to shorten extended labor or
to quickly deliver a baby in fetal distress. A baby's head may become lodged in
the birth canal in an inappropriate transverse or posterior position. Often gentle
rotation of the head by forceps solves the problem.

fossa

fossa Latin, ditch, trench; plural fossae

In anatomy, a fossa is a furrow or shallow depression in a body structure, for
example, the amygdaloid fossa contains the tonsil (*amygdal-oides* Greek,
almond-shaped, or as here, tonsil-shaped). The glenoid fossa is a shallow
depression on the shoulder blade where the head of the humerus articulates with
the shoulder blade (*glen-oides* Greek, socket-like).

fracture

fractura Latin, a breaking, a splintering

A simple or closed fracture has the bone broken, but no open wound. A
compound or open fracture has the bone broken with an open wound. A
comminuted fracture has the bone crushed or split into many pieces (*com* > *cum*

with + *minutus* small). A greenstick fracture has the bone not broken off cleanly. Greenstick is seen in children's fractures where the bone is still cartilaginous and bends like a green twig in the spring.

frenulum

fraenulum Latin, a little bridle < *fraenum* bridle, brake, thing that stops an action + *ulum* small

A frenulum is a small fold of ligament that limits movement of a body part. The frenulum of a lip is a fold of mucous membrane that connects the inside of each lip to the gums. The frenulum of the penis is the fold under the penis that connects it to the foreskin. The frenulum of the tongue, also called the lingual frenulum, is the vertical fold of mucous membrane under the tongue that anchors the tongue to the floor of the mouth.

functional

functionalis scientific Latin, pertaining to performance of an action or actions

Functional has a special use in medicine, where it means disturbed function but with no organic cause. A functional disease of an organ shows disturbed function but no structural or physiological changes to the organ itself. Compare the term functional psychosis, a mental disorder with no pathology of the central nervous system.

funis

funis Latin, rope, cord

The formal anatomical name for the umbilical cord is funis umbilicalis. Funic presentation in obstetrics sees the umbilical cord appear before the main presenting part of the fetus. Funic souffle (*souffle* French, a breath) is sometimes heard during fetal stethoscopy as a soft, muffled whooshing sound, the sound of blood flowing through the umbilical vessels in time with the fetal heartbeat.

galacto-

gala, galaktos Greek, milk; compare the Latin word *lac, lactis*
Galaxy in English was first applied to the Milky Way, a milky blur of stars across the heavens. Its adjective galactic can refer now to anything in outer space.

galact-agogue

gala, galaktos milk + *agogue* leading, inducing, from *agogia* Greek, a leading, a guiding
A galactagogue is a chemical agent, often a hormone supplement, that helps promote the flow of milk in the breasts of nursing mothers by increasing milk secretion. A synonym is a galactopoietic (*poietikos* Greek adjective, making). The chemical opposite is a galactostatic (*stasis* Greek, a stopping of). See note under *agog* entry for other medical words with this ending, like emmenagogue and hypnagogue.

galact-ase

gala, galaktos milk + *-ase* chemical suffix for names of enzymes. This ending is added to word roots that name the substance on which the enzyme acts. Thus sucrase is a catalyst in the breakdown of complex sugars, amylase of starches (*amylon* Greek, starch), and lipase of fats or lipids (*lipos* Greek, a fat). Galactase acts during the digestion of milk to catalyze the breakdown of its proteins.

galacto-cele

gala, galaktos milk + *kele* Greek, swelling
A galactocele is a swelling caused by obstruction of one or more milk ducts.

galacto-rrhea

gala, galaktos milk + *rrhoia* Greek, a flowing through, a discharge

Galactorrhea is excess flow of milk from the breast, possibly due to a pituitary tumor that causes the secretion of excess milk-stimulating hormones. The symptom is sometimes referred to as incontinence (see entry) of milk.

galact-ose

gala, galaktos milk + *-ose* chemical suffix for names of sugars like glucose, sucrose, fructose, lactose

Galactose is a simple milk sugar metabolized from lactose.

gallbladder

The gallbladder is a storage sac for bile made by the liver. The gallbladder is located under the right lobe of the liver. Gall has some of its water content removed while in the gallbladder. Pathologies of the gallbladder are named using the prefix *cholecysto-* (Greek for bile-sac). See the *cholecysto* entry. The Latin word for gall forms medical terms like biliary (*bilis* Latin, bile, gall). See *bile* entry.

ganglion

gagglion Greek, encysted tumor on leg, head, etc.; plural ganglia

The Greek-speaking Roman physician and medical writer Galen (AD 129–199) first compared these knots of nerve tissue to tumors. Ganglia are masses of nervous tissue lying outside the brain and spinal column. They may be thought of as substations for the routing of nerve impulses, receiving, collecting, and sending impulses from nerve tissue throughout the body. Sometimes the original Greek meaning of ganglion is used in modern medicine too, where a ganglion is a cystic tumor on a tendon, sometimes a tendon on the back of the wrist.

gangrene

gaggraina Greek, a sore or severe ulcer in which the tissue dies < *gran* Greek, to gnaw

Gangrene is tissue death or necrosis (*nekros* Greek, dead) when that tissue loses adequate blood supply. Gangrene may be due to diseases like diabetes, trauma, embolisms, frostbite, an improperly affixed tourniquet, severe burns, or bacterial infection. The most common sites of gangrene in humans are the arms and legs. Treatment may include antibiotics, a hyperbaric chamber (see *hyperbaric* entry), and surgical excision of necrotic tissue and occasionally of severely gangrenous limbs.

gastri-, gastro-

gaster, gastros Greek, belly, stomach

gastric

gastrikos Greek, of the stomach

Gastric juices secreted in the stomach include enzymes like pepsin, protease, lipase, and also hydrochloric acid to help churn food to a goopy chyme (*chymos* Greek, juice) ready to enter the small intestine for further digestive processing.

gastro-intestinal

The gastrointestinal tract is a common name for the digestive system, also known as the alimentary canal, where food is taken in, digested, and absorbed, and solid waste is eliminated. Its major parts are the mouth, throat, stomach and intestines. A gastrointestinal series is a group of diagnostic tests to detect abnormalities of the stomach or intestines. Often a barium enema introduces a contrast medium so that X-rays are clear. A GISA (gastrointestinal system assessment) is a more extensive diagnostic survey of a patient's digestive system and symptoms.

gastro-gavage

gavage French, a stuffing, a cramming

Gastrogavage is artificial feeding through a tube passed into the stomach through a small surgical incision. The procedure is a gastrostomy (*stoma* Greek, mouth), the making of a small opening in the stomach, sometimes necessary in cases of prolonged loss of consciousness or pathologies like cancer of the esophagus.

gastric lavage

lavage French, a washing

Gastric lavage has a common synonym, 'pumping out the stomach'. Sterile water or a saline solution is instilled through a tube put through the nose and gently guided by nurse and patient down to the stomach. A bulb syringe removes the aspirant specimen. Gastric lavage may be used to wash out the stomach when its contents are irritating or poisonous, in pre-operative cleansing, or to remove a test meal in certain digestive diagnostic procedures.

genu

genu Latin, knee, or any structure resembling a knee

genu recurvatum

recurvatum Latin, bent backward
In genu recurvatum the knee joint is hyperextended or bent backward, due to injury or, less often, congenital deformity.

genu valgum

valgus New Latin, knock-kneed
Genu valgum is a deformity in which the knees are too close together, and the ankles are too far apart.

genu varum

varus Latin, bow-legged
Genu varum is the anatomical name for being bowlegged, that is, with outward curving of one or both legs near the knee.

genu-flect

flectere Latin, to bend
To genuflect is to bend the knee, often part of a general physical examination. In extramedical English, it means to kneel, often as a sign of obeisance to a ruler or potentate.

gen-icul-ate ganglion

genu knee + *iculum* little + *ate* adjectival suffix, similar to, like a
The geniculate ganglion is a mass of neural tissue where the facial nerve makes a knee-like bend.

geri-, geronto-

geron, gerontos Greek, old person

ger-iatric

geron old person + *iatros* Greek, doctor + *ikos* adjective ending
The root *iatros* appears in several medical specialties: pediatrics (*paidos*, of the child), podiatry (*pos, podos* foot), and psychiatry (*psyche* soul, mind). Geriatrics is the branch of medicine that treats the problems and diseases of old age.

geronto-logy

geron, gerontos old person + *logos* study of
Gerontology is the scientific study of aging, by a researcher called a gerontologist.

pro-geria

pro Greek, before, in front of + *geras* old age
Progeria is a rare childhood retardation characterized by premature aging symptoms like wrinkled skin, gray hair, small stature and hardening of the arteries. This progressive and early senility contributes to a shortened life span.

gingiva

gingiva Medieval Latin, the gums
The gingiva is the gum, the fibrous tissue surrounding the necks of the teeth and covering the alveolar processes of the jaws. The gums are themselves covered with a mucous membrane.

gingiv-itis

gingiva the gums + *itis* inflammation of
Most inflamed, bleeding gums are due to sticky plaque and bacterial build-up brought on by negligent dental hygiene, although some drugs like Dilantin™ may make gum margins swell. Trench mouth is a severe necrotizing, ulcerative gingivitis, in which débridement of the dead gingival tissue is indicated along with saline rinsing or hydrogen peroxide rinsing.

gingiv-ec-tomy

gingiva the gums + *ex* out + *tome* a cutting
Gingivectomy is a surgical cutting out of gum margins afflicted with severe gingivitis.

163

glaucoma

glaukos of gray-green color + *oma* swelling; Hippocrates and Aristotle used *glaukoma* to mean 'cataract'

Glaucoma is not a cataract of the lens, as the ancients supposed. It was not until modern times that glaucoma was recognized as a disease caused by elevated pressure of the aqueous humor, pressing on and damaging the optic nerve. Glaucoma is often hereditary, sometimes congenital, and infrequently the sequela of some other eye disorder (*sequela* Latin, sequel, thing that follows after something).

-glia, glio-

glia Medieval Greek, glue

gli-oma

glia glue + *oma* tumor

A glioma is any tumor made of neuroglia. For example, one composed of astrocytes (see next definition) is an astrocytoma.

neuro-glia

neuron nerve + *glia* glue

Neuroglia, literally 'nerve glue', is the varied supporting and connecting cells of nerve tissue, also called glial cells. One particular kind of glial cell, with fibrous or protoplasmic processes that give it the microscopic appearance of a little star is an astrocyte (*aster* star + *kytos* cell). When astrocytes together are considered as a tissue, they are named astroglia.

glossa-, glosso-

glossa Greek, the tongue

glossal

glossalis scientific Latin, lingual, pertaining to the tongue. *Lingua* is the Latin word for tongue.

glosso-plasty

glossa tongue + *plastia* a shaping, a forming by means of surgery

Glossoplasty is plastic surgery of the tongue, often to repair cleft tongue. See *schistoglossia* entry below.

glosso-rrhaphy

glossa tongue + *rrhaphe* surgical suture + *y* noun ending
Glossorrhaphy is suturing the tongue, often part of glossoplasty, and also done to repair wounds to the tongue.

schisto-glossia

schistos split + *glossa* tongue + *ia* medical condition
Schistoglossia is split tongue, a birth defect, also called cleft or bifid tongue, or lingua bifida.

glottis

glottis, glottidis Greek, mouth of the windpipe
The glottis is the slit or cleft between the true vocal cords. Cord here is a misnomer. They are really vocal folds, and the anatomical name for the vocal cords makes this clear: plicae vocales, 'vocal folds of tissue'. The glottis includes the opening, its walls and boundaries. The median slit itself has its own anatomical name: rima glottidis (*rima* Latin, a slit).

As well as in breathing, the glottis also opens and closes in the production of certain speech sounds. For example, the glottal stop that is heard in the Cockney pronunciation of the word 'bottle'; instead of a *t*-sound, the glottis closes quickly, so 'bottle' sounds like 'bo'l'.

gluco

glykys Greek, sweet

gluc-ose

glykys sweet + *ose* chemical suffix in names of sugars like sucrose, fructose, lactose
Glucose is the simple sugar found in human blood, and the main source of energy for all living organisms.

glucos-uria

glucose + *ouron* Greek, urine + *ia* medical condition

Glucosuria is the presence of high glucose levels in the urine, often indicating diabetes.

glucose tolerance test (GTT)

A glucose tolerance test is a part of blood work. A patient fasts for several hours, then the blood sugar level is measured. Glucose is then given orally or by injection, followed by more blood tests, possibly to diagnose diabetes mellitus.

gluteus

gluteus Latin spelling of *gloutos* Greek, buttocks

Three muscles form the human buttocks. The gluteus maximus (Latin, largest) muscle extends movements of the thigh. The gluteus medius (Latin, middle) abducts and rotates the thigh. The gluteus minimus (Latin, smallest) also helps abduct the thigh (see *abduct* entry). The Latin word for the buttocks is nates (singular, natis) and this word applies in medicine to the gluteal muscles and the fat stored under them, both of which make the large, fleshy pads that comprise the buttocks.

gluteal tuberosity

glutealis New Latin, pertaining to gluteal muscles + *tuberosity* an elevation or protuberance on a bone < *tuberosus* full of bumps < *tuber* bump, swelling, hump

The gluteal tuberosity is a small ridge on the lateral posterior surface of the femur where the gluteus maximus is attached to the femur.

glyco-

glykys Greek, sweet

glyco-gen

glykys sweet + *gen* Greek, making, producing

Glycogen is the chemical called animal starch, as which the human body stores carbohydrate to be converted into glucose to move muscles and make heat. Glycogen storage is complex and subject to several inherited abnormalities, usually tagged as glycogen storage diseases, types I to VII.

glyc-em-ia

glykys sweet + *em* short for *haima* blood + *ia* medical condition

Glycemia or glycosemia is an abnormal amount of sugar in the blood. Hypoglycemia is abnormally low blood sugar (*hypo* Greek, under, below). Hyperglycemia is too much sugar in the blood (*hyper* Greek, over, above). Both conditions are seen in forms of diabetes.

glycos-uria

glykys + *ouron* Greek, urine + *ia* medical condition

A synonym for glucosuria (given above). Abnormal amounts of glucose in the urine may indicate diabetes mellitus, but other causes including excessive carbohydrate intake can produce this oversupply.

-gnosis

gnosis Greek, a knowing, knowledge, telling what is known

dia-gnosis

dia Greek, through + *gnosis* knowledge

Diagnosis is finding the cause of a disease; the plural is diagnoses. So the sense of diagnosis is distinguishing one from many causes. Diagnostics is the science and practice of diagnosis, as conducted by a physician in his role as diagnostician. A differential diagnosis tries to pinpoint which precise disease of several is causing symptoms. Other phrases sometimes heard are: clinical diagnosis, based on the signs and symptoms exhibited by the patient; and laboratory diagnosis, based on analysis of X-rays and tests like blood work and urinalysis.

pro-gnosis

pro Greek, beforehand + *gnosis* knowledge, knowing, telling

Prognosis is predicting the course and outcome of a disease.

gonad

gonas, gonadis New Latin, sex gland, based on *gonos* Greek, seed, offspring

Gonad is a generic term for human sex glands. The female gonad is the ovary, the male is the testis. But also in loose clinical parlance, the gonads can refer to private parts, to sex organs. In embryology, the gonad is the undifferentiated sex gland before it is definitively a testis or an ovary.

gonado-tropin

gonadis of a sex gland + *tropos* Greek, a turning, a changing, an affecting of

A gonadotropin is any hormone whose presence produces changes in the sex glands, for example, luteinizing hormone (see entry) or follicle-stimulating hormone.

gono-

gone Greek, seed, offspring, sex organs

gono-coccus

gone Greek, sex organs + *kokkos* Greek, berry

Gonococcus is a species of bacterium, *Neisseria gonorrhoeae*, that causes gonorrhea (see next entry). It is found on the surface of the genitals, inside the genitals, in blood, in joints, in the heart, the eye, in feces and in boils.

gono-rrhea

gone Greek, sex organs + *rrhoia* Greek, a discharge

Gonorrhea is a widespread contagious inflammation of genital mucous membranes in the male and female, caused by *Gonococcus* bacteria. In the male, symptoms include the discharge of yellow pus from the penis, difficult urination, and sometimes prostatic involvement. In the female, gonorrhea may be asymptomatic but can include painful urination, abnormal vaginal discharge, and, possibly, acute pelvic inflammatory disease. Condoms are a useful precaution in the prevention of gonorrhea.

-gyn-, -gyne, gyneco-

gyne, gynaikos Greek, a female, a woman

andro-gyn-oid

andros Greek, of a male + *gyne* female + *eides* formed like

Synonyms are androgyne and androgynous person, a person with ovaries but with the secondary sexual characteristics of a male. Also called a female pseudohermaphrodite (*pseudos* Greek, false). See the *hermaphrodite* entry.

gyn-ander

gyne female + *aner, andros* male
A gynander is a person possessing both male and female characteristics. Gynandrism is male hermaphroditism.

gyneco-logy

gyne, gynaikos woman + *logos* study of
Gynecology is the study and treatment of diseases of the female reproductive organs, including the breasts.

gyneco-mast-ia

gyne, gynaikos female + *mastos* Greek, breast + *ia* medical condition
Gynecomastia affects males. It is excessive development of the male mammary glands.

gyne-phobia

gyne woman + *phobos* fear + *ia* medical condition
Gynephobia is a morbid dread of women, including a fear of their company.

gyn-iatrics

gyne female + *iatros* Greek, doctor + *ikos* adjective ending
Gyniatrics is the treatment of diseases of women.

miso-gyny

misos Greek, hatred + *gyne* female
Misogyny is a pathological hatred of women. Hatred of males is misandry.

gyrus

gyros Greek, circle

The cortex that covers the hemispheres of the brain has many complex infoldings. Many of these curved portions or convolutions (plural *gyri cerebri*) are named after their cerebral location, for example, hippocampal gyrus and parietal gyrus. The shallow grooves that separate gyri are sulci (singular sulcus). The deeper grooves are fissures (see *sulcus* and *fissure* entries).

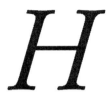

H

h.s.

hora somni Latin, literally, at the hour of sleep, i.e. before bedtime

H.s. is a common pharmacological abbreviation seen in prescriptions.

hal-

halare Latin, to breathe

ex-hale

ex Latin, out + *halare* to breathe

Exhalation is the process of breathing out, the opposite of inhalation.

hal-itus

halare to breathe + *itus* Latin noun suffix, the act of

Halitus means 'the breath' in medicine, or a warm vapor.

halit-osis

halitus breath + *osis* abnormal condition of

Halitosis is bad breath, foul and offensive, usually due to poor oral hygiene or dental infections, but halitosis may be of diagnostic importance in certain disorders too: in some patients with certain forms of diabetes the breath can smell of acetone; in some liver diseases, the breath can smell of ammonia.

in-hal-ator, inhaler

in Latin, in + *halare* to breathe + *ator* Latin agent noun suffix meaning here 'device which'

An inhalator or inhaler is a device for delivering vaporous medication to be inhaled, including certain gases used in anesthesia. Inhalation therapy is a term for such delivery of medications and gases like oxygen, carbon dioxide and helium. Inhalants are often turned into very small particles by a nebulizer before being inhaled (*nebula* Latin, cloud, mist).

hallucination

alucinari Latin, to wander in the mind > *hallucinatio,*
hallucinatonis Late Latin, delusion

Hallucination is a term in psychology for a false sense perception. An auditory hallucination is imaginary sounds heard as part of a psychotic disorder or subsequent to an organic disorder like inflammation of the inner ear producing a tinnitus (Latin, a ringing sound). Gustatory hallucination involves imaginary tastes. Olfactory hallucination produces imaginary smells. And hallucinations may involve the senses of touch, body movements and sight.

hallucino-gen

alucinari to wander in the mind + *gen* Greek, making,
producing

A hallucinogen such as LSD or peyote produces imaginary responses of the senses.

hallux, hallex, hallus

hallux, hallucis Latin, big toe

Hallux is the anatomical name of the great toe. Hallux flexus is hammertoe or claw toe in which the phalangeal joints of the big toe are bent in inappropriate flexions.

hemi-

hemi Greek prefix, a half; akin to Latin *semi-*, half

hemi-an-opia, hemi-an-opsia

hemi half + *an* not + *ops, opos* Greek, eye, or + *opsis* Greek,
vision, sight

Hemianopia is blindness in half the field of vision for one or both eyes. There are varieties of the disorder like binasal hemianopia, in which the nasal half of the field of vision in both eyes is affected.

hemi-facial

hemi half + *facialis* scientific Latin, of the face
A hemifacial paralysis affects half of the face.

hemi-pleg-ia

hemi half + *plege* Greek, a stroke + *ia* medical condition
Hemiplegia is paralysis of one side of the body. Cerebral hemiplegia (*cerebrum* Latin, brain) is a paralysis on one side of the body due to a brain lesion.

hemi-sphere

hemi half + *sphaira* Greek, globe, ball, sphere
A hemisphere is half of a spherical structure or organ, like a cerebral hemisphere, one of the paired structures forming most of the human brain.

hem-, hema-, hemato-

haima, haimatos Greek, blood

hem-angi-oma

haima blood + *angeion* Greek, blood or lymph vessel + *oma* tumor
An hemangioma is a benign tumor of dilated blood vessels.

hemat-emesis

haima, haimatos blood + *emesis* Greek, vomiting
Hematemesis is a medical emergency, the vomiting of blood, a sign of serious internal hemorrhage. Gastric blood is dark and acid; pharyngeal blood is bright red and alkaline.

hemato-crit

haima, haimatos blood + *kritikos* Greek, separating, judging
An hematocrit is a centrifuge that separates blood solids from the liquid plasma. Hematocrit is also used in blood work to label the measurement of red blood cells in a given volume of blood. For example, a normal hematocrit for an adult female at sea level is 42%, with a range of 5% lower or higher.

hemo-globin

haima blood + *globus* Latin, ball, clump, globe + *in* ending for organic chemical compounds

Hemoglobin is the pigment of red blood cells that contains iron. It carries oxygen from the lungs to individual cells of the body via the blood's circulation. The molecule of hemoglobin is a large one, subject to mutation. Some of the diseases caused by hemoglobin abnormalities are sickle cell anemia, hemolytic anemia, and congenital cyanosis (see *anemia* and *cyanosis* entries).

hemo-lysis

haima blood + *lysis* Greek, a breaking up of

Hemolysis is the destruction of red blood cells in which hemoglobin seeps into surrounding tissues and fluids. Hemoglobinuria is red-colored urine, stained by hemoglobin which has been lost due to hemolytic action inside the blood vessels.

hemo-philia

haima blood + *philia* Greek, fondness for, a loving of

Hemophilia is bleeder's disease, an heriditary slowness of the blood to coagulate when its vessels are ruptured. The blood of hemophiliacs lacks certain clotting factors and serious, sometimes fatal internal hemorrhage may occur. While there is no cure for hemophilia, various coagulants are administered to help the blood clot in a normal time period.

hemo-rrhage

haima blood + *rrhagia* Greek, bursting, gushing forth

Hemorrhage is abnormal bleeding, the internal and external escape of blood from vessels.

hemo-stasis

haima blood + *stasis* Greek, stopping, standing still

Hemostasis is the stopping of bleeding, either naturally or by hemostatic surgical means. A hemostat is a little surgical clamp used to constrict a blood vessel.

hepato-

hepar, hepatos Greek, the liver

hepat-itis

hepar, hepatos liver + *itis* inflammation of

Hepatitis is inflammation of the liver due to toxins like excessive alcohol, or in acute forms, infection by hepatitis viruses A, B, C, D, and E. Hepatitis B is more prolonged than A, and may be caused by dirty needles used by drug addicts, contaminated blood, or oral intake of virally infected materials.

hepato-megaly

hepar, hepatos Greek, the liver + *megale* enlargement < *megas* big

Hepatomegaly is abnormal enlargement of the liver. It may be part of cirrhosis, a group of chronic liver diseases in which hepatic functions and structures degenerate.

hernia

hernia Latin, a rupture, a protruding

Hernia is the abnormal protruding of an organ or body part through a muscular wall that usually contains the organ.

hiatus hernia

hiatus Latin, gap, opening

Hiatus hernia is a protruding of part of the stomach upward through the diaphragm, often with the result that some acid contents of the stomach flow back up into the esophagus. This symptom is called gastroesophageal reflux (*gaster* Greek, stomach). *Reflux* is Latin for 'a flowing back'.

inguinal hernia

inguen, inguinis Latin, groin; the adjective is *inguinalis*, of the groin

Inguinal hernia is the most common rupture in the male: a loop of intestine slips into a gap in the abdominal muscles where the testes descended into the scrotum (in most males before birth). Sometimes this prenatal descent of the testes pulls down a bit of the peritoneal lining of the abdomen, and a loop of intestine can herniate into this space. Herniorrhaphy is the suturing repair of a hernia (*rrhaphe* Greek, surgical suture).

herpes

herpes Greek, literally 'the creeps', shingles, from *herpein* to creep

Herpes is a persistent, recurrent viral skin disease marked by clusters of painful blisters. Herpes simplex virus, or HSV-1, is the virus that causes brain, eye, mouth and skin herpes. HSV-2 causes genital herpes. Herpes labialis is the common cold sore (*labium* Latin, lip). Herpes zoster (*zoster* Greek, girdle) attacks sensory neurons near the spinal cord causing painful skin blisters above the course of the infected nerve. These eruptions may girdle the body on one side only.

hetero-

heteros Greek, different, opposite

Two confusible adjectives derived from this Greek root are used in medicine. Heterogeneous means 'consisting of different parts, unlike', or 'not of uniform composition' (*genos* Greek, kind, type). Heterogenous means 'not from the same source' or 'from two different sources'. A heterogenous vaccine would be one not produced from a patient's own tissue. A heterograft is transplant tissue taken from a different species than the patient. A homograft is transplant tissue from the same species as the patient (*homoios* Greek, similar, the same, like). A heterosexual is attracted to persons of the opposite sex.

hiatus

hiatus Latin, a gap, a yawning hole < *hiare* to gape, to yawn, to open

A hiatus can be a natural or a pathological opening in a membrane or body tissue. Hiatus hernia (see entry above) is pathological. The hiatus aorticus is the natural opening in the diaphragm through which passes the aorta and the thoracic duct. The hiatus esophageus is the opening in the diaphragm for the passage of the esophagus.

hidro

hidros Greek, sweat, perspiration

an-hidro-sis

a not + *hidros* sweat + *osis* diseased condition

Anhidrosis is an abnormally low volume of sweat, or absence of sweating. Hidrosis is the normal secretion of perspiration.

hidr-aden-itis, hydradenitis

hidros Greek, sweat + *aden* Greek, gland + *itis* inflammation of

Hidradenitis is inflammation of the sweat glands. There are two kinds of sweat glands. Eccrine or exocrine sweat glands secrete through pores on most of the body surface. Sweating helps cool the body through surface evaporation of the sweat. Apocrine sweat glands empty a secretion thicker than normal sweat into hair follicles.

Hippocratic oath

Hippokrates ancient Greek personal name that means 'he who rules horses'

Hippocrates, often called the father of medicine, was a Greek physician born around 460 BC. He was famous in his lifetime as a doctor and teacher of medicine at an academy that he founded on the Greek island of Cos where he introduced a scientific method of studying diseases and healing. His own medical writings survive in part, along with papers written much later by his students and by physicians who lived many centuries after him. The famous Hippocratic oath begins, 'I swear by Apollo the physician...'. Its most famous line is usually found in Latin: *Primum non nocere,* 'First, do no harm'.

histo-

histos Greek, something woven, a web, a tissue

To the very earliest Greek physicians, skin appeared as if it might be woven like certain fine textiles; indeed the entire structure of the human body seemed like some complex tapestry. Around 1800, a French physician named Bichat simply translated this Greek concept into French and began to use a French word for a rich fabric, *tissu,* to refer to groups of cells specialized to perform particular functions. From French, English acquired its word *tissue.* 'To weave' in French is *tisser,* from Latin *texere,* 'to weave'. Compare *textilis,* 'capable of being woven', which gives the English word *textile.*

hist-amine

histos tissue + *amine* from Latin, *am (monia)* + *ine* biochemical suffix indicating compound substance

In biochemistry, an amine is a type of organic compound, a derivative of ammonia. Histamine is a chemical, an amine found in all cells, that assists in gastric secretion, widening capillaries, and contracting the smooth muscle layers of the bronchi. An anti-histamine is any drug that counteracts the effects of histamines. Anti-histamines, for example, widen small blood vessels that are constricted and inflamed.

histo-compatibility

In tissue transplanting, histocompatibility is the measure of how the recipient's defense system (antigens) will tolerate foreign material such as the donor's tissue. Histocompatibility antigens on the cell surface in the recipient cause most rejection of grafted tissues. When the recipient and the donor have tissues of different genotypes, they are said to be histoincompatible.

histo-logy

histos tissue + *logos* study of

Histology deals with the microscopic form, function, and identification of tissues. A tissue is a group of cells which together perform a special function.

HIV

HIV is human immunodeficiency virus, a type of retrovirus that causes AIDS, acquired immunodeficiency syndrome.

homo-, homeo

homoios Greek, similar, the same, alike

homeo-stasis

homoios the same + *stasis* Greek, stopping, standing still

Homeostasis is the internal state of balance in the human body. This healthy 'steady-state' is achieved by sensory circuits, feedback and control systems. Examples of homeostatic processes are heartbeat, blood-making, blood pressure and body temperature regulation, breathing and secretion of hormones by various glands.

homo-logue, homolog

homoios the same + *logos* Greek relationship, proportion

A homolog is an organ or body part common to a number of species, or an organ that corresponds to an organ in another structure. The arm of a human, the flipper of a seal, the wing of a bird, and the forelimb of a dog are homologous structures. The clitoris in the human female is a homolog of the corpus cavernosus in the penis of the human male.

In biology and anatomy, the opposite of homolog is analog or analogue. Analogous organs in different species or sexes are similar in function, but different in structure and origin (*analogos* Greek, relation, analogy). The eye of a grasshopper and the eye of a human are analogous, but not homologous.

homo-sexual

homoios the same + *sexualis* scientific Latin, pertaining to gender

As an adjective, homosexual denotes the same sex. As a noun, it is a person sexually attracted to members of the same sex. Homosexual panic is a psychological term for anxiety arising from gender identity conflict and fear of being homosexual.

hordeolum

hordeolum Latin, a grain of barley; in medicine, a stye in the eye

The name derives from the supposed resemblance of a stye to a grain of the cereal barley. A ripe head of barley, also called a barleycorn, is reddish and puffed-up.

A hordeolum is a stye. One or more of the sebaceous glands at the base of the eyelid becomes infected, usually by staphylococcic bacteria. The cyst formed is red, filled with pus, warm to the touch, and painful. Therapy includes hot compresses and antibiotics. An external hordeolum is on the skin surface at the edge of the eyelid. An internal hordeolum is on the conjunctival surface.

hormone

hormon Greek present participle, setting in motion, urging forward, speeding up

Hippocrates used the word *hormon* to mean a principle of vitality and considered certain body secretions to be 'rousers'. The word was redefined and reintroduced to medicine in 1905 by Ernest Starling, a British physiologist.

A hormone is a complex biochemical stimulant originating in one organ and traveling through body vessels to another body structure where it acts to begin a function or to initiate or inhibit the secretion of another hormone. Dozens of hormones are necessary for healthy functioning of the human body.

humerus

humerus Latin, bone of the upper arm, akin to *omos* Greek, shoulder

The humerus is the largest bone of the upper arm. Proximally, the humerus articulates with the shoulder blade in the glenoid cavity. Distally, the humerus has a condyle (see entry) with several depressions where it articulates with the two long bones of the forearm, the radius and the ulna. Humeral articulation may be adversely affected in chronic arthritis.

hyal-

hyalos Greek, glass

hyaline bodies

Hyaline meaning 'clear and glassy' has a pathological meaning and also refers to healthy tissue (see next entry). Hyaline bodies or hyalins are clear, glassy deposits caused by the breakdown of connective tissue and colloids or, in the tubes of the kidneys, due to protein molecules that cannot be processed. Pale, transparent hyaline casts (mineral deposits) may be found in the urine of patients suffering from certain kidney diseases or nephropathies (*nephros* kidney + *pathos* disease).

hyaline cartilage

Hyaline cartilage is also called true cartilage, the bluish-white, smooth, pearly, elastic tissue that covers the articulating ends of bones and connects the ribs to the breastbone. Hyaline cartilage also helps support the nose, the trachea and part of the larynx.

hyaloid

hyalos glass + *eides* Greek, form, hence *-oid* means 'formed like'

The hyaloid membrane, clear and glassy, surrounds the vitreous humor of the eyeball and separates the vitreous humor from the retina. When this membrane becomes inflamed, the pathology label may be hyaloiditis. Inflammation of the vitreous humor itself is hyalitis.

hydatid

hydatis, hydatidis Greek, cyst filled with watery fluid < *hydor, hydros* water

Hydatids are fluid-filled cysts, chiefly found in the liver, caused by parasitic infestation by the larvae of the dog tapeworm. Hydatids can attain large size over time and must be removed surgically.

hydro-

hydor, hydros Greek, water

hydro-cele

hydor, hydros water + *kele* swelling

Hydrocele is an abnormal fluid accumulation in the tunica of the testes or along the spermatic cord, caused by clogged lymph ducts or veins in the cord. It may also accompany inflammation of the testis or epididymis (see *epididymis* entry).

hydro-cephalus

hydor, hydros water + *kephale* Greek, head

Hydrocephalus is 'water on the brain' in common speech, an abnormal retention of cerebrospinal fluid within the vault of the cranium. Obstructions, increased fluid secretion, or faulty re-absorption of cerebrospinal fluid may cause this pathological condition, those causes themselves being due to infection, trauma, tumors, or developmental irregularities of brain structure. Congenital hydrocephalus is fatal in half of patients. The surgical remedy of hydrocephalus usually involves a shunt to divert the excess cerebrospinal fluid to a cavity such as the peritoneum where it can be safely absorbed and eliminated.

hydro-meter

hydor, hydros water + *metron* Greek, device that measures

An hydrometer is an instrument that measures the density or specific gravity of a fluid.

hydro-nephr-osis

hydor, hydros water + *nephros* Greek, kidney + *osis* diseased condition

Hydronephrosis is a swelling of the kidney through flow-back pressure from an obstruction such as a calculus or stone in the urinary tract, a urethral tumor, prostatitis (see entry), or edema.

hydrops, hydropsy, dropsy

hydor, hydros water

Hydrops is the word origin of 'dropsy', an edema, a condition in which body tissues retain an excessive amount of fluid. Examples are hydrops fetalis, a massive edema in the fetus or newborn, and hydrops gravidarum (Latin, of pregnant women), a generalized edema caused by pregnancy.

hydro-phobia

hydor, hydros water + *phobos* fear + *ia* medical condition

Hydrophobia is an old name for rabies, an acute, dangerous viral infection passed to humans by animal bites. Exposed victims need immediate vaccination. French scientist Louis Pasteur invented the vaccine in 1885. But hydrophobia means 'fear of water'. During the crisis of rabies, which can be fatal within a few days if not treated, fever, delirium, paralysis and muscle spasms may occur. The patient is thirsty because of the fever, but severe spasm of the throat muscles makes the patient terrified to drink water – hence 'fear of water' to label the disease.

hydro-salpinx

hydor, hydros water + *salpinx* Greek, trumpet; in medicine, a Fallopian tube

Hydrosalpinx is an abnormal fluid accumulation in an encysted Fallopian tube, due to a previous infection that blocked the tube at both ends.

hymen

hymen Greek, any body membrane, also Hymen, ancient Greek god of marriages

The hymen is a fold of mucous membrane, skin and fibrous tissue partly covering – or more rarely totally covering – the vaginal orifice. In old English, the hymen was the maidenhead; in modern English slang, it is called 'the cherry'. Normally the hymen has some openings. Vigorous exercise, petting, and masturbation usually succeed in breaking it well before menarche or before initial sexual intercourse. Hymenal tags are bits of hymenal tissue protruding from the floor of the vagina, seen normally for a few weeks after birth.

hymeno-tomy

hymen maidenhead + *tome* surgical incision of
Hymenotomy is the rare surgical perforation of a thick or complete hymen.
Even rarer is a surgical excision of the hymen, called a hymenectomy.

hyoid

hyoeides Greek, U-shaped < *hy* or *hu*, colloquial name for the
Greek letter upsilon whose lower-case form resembles a U or a
horseshoe + *eides* Greek, form, hence -*oid* means 'formed like'
The hyoid bone is a small, isolated, U-shaped bone at the base of the tongue.
The hyoid is suspended from two little processes of the temporal bones. It is
attached to various muscles and works with them to move the tongue. For
example, one of these muscles is the hyoglossus (*glossa* Greek, tongue) which acts
to draw down the sides of the tongue and to retract the tongue back into the
mouth.

hyper

hyper Greek, over, above, abnormally increased, excessive; akin
to Latin *super*, German *über*, English *over*

hyper-active

hyper over + active
Hyperactive is the source of the slang adjective 'hyper'. Hyperactive child
syndrome is a much abused label for normally lively youngsters in the care of
adults with no tolerance or sympathy or understanding of childhood.
Hyperactive child syndrome could, in many cases, be more accurately labeled
'bad parent syndrome'. Notwithstanding its abuse, there is a legitimate
syndrome of disturbed, overactive, aggressive, impulsive behavior in children
due to severe emotional disorders, retardation, and, rarely, central nervous
system disorders. By adolescence, most children outgrow hyperkinesis (*hyper*
excessive + *kinesis* Greek, movement).

hyper-beta-lipo-protein-emia

hyper over + *beta* second letter of the Greek alphabet, used in
listing: type one is alpha, type two is beta, type three is gamma,
etc. + *lipos* Greek, fat + protein + *em* short for *haima*, Greek,
blood + *ia* medical condition

Hyperbetalipoproteinemia is often cited by beginners as the kind of polysyllabic horror that makes learning the technical terms of medicine such a daunting task. Nonsense, of course. By now the attentive student can see how even this so-called 'jaw-breaker' is itself broken up into its parts, simply and easily. Hyperbetalipoproteinemia is a genetic disorder of fat metabolism in which very high levels of serum cholesterol are found in the blood. Young people so afflicted have a tendency to very early hardening of the arteries and heart disease. You should be able to guess the meaning of the next ten-dollar word. Try. Then look at the roots of the word.

hyper-bilirubin-emia

hyper excessive + bilirubin, a bile pigment + *em* short for *haima*, Greek, blood + *ia* medical condition

Hyperbilirubinemia is excessive amounts of the bile pigment, bilirubin, in the blood (*bilis* bile + *rubus* Latin, red + *in* organic compound). Bilirubin is a product of the breakdown of hemoglobin in old red blood cells. So this pathology indicates excessive destruction of red blood cells. It is accompanied by jaundice, loss of appetite and a general malaise. Hyperbilirubinemia is common in newborns.

hyper-sensitivity

hyper excessive + sensitivity

Hypersensitivity reaction is an excess immune response by the body to invasive foreign cells. Common allergens producing it are weed pollen, dust, animal hairs breathed in or touching the skin and certain foods. Symptoms can be mild, like a runny nose, or severe like anaphylactic shock (see entry).

hyper-tension

hyper excessive + *tensio, tensionis* Latin, the action of being stretched out, as vessels are by blood

Hypertension is high blood pressure. It is without symptoms. Essential hypertension has no known causes, although obesity and high sodium levels in the blood predispose one to it. There are many drugs to treat it, including diuretics, vasodilators, beta blockers, etc. Rest and a low-salt, low-fat diet help too.

hyper-trophy

hyper excessive + *trophe* Greek, nourishment, feeding

Hypertrophy is excess growth of tissue due to increase in the size of tissue cells. Therefore hypertrophied organs are abnormally enlarged ones. Hypertrophy is not the result of tumor formation, hence a name like benign prostatic hypertrophy to label a common enlargement of the prostate gland in men over 50 years old. It is not malignant and not inflammatory.

hyper-plasia

hyper excessive + *plasia* Greek, a forming (of cells)
Hyperplasia is excess growth of tissue due to an increase in the number of cells. Thus note the difference between this word and hypertrophy. For example, hyperplastic gingivitis is an inflammation of gum tissue with an increase in the number of cells in the gum tissue. It is caused by a build-up of dental plaque. Following inflammation, some tissues and organs exhibit fibrous hyperplasia, an increase in the number of cells of connective tissue.

hyper-ventilate

hyper excessive + *ventilare* Latin, to breathe loudly, making a sound like the wind < *ventus* wind
In Classical Latin, *ventillare* meant 'to produce a *ventilla* (little wind)', hence, to fan oneself. To hyperventilate is to breathe faster than necessary for the normal inhaling of oxygen and exhaling of carbon dioxide, often due to acute anxiety. Hyperventilation causes a low level of carbon dioxide in the arteries and an increase in blood pH (see *pH* entry), with resultant chest pain, dizziness and numbness of the digits, among other symptoms.

hypno-

hypnos Greek, sleep

hypn-osis

hypnos Greek, sleep + *osis* diseased condition
Hypnosis is an artificially induced sleep-like state, where the hypnotized subject is often responsive to suggestion, hence the term 'hypnotic suggestion'.

hypno-therapy

hypnos Greek, sleep + *therapeia* Greek, healing the sick; in modern English therapy means 'the treatment of disease'

Hypnotherapy is a curative or psychological technique to relax, re-educate, or assist self-analysis by hypnosis.

hypn-odontics

hypnos sleep + *odontikos* Greek, pertaining to teeth
Hypnodontics is using hypnosis in dentistry.

hypo

hypo Greek, under, below, abnormally low; akin to Latin *sub*

hypo-dermic

hypo under + *derma, dermatos* Greek, the skin
Hypodermic is, first, an adjective that means 'applied under the skin'. Often in common clinical parlance, the syringe or the injection itself is called a 'hypo'. A hypodermic implantation is the placing of a solidified drug under the skin of the chest or abdomen to produce a local effect or to slow the rate of the drug's absorption. If you translated 'under the skin' into Latin, you would have the adjective *subcutaneus* (*sub* under + *cutaneus* New Latin, pertaining to the *cutis*, skin). A hypodermic injection is usually a subcutaneous one.

hypo-tension

hypo abnormally low + *tensio, tensionis* Latin, the action of being stretched out, as vessels are by blood
Hypotension is abnormally low blood pressure, too low to get sufficient oxygen to all the tissues of the body. Decreased thrust of the beating heart and dilated blood vessels are often immediate causes.

hypo-therm-ia

hypo abnormally low + *thermos* Greek, heat + *ia* medical condition
Hypothermia is an abnormally low and potentially injurious body temperature below 95°F (35°C), often induced by long exposure to cold.

hypo-glyc-emia

hypo low + *glykys* Greek, sweet + *em* short for *haima* blood + *ia* medical condition

Hypoglycemia is abnormally low blood sugar. If the glucose level in the blood falls too low, hypoglycemic coma may follow. Immediate intake of sugary juices or candy bars by conscious patients can alleviate the symptoms of fatigue, general malaise and weakness.

hysteri-, hystero-

hystera Greek, uterus

hyster-ec-tomy

hystera uterus + *ek* out of + *tome* a surgical cutting
A hysterectomy is a surgical cutting out of the uterus, usually because of malignant uterine tumors or many benign tumors.

hyster-ia

hystera uterus + *ia* medical condition
Ancient Greeks had the sexist notion that nervous afflictions were peculiar to women. They imagined that the uterus was a separate spirit and an animal part of a woman that only wanted to become pregnant. If it did not, this imaginary uterus-spirit wandered through the body causing trouble. When it arrived at the brain, it caused hysterics. For such reasons, and because its diagnosis had much to do with misogynist feelings on the part of male psychiatrists, nowadays hysteria is not generally accepted as a legitimate term for a mental disorder. But it is still widespread in ordinary speech, and seen in historical medical literature.

I

-iasis

-iasis Greek noun suffix indicating a pathologic condition, similiar to *-osis*

-Iasis was a common Greek noun suffix that indicated process or action in time. Hypochondria was the disease; hypochondriasis is the pathological condition with all its signs and symptoms. Elephantiasis is enormous enlargement of a limb with hard, rough, fissured skin like an elephant's. Satyriasis is pathologically excessive and constant sexual desire in a male, supposedly like the randy hanky-panky committed by those imaginary creatures of Greek mythology, the goat-like satyrs. In the formation of such medical words, the suffix *-iasis* was influenced by its similarity to an actual Greek word *iasis* which means 'cure, medical procedure'. It is related to Greek *iatros* 'doctor' (see next entry).

candid-iasis

candidus white + *iasis* < *osis* diseased condition

Candidiasis is infection by candida fungi. A former name is moniliasis, itself from the former name of the fungi genus *Candida*.

-iatric, iatro-, -iatry

iatros Greek, physician, doctor; *iatrikos* pertaining to a doctor; *iatreia* doctoring, healing, curing

The root appears in several medical words: pediatrics (*paidos*, of the child), podiatric (*pos, podos* foot), and psychiatric (*psyche* soul, mind). Geriatrics (*geron* old person) is the branch of medicine that treats the problems and diseases of old age.

iatro-genic

iatros physician + *gen* Greek, produced by

Iatrogenic conditions are produced by the patient's contact with medical diagnostic procedures, or by exposure to diseases while being treated in hospitals and clinics, or infections passed by health services personnel during their contacts with the patient. Adverse reactions to certain drugs may be labeled iatrogenic. Certain mental states may be iatrogenic also. Proper procedures and care by the health professionals involved prevent many of these adverse effects.

psych-iatry

psyche Greek, soul, mind + *iatreia* doctoring

Psychiatry studies and treats mental disorders, while psychology studies the mind and mental processes (*logos* study).

icter-

ikteros Greek, a yellow bird, an Hellenic species of oriole or golden thrush whose yellow feathers resembled the yellow skin discoloration of jaundice

Icterus is jaundice (*jaunisse* French, yellowness, jaundice), yellow discoloration of the skin, of the sclerae (whites) of the eyes, of mucous membranes, and of body fluids caused by excess deposits of bilirubin, a bile pigment. Jaundice is a symptom of many liver diseases and several other disorders, most commonly of a bile duct blocked by a gallstone. Icterus neonatorum (of neonates or newborns) is also called physiological jaundice of the newborn, a mild, self-limiting (usually clears up in three days) breakdown of excess hemoglobin in red blood cells. Icterohepatitis is inflammation of the liver with jaundice. Icteroanemia is anemia with jaundice, enlarged spleen, and destruction of red blood cells.

idio-

idios Greek, of an individial, peculiar to one person; compare *idiotes,* a private person

Idiot and idiocy obviously contain this root. They derive from *idiotes* which was the word for a private person, as opposed to a person of rank and influence holding public office in ancient Greece. Hence, it was supposed, an *idiotes* was ignorant and stupid. The ancient Greeks were rather free in their putdowns of common people. Consider hoi polloi (*hoi polloi* Greek, the many), a phrase referring to the general mob of humanity, and still used in English today.

idio-pathic

idios of an individial + *pathos* Greek, disease

Idiopathic in medicine means 'pertaining to a disease of unknown cause'. Thus, an idiopathic cardiomyopathy is any heart-muscle disease of unknown cause (*cardio-* heart + *myos* of a muscle + *pathos* Greek, disease). Idiopathic pulmonary fibrosis is a serious lung disease, with no known etiology (cause).

idio-syn-crasy

idios of an individial + *syn* together + *krasis* Greek, mixture

An idiosyncrasy in common speech is a pecularity of an individual. In medicine, it is used to label an unusual response to a drug. An idiosyncratic effect of taking a drug might be the patient's toxic response to a dosage normally considered safe.

ileum

ileum 17th Century medical Latin, from *eileos* Greek, twisted, because first used to describe a pathological bowel condition like colic

In modern anatomy, the ileum is the lower part of the small intestine.

ileo-stomy

ileum + *stoma* Greek, mouth + *y* noun ending

Ileostomy is making an opening in the ileum, with the mouth or stoma on the abdominal wall. An ileostomy is done when the entire large intestine is removed in a colectomy, due to a severe ulcerative colitis. An ileostomy bag must be attached to the stoma to collect feces.

ileus

eileos Greek, twisted

An ileus is any temporary bowel obstruction, often due to the bowel's post-operative paralysis, usually lasting 3 to 4 days. Other causes are bowel spasm and other irregular muscle contractions in the intestines, and pregnancy.

ilium, combining forms ilio-, ilia-

ilium Medieval Latin, hipbone < Classical Latin *ilia* flanks, soft parts < *ilis*, soft

The ilium is the largest part of each hipbone. It forms a bony wall between the abdomen and the buttock and thigh muscles. Each ilium supports the sides of the abdomen. The other two parts of the hipbone are the ischium and pubis. All three parts help to form the large socket joint called the acetabulum where the upper leg bone or femur articulates with the hipbone.

iliacus, iliac muscle

iliacus Medieval Latin, pertaining to the ilium
The iliac muscle covers the concave inner surface of the ilium, providing the muscular floor of the abdomen.

immune

in > im not + *munis* Latin, serving, defending
Immunis began in Latin as a military adjective that meant 'not drafted, not called up to service in the Roman army, exempt from military service'. Then *immunis* came to mean 'safe' because one was not going to be killed in wartime service. The medical meaning followed, in which immune means safe from or resistant to disease and infection because of the body's production of antibodies.

The immune system is the organs, tissues, and processes by which the body identifies a foreign or abnormal protein and attacks it chemically to prevent harm to the body. Immunity is the state of being so protected.

immuno-globul-ins

immuno + *globulus* Latin, little ball + *in* noun ending for organic chemical compounds
One of five classes of proteins that act as antibodies. Immunoglobulins are present in all body secretions, internal and external.

impetigo

impetigo Latin, infestation < *impetus* attack
Impetigo is a contagious bacterial infection of the skin, common in children. The symptoms are redness of the skin, then pus-filled blisters that crust. The treatment is antibiotics and careful washing.

im-potence

in > im not + *potentia* Late Latin, power
Impotence is inability of the adult male to achieve a useful erection. Causes may be psychological, diseases like diabetes mellitus, or the effect of certain drugs.

in-

The prefix has two distinct meanings in English medical words: *in* Latin preposition and prefix, into, inside, towards, on; and *in* Latin negative prefix, not, akin to English *un* in 'undo, untie'

in situ

Latin 'in its *situs*', original position, normal site

In situ means in its normal place, or confined to the site of origin. For example, a carcinoma may be *in situ*. It has not yet spread (metastasized), and is at its original site. In cervix or bladder cancer, *in situ* means confined to the epithelium. A Pap test may detect such a cervical cancer. A site in medicine is a position or a locus, a location. To situate in everyday English is a verb, but in medical description situate is also an adjective meaning 'located' or 'beside'.

in utero

Latin, inside the uterus

The Latin phrase is seen in expressions like fetus *in utero*, and an *in utero* anomaly, to describe an intrauterine irregularity.

in vitro

in Latin, in, on + *vitrum* Medieval Latin, glass; literally, in or on glass; modern meaning 'in a glass laboratory container or apparatus' like a test tube, a flask, or a glass slide

An *in vitro* test is performed in a pathology laboratory on a small tissue or cell sample. *In vitro* fertilization (IVF) is done outside the body, often in a glass Petri dish, where extracted ova are placed with spermatozoa. The fertilized ova are then injected into the uterus through the cervix.

in vivo

in Latin, in + *vivus* Late Latin, a living person, the living body

An *in vivo* test is performed in a living body. For example, in nuclear medicine, an *in vivo* tracer study is a diagnostic procedure in which a radioactive tracer is introduced into a patient's body, and radiograms are taken to show internal structures and processes.

in-competence

in Latin, not + *competentia* Late Latin, capability, adequacy

In medicine, an organ or structure may be incompetent if it does not function adequately. Aortic incompetence is one example. An incompetent cervix dilates before labor begins, resulting in possible miscarriage or premature delivery. The legal word *incompetency* refers to a patient unable to look after himself or herself and hence one in need of legal protection.

in-continence

in Latin, not + *continentia* Late Latin, retention, containment

Incontinence is not being able to control urination, defecation and discharge of semen. The loss of sphincter and neural control may be due to lax muscles or cerebral or spinal lesions. Also, galactorrhea (see entry) is sometimes spoken of as incontinence of milk. Reflex incontinence is the involuntary loss of urine whenever a specific bladder volume is attained. Urinary stress incontinence is the loss of small amounts of urine during laughing, coughing, sneezing, lifting, or other sudden movements that produce normal abdominal muscle contractions.

incus

incus, incudis Latin, anvil

The incus or anvil is one of the three tiny bones or ossicles (*ossiculum* Latin, tiny bone) of the middle ear. Incudal is the adjective. Surgical excision of all or part of the anvil is incudectomy.

The other two auditory ossicles of the middle ear are the malleus (Latin, hammer) and the stapes (Latin, stirrup of a saddle), and so there are adjectives like incudomalleal 'pertaining to the incus and the malleus' and how they articulate in the middle ear, and incudostapedial 'pertaining to the incus and the stapes' and their articulation.

in-duration

in Latin, intensive prefix whose sense is 'thorough' + *duratio, durationis* Late Latin, a hardening

Induration is a hardening of tissue, usually said of the skin, due to inflammation, edema, or other disorders. Indurated lung tissue has informal medical labels like black induration for 'black lung' disease of miners, gray induration for fibrotic pneumonia, etc. Indurative myocarditis is inflammation that hardens the muscles of the heart walls.

in-farct

in Latin, intensive prefix, thoroughly + *farcire* Latin, to stuff
An infarct is an area of tissue that dies because its blood supply stops.

myo-cardial infarction

mys, myos muscle + *kardia* heart > *myocardialis* scientific Latin, of the heart muscle; *infarctio, infarctionis* Latin, stuffing a sausage until it is full
A myocardial infarction is a heart attack due to the closing off of a coronary artery that causes an infarct of the heart muscle. In an infarct, part of the heart muscle dies from lack of oxygen because blood supply via the coronary artery has been interrupted. Infarction is a 17th-Century coinage belonging to the discredited theory of humors, and so the word is not truly appropriate to modern cardiology – but some old words die slowly. Originally, infarction referred to a 'thorough stuffing together' of bodily humors. Myocardium is heart muscle, cardiac muscle that surrounds the heart in a thick layer.

infection

infectio, infectionis Late Latin, a tainting
Infection is invasion into a body by disease-producing micro-organisms like bacteria. An infectious disease is caused by a pathogenic agent, like a virus or bacterium. Thus an infectious disease may or may not be contagious. An opportunistic infection is one caused by a micro-organism that does not normally produce disease in humans. Opportunistic infections occur in patients whose resistance has been lowered by faults in their immune systems, for example, persons with full-blown acquired immune deficiency syndrome. Advanced AIDS sufferers are subject to otherwise rare cancers like Kaposi's sarcoma, to parasitic pneumonias, and rare opportunistic viral infections.

inferior

inferior Latin, lower, in a lower place
Inferior pertains to the lower portion of a body part, situated below, or the lower of two similar structures, e.g. the inferior vena cava. For example, inferior conchae are thin bones forming the lower part of the side wall of the nasal cavity. They are shaped like conchs, scrolled sea-shells. They are termed inferior because there are other conchae, and these shell-shaped bones of the nose are located above or superior to the lower conchae. Superior (Latin, higher) is the opposite of inferior. The eyes are superior to the mouth, but inferior to the scalp. The two venae cavae are the large veins that bring deoxygenated venous

blood back to the heart. The superior vena cava, above the heart, more toward the top of the body, returns blood from the upper part of the body. The inferior vena cava, below the heart, returns blood from the lower part of the body.

influenza

Italian, influence

The short form of the word *influenza* is flu. Influenza is an acute viral infection of the respiratory tract, highly contagious. The flu normally runs its course in a week. Very young and very old patients and those weakened by poor health are at risk of complications like bacterial pneumonia. Influenza-virus vaccine is an often effective immunizing agent.

The Italian word, in print as early as AD 1375, refers to the mistaken medieval notion that the infection was 'influenced' by unfavorable stars and planets. This horoscopic poppycock lingered for almost 500 years until modern theories of disease and the identification of viruses. During that half-millennium, nations blamed one another for the malady. In Russia, the flu was called 'the Chinese disease', in Germany 'the Russian pest', and in Italy the flu was 'the German disease'. In a similar manner, the English called syphilis 'the French disease' and the French termed it *'la maladie anglaise'*.

infra

infra Latin, below, under

Infrared light rays are invisible waves that lie beyond the red end of the spectrum. When infrared radiation strikes the human body, it is perceived as heat. Ordinary English refers to something very vulgar as *infra dig*, a contracted form of the Latin phrase *infra dignitatem* 'beneath one's dignity' (to acknowledge).

infra-orbital

infra Latin, below + *orbis, orbitis* Latin, anything globular, eye socket + *al* common adjectival suffix

Infraorbital pertains to the area under the eye socket. The infraorbital foramen is an opening on the anterior of the upper jawbone through which pass some nerves and blood vessels that supply the skin of the cheek and the upper teeth except for the molars.

insulin

insula Latin, island, islet: small island; named from the fact that insulin is secreted in the islets of Langerhans in the pancreas + *in* noun ending for organic chemical compound

In 1921, four scientists at the University of Toronto (Banting, Best, MacLeod and Collip) first isolated this pancreatic hormone. That year when they published their research in the American Journal of Physiology (Proceedings of the American Physiology Society, December 1921) they wrote 'we suggest the name insulin'. Nine years earlier, Sir Edward Schafer, a noted British physiologist, had suggested in print the existence of the chemical and he had named it insulin, from its secretion in the islets of Langerhans in the pancreas. Even Schafer may have seen a journal article by the French biologist De Meyer who suggested the name *insuline* in a 1909 publication. Did all these separate instances of the word insulin spring up independently, by the merest scientific serendipity, as the result of simultaneous discovery? The progression of publication dates suggests they did not.

Insulin is a hormone that helps regulate how the body metabolizes carbohydrates, fats and amino acids; specifically it manages the carrying of the simple body sugar, glucose, to individual cells. Insulin is secreted by glands spread throughout the tissues of the pancreas, and emptied into the bloodstream. These glands are called the islets of Langerhans. When insulin is low or absent, high blood sugar and diabetes result. Insulin injections are often used to treat diabetes. Too much insulin results in dangerously low blood sugar levels and insulin shock.

inter

inter Latin, between, among

inter-costal

inter between + *costa* Latin, rib

Intercostal is between the ribs, hence the intercostal muscles that help expand the rib cage when one breathes in and out. Nerve pain in this same area is intercostal neuralgia (see entry).

inter-mittent

inter in between + *mittens, mittentis* Latin present participle, sending

Intermittent pertains to actions or processes that stop and start at intervals. Intermittent fevers like malaria occur in cycles of acute symptoms followed by periods of remission. Rheumatoid arthritis symptoms are often intermittent, a time of symptomatic distress followed by a period of remission of symptoms. Intermittent assisted ventilation (IAV) is a respiratory therapy that involves the patient breathing on his own and then being assisted by a mechanical respirator.

inter-val

intervallum Latin, the space between the ramparts of a fort. The Latin *vallum* is akin to English *wall*.
An interval is a space between two parts, or time between two events. Interval health history notes the patient's general condition between clinical visits.

inter-stice, interstitium

inter between + *stitium* Latin, a standing, a placement < *sistere* to put, to place
An interstice is a space or gap in a structure or tissue.

interstitial fluid

Interstitial fluid is the watery substance that fills the spaces between all the cells in the body. It is the liquid that filters through blood capillaries and is drained off as lymph.

interstitial lung disorders

Interstitial lung disorders are a group of almost 200 pulmonary disorders in which the chief symptom is limited ability of the lungs to transfer oxygen from the alveoli to the lung capillaries. Inflammation and fibrosis of the walls of the alveoli are produced by many causative agents, such as inhaled toxins.

intestine

intestinus Latin, internal > *intestini* guts, internal organs
The intestines are all the structures of the digestive tract from the pylorus of the stomach to the anus.

intestinal flora

flora Latin, literally, flowers
Intestinal flora are the natural, healthy and essential bacteria that grow inside the digestive tract. In biology, flora are forms of plant life, as opposed to fauna, or animal life. At one time, bacteria were considered part of the plant kingdom.

intra

intra Latin, inside of, within

intra-muscular

Intramuscular is within the substance of the muscle. Medication may be given intramuscularly (i.m.). Note the difference between intramuscular and intermuscular, the latter meaning 'between muscles'.

intra-uterine

intra within + *uterinus* of the uterus

Intrauterine is within the uterus. The IUD (intrauterine device) is a form of birth control, in which a plastic device, inserted into the uterus, prevents implantation of the fertilized egg. The many undesired side-effects of the device have caused its use to decline in the United States.

intra-venous (IV)

intra inside + *vena* Latin, vein

Fluids like glucose and saline are often given within the vein. Intravenous medication is injected or infused into a vein. Intravenous feeding may be delivered also, usually through a major vein like the subclavian or jugular. An intravenous infusion pump helps maintain an adjustable rate of flow of solutions.

ischium

iskion Greek, rump bone < *iskys* strength, hence strong bone; borrowed into Latin as *ischium*

The ischium is the rump bone, the bone one sits on. The lower part of the pelvic girdle is composed of the two ischia. An ischium is thick and three-sided and is fused together with the ilium and the pubis at the big hip socket or acetabulum.

ischio-coccygeal

ischio combining form of ischium + *kokkyx, kokkygis* Greek, the cuckoo bird

Ischiococcygeal pertains to the ischium and the coccyx or tail bone. The little triangle of fused, rudimentary tail vertebrae which ends the human spinal column is named after a supposed resemblance of the bone to the bill of a cuckoo.

iso-

isos Greek, equal

This prefix is widespread in English scientific vocabulary: isocaloric 'with equal calories'; isodiametric 'with equal diameters'; isodontic 'with teeth of equal size'; and isotherms 'lines on a chart that connect areas having the same temperature'.

iso-metric

isos equal + *metrikos* Greek, pertaining to measurement or dimension

The isometric contraction phase of the human heartbeat is the first part of the contraction of the ventricle, when blood pressure in the ventricle increases but volume of blood does not because the semilunar valves are still closed.

iso-tonic

isos equal + *tonos* Greek, the quality of being stretched, like a musical note (tone) or a muscle < *teinein*, to stretch

Isotonic contraction has the muscle shortening against a pulling resistance, but the muscle tone stays the same.

-itis

-itis Greek suffix now denoting inflammation and infection

In Classical Greek, *-itis* began as the feminine singular of adjectives ending in *-ites*. When used in ancient Greek medical vocabulary, the feminine noun *nosos* 'disease' was understood. Thus arthritis in ancient Greek was *he arthritis nosos* 'the disease of the joints'. From this use developed the common noun suffix, later added to the end of disease names to indicate inflammation or disorder. There are thousands of words in medicine ending with *-itis*, such as appendicitis, inflammation of the appendix, and cystitis, inflammation of the urinary bladder. There is a plural form of *-itis* words that should be recognized. The plural of cystitis is cystitides. Likewise, arthritides, appendicitides and hepatitides. The more conventional, English-style plural ending is seen frequently, for example, hepatitises, cystitises.

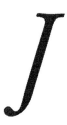

jaundice

See *icterus* entry

jejunum

ieiunus Latin, empty

The jejunum is the middle portion of the small intestine. The first part is the duodenum, the third is the ileum. The jejunum has thick walls with many circular folds for absorption. The name was applied because ancient Greek and Roman physicians noted that it was usually empty after death.

jejunal feeding tube

A jejunal feeding tube is created surgically by a jejunostomy, making a mouth-like opening to the jejunum through the abdominal wall, to introduce liquified foods via the tube.

jejuno-ileitis

jejuno of the jejunum + *ileo* of the ileum + *itis* inflammation of

Jejunoileitis is the better medical term for Crohn's disease, an inflammation of the jejunum and ileum, a chronic, idiopathic bowel disorder with frequent diarrhea, severe local pain, fever, chills, nausea, anorexia and subsequent weight loss.

jugular veins

iugulum Latin, neck, literally, part that joins (Latin root *iug;* compare English *yoke*) the head to the body

The external jugular vein receives deoxygenated blood from the outside of the skull and the deep areas of the face. It passes down the neck to join the subclavian vein. The internal jugular vein takes blood from the brain and the surface of the face and neck. It passes down the neck beside the internal carotid artery and also joins the subclavian. The jugular pulse is useful diagnostically, indicating the actions of the right side of the heart. Jugular venous pressure (JVP) also reflects the activity of the heart's right side.

kel-oid

kele Greek, tumor + *eides* Greek, form, hence *-oid* means 'formed like'

A keloid is an abnormally large scar formation in the skin following injury or surgery. Excess amounts of collagen are deposited, and therefore drugs that interfere with collagen synthesis may prove effective. Corticosteroids help some patients.

kerato-

keras, keratos Greek, horn, cornea of the eye, horny body tissue

kerat-in

keras, keratos horn + *in* noun ending for organic chemical compounds

Keratin is a tough, horny protein found in fingernails, toenails and in the horny layer of the skin.

kerato-malacia

keras, keratos cornea + *malakos* Greek, soft, degenerated + *ia* medical condition

Keratomalacia is a softening and necrosis of corneal tissue due to vitamin A deficiency.

kerato-scopy

keras, keratos cornea + *skopeia* Greek, a viewing

Keratoscopy is inspection of the cornea with any of several ophthalmoscopic devices (*ophthalmos* Greek, eye).

kerat-osis

keras, keratos horn + *osis* diseased condition

Keratosis is any horny skin growth, like a wart or a callus, or the condition of having such growths.

kyph-osis

kyphos Greek, bent forward, stooping + *osis* diseased condition

Kyphosis is hunchback, humpback, or Pott's curvature, in which the upper curve of the spine increases, so the back has a hump.

L

labia, labio-

labium Latin, a lip or liplike structure, plural labia

labia majora

labia lips + *maiora* Latin, larger, greater
The labia majora are two long folds of skin, one on each side of the vaginal opening, that make up the outer, larger lips of the external female genitalia.

labia minora

labia lips + *minora* smaller, lesser
The labia minora are the smaller skin folds at the vaginal opening, inside the labia majora, extending back from the clitoris.

labial

labialis New Latin, of the lips
Labial refers to the lips of the mouth or the vagina. Labial is said of a sound made by the lips, and is also a noun used in speech pathology and linguistics. Labiodental pertains to a speech sound made by the lips and the teeth.

lacrima

lacrima Latin, tear

lacrimal apparatus

lacrimalis Latin, pertaining to structures that secrete, hold, or transport tears; *ad* > *ap* to + *paratus* Latin, ready > *apparatus* Latin, literally 'something prepared for a special purpose' like a medical instrument. Compare the motto of the Boy Scouts: *Semper Paratus,* 'always prepared'.

The lacrimal structures are those that secrete and drain tears from the eyes, e.g. the lacrimal gland, an oval exocrine gland on the upper, outer side of each eye which secretes tears to moisten the conjunctiva. The lacrimal duct or lacrimal canaliculus (Latin, little canal) is a drainage tube that empties tears into the nasal cavity. The lacrimal sac is an enlargement of a lacrimal duct where tears are stored before they drain into the nasal cavity.

punctum lacrimale

punctum Latin, literally, a hole pricked out of some material, a point; compare 'puncture'

The punctum lacrimale is the tiny opening at the inner corner of each eye through which tears enter the lacrimal sac.

lac

lac, lactis Latin, milk; akin to *galas, galaktos* Greek, milk; from the Latin root is French *lait,* Spanish *leche,* and the original form of the word lettuce, *lactuca,* because of its milky juice

ab-lact-ation

ab away from + *lac, lactis* milk + *ation* noun ending > *lactatio, lactationis* Latin 'secreting milk'

Ablactation is weaning, getting an infant used to taking solid food instead of breastfeeding. Ablactation also means cessation of maternal milk secretion.

lact-ase

lac, lactis milk + *-ase* common ending for name of an enzyme

Lactase is an enzyme found in the small intestine that converts lactose into simpler sugars used by the body.

lact-ose

lac, lactis Latin, milk + *-ose* chemical suffix for names of sugars like glucose and sucrose

Lactose is the sugar found in milk.

lacti-ferous ducts

lac, lactis milk + *ferre* Latin, to carry + *ous* adjectival suffix; *ductus* Latin, canal, channel, any hollow tube which conveys liquids < *ducere* to carry, to lead

The lactiferous ducts carry milk from the lobes of the breast to the nipple.

pro-lact-in

pro Latin preposition, in front of, in favor of, promoting + *lac, lactis* milk + *in* noun ending for organic chemical compounds

Prolactin is a pituitary hormone that acts with other hormones to begin development and growth of the mammary glands. After childbirth, prolactin helps begin milk production.

laparo-

lapara Greek, loins, but literally 'the soft parts'

This is a common ploy of languages in naming especially the female genitalia. Compare *die Weiche* in German, literally 'the soft parts', the loins, the flank, the pudendum.

laparo-scop-y

lapara loins + *skopein* to examine + *y* noun ending

Laparoscopy is a surgical procedure to view internal organs. A local or general anesthetic is given, then a small abdominal incision is made, often below the navel so that no scar is seen later. Carbon dioxide gas is pumped into the abdomen to inflate it and allow better viewing. Passed in through the tiny incision is a laparoscope, a metal tube with lens and light at one end, and a telescope at the other. Laparoscopy helps discover reasons for problems like vaginal bleeding or abdominal pain, and is used during tubal ligation as well.

-lapse

lapsus Latin, a slipping, a falling. The root appears in several common English words: e.g. collapse, 'to fall together' and elapse, 'to slip out, to slip past', like elapsed time

The Greek translation of *lapsus, ptosis* (see entry) is widely used in medical words and lies slightly disguised in the word symptom (*syn* together + *ptoma* a falling, a slipping, something that befalls a person).

lapsus linguae

lapsus Latin, a slip; *linguae* of the tongue

A lapsus linguae is a slip of the tongue. In Freudian psychoanalysis for example, it is saying 'bother' when you mean to say 'father'. The phrase also refers to everyday, more innocent mistakes in the articulation of speech sounds. And compare a literary term, *lapsus calami*, a mistake made while writing, literally 'a slip of the pen'.

pro-lapse

pro in front of + *lapsus* a slipping

Prolapse is a slipping forward or falling of an organ from its normal position, e.g. prolapse of the uterus or prolapse of the rectum, due to muscular laxness in herniation, and other causes.

re-lapse

re Latin prefix, again, back, repeated + *lapsus* a slipping

Relapse is a slipping back into a previous condition, i.e. the return of a disease after its apparent end.

larynx, laryngo-

larynx, laryggis Greek, the upper part of the windpipe

The larynx is an organ that contains the vocal cords (better, vocal folds). It is part of the air passageway that connects the pharynx with the trachea (see entries). The bump in the front of the throat called the Adam's apple is made by the thyroid cartilage which serves to protect the larynx.

laryng-ec-tom-y

larynx, laryggis + *ek* out + *tome* a surgical cutting + *y* noun ending

After surgical removal of all or part of the larynx, often due to cancer, the patient must acquire the ability to produce esophageal speech by modifying the way air is expelled from the esophagus. The mouth, tongue and pharynx must be trained anew as well.

laryng-ismus

larynx, laryggis + *-ismus* Latin form of a Greek noun suffix (*ismos*) used in medicine often to denote sudden occurrence of violent muscular contractions, as in words like paroxysm and bruxism (grinding the teeth)

Laryngismus is sudden contraction of the laryngeal muscles, marked by raspy intake of breath, often due to croup, laryngitic irritation, or a foreign body caught in the throat. Complete spastic closure of the airway of the larynx is laryngospasm, seen in severe allergic reactions and in young children with severe laryngitis.

laser

The word laser is an acronym formed from the initial letters of the phrase 'light amplification by stimulated emission of radiation'. A laser is a device that emits coherent light waves of great intensity. Their power makes lasers useful in modern surgery for division of tissue, destruction of tissue and for making adhesions and fixing tissue in place. Laser bronchoscopy uses a carbon dioxide laser beam conducted to bronchial sites by fiberoptic cable, to diagnose and treat bronchial disorders.

lateral

lateralis Latin, of a side, on the side < *latus* side

Lateral as an anatomical position means on the side, toward the side, or more away from the center of a body.

bi-lateral

bis Latin, twice, two + *lateralis* of a side

Bilateral is two-sided, or affecting both sides. Bilateral strabismus is squinting in both eyes due to faulty eye accommodation.

lateral-ity

lateralis of a side + *ity* noun suffix derived from Latin noun suffix *-itas*

Laterality is literally sidedness. Left-handedness is a laterality, a tendency to favor in use the organs on one side of the body.

col-lateral

cum > cul > col Latin, with + *lateralis* of a side

The literal sense of collateral is 'sharing a side with'. Its developed meanings include 'secondary, accessory, parallel, lying beside'. In anatomy, a collateral vessel is the branch of an artery or vein used as an accessory by the main vessel. Collateral ligaments in fingers and at the elbows, knees and ankles support and stabilize joints at their sides.

lesion

laesio, laesionis Latin, damage, injury

Lesion is a general word in medicine for any abnormal change in the structure or function of tissue because of injury or disease; a lesion is always a visible change, with a well defined limit, like a wound, a blister, a rash, an abscess, or a tumor. An example of a pre-cancerous lesion is cervical dysplasia, an abnormality in cells of the cervix. A primary lesion is the original invading site of a disease. For example, the primary lesion of syphilis might be a genital chancre, a small hard lump on the genital skin that may form an ulcer.

leuco-, leuko-

leukos Greek, white

leuk-emia

leukos white + *em* short for *haima* blood + *ia* medical condition

Leukemia is blood cancer – a progressive, malignant neoplasm of leukocyte-forming elements in the blood and bone marrow.

leuko-cyte

leukos white + *kytos* cell

A leukocyte is a white blood cell, or in its older, obsolescent name, a white corpuscle (*corpusculum* Latin, little body). The many kinds of leukocytes fight disease by ploys such as engulfing germs, dead cells and other hematic debris. Leukocytosis is an abnormal increase in the number of white cells in the blood, often seen in bacterial, but not viral, infections.

leuko-rrhea

leukos white + *rrhoia* Greek, a flowing through, a discharge
Leukorrhea is any white, thickish vaginal discharge, often indicating vaginal or
uterine infections and other disorders.

levator

levator Latin, lifter; in medicine, a muscle that lifts or elevates a
structure; compare elevator, literally 'outlifter'

levator anguli oris

Anatomical Latin, literally, lifter of the corner of the mouth
This is the anatomical name of the smile muscle. The levator anguli oris also
helps in eating and making speech sounds.

levator palpebrae superioris

Anatomical Latin, literally, lifter of the upper eyebrow. From
palpebra Latin, eyelid, comes the medical verb, palpebrate, to
wink or to blink.
This levator is a muscle that raises one eyebrow, e.g. when one is surprised.

levator scapulae

Anatomical Latin, literally, lifter of the scapula or shoulder blade
The two levators lift the shoulder blades when one shrugs in the common
gesture to indicate 'I don't know'.

lig-

ligare Latin, to tie up, wrap, bind, constrict, pull tight

ligament

ligamentum Latin, rope, bandage, tie
A ligament is a fibrous band of connective tissue that joins bones where they
articulate with other bones. Ligaments help keep joints together, and they set
the limits of joint movement. They are not tendons, which are bands of fibrous
tissue that attach muscles to bones.

ligation

ligatio, ligationis Latin, a tying off with string or wire

Ligation is the act of binding or tying off a tube, a blood vessel, or a duct. Tubal ligation is a birth control method in which the Fallopian tubes are tied off or ligated by means of a wire or thread called a ligature.

lipi, lipo-

lipos Greek, a fat

lip-ase

lipos fat + *-ase* common chemical ending for the name of an enzyme

Lipase is a stomach enzyme that helps split up fat, that takes part in natural lipolysis (*lysis* Greek, loosening, breakdown), the digestive breakdown of fats.

lipid

lipos fat + *eides* Greek, form, hence *-id* here means 'formed like'

A lipid is any fat chemical of the body, such as fatty acids, waxes, and steroids. Lipids are an important constituent of cells. Lipids provide body fuel. Lipid tests, a part of blood work, determine cholesterol and triglyceride levels in blood.

lipo-cyte

lipos fat + *kytos* cell

A lipocyte is a fat cell located in the hypodermis where it makes and stores fat.

lipo-suction

lipos fat

Liposuction is removal of fat under the skin by suction. The procedure is also called suction-assisted lipectomy.

litho-

lithos Greek, stone; the Latin translation *calculus* 'stone, pebble' is frequently used in medicine

211

litho-tripsy

lithos stone + *thrypsis* Greek, a breaking into small pieces, a crushing + *y* noun ending

Lithotripsy is the crushing of kidney stones, often by extracorporeal shock-wave lithotripsy (*extra-corporealis* New Latin, outside the body). Sound waves conducted through water disintegrate the stones, and the debris is washed out of the system. The shock wave generated is similar to that produced by a 'depth charge'. A popular name for the device is the stone-crushing machine.

livid

lividus Latin, of a black-and-blue color

An interesting cognate is the Old Slavic *sliva*, a word for 'plum' named for the lead-colored bloom or powdery protective coating on the ripe fruit. There is a popular plum brandy called Slivovitz.

lividity

lividitas Latin, a black-blue quality of color

Lividity is the black and blue discoloration of a body after death. Post mortem lividity, or livor mortis, may aid a coroner in determining the time of death. As blood cells die, and hemoglobin gives up oxygen, the blood darkens and collects in lower body parts. The amount and the site of lividity are markers as to the time elapsed since death occurred.

lordosis

lordosis Greek, a bending backwards < *lordos* adjective, bent backwards. This was Hippocrates' term for convex curvature of the spine.

Lordosis is swayback, a spinal condition in which the lower or lumbar curve of the spine increases, so that the belly protrudes.

lumbar

lumbus Latin, loin; the adjective is lumbar, pertaining to the loins. Latin *lumbi* entered Medieval French as *loigne*, which became loin in English. A cut of meat over that area was a *sur-loigne* or sirloin.

lumbago

lumbago Latin, lower-back ache
Lumbago is a general term for rheumatic, arthritic, or muscular pain in the lower back muscles, often caused by decreased blood supply to the affected parts.

lumbar puncture

lumbaris Late Latin, of the loins + *punctura* a piercing
A lumbar puncture is a spinal tap, tapping the subarachnoid space between the 3rd and 4th lumbar vertebrae with a hollow needle, usually to draw off a small quantity of cerebrospinal fluid for analysis.

lumen

lumen, luminis Latin, light, or an opening that light comes through, then the hollow part of any tube
A lumen is the hollow channel or cavity of a tubular organ, through which air or blood may flow. One might refer to the blocked lumen of an artery, or the lumen of a bronchiole.

trans-luminal

trans Latin, across, through + *lumen, luminis* the hollow of a tube
Transluminal means ' through a lumen'. In percutaneous transluminal coronary angioplasty (see *angioplasty* entry), a tiny balloon at the end of a catheter is inserted through the skin (percutaneous) and through the lumen of a blocked heart artery; then the balloon is dilated and helps open up the blocked artery, and makes the lumen patent (*patens, patentis* Latin, wide-open).

luteus

luteus Latin adjective, yellowish

lute-in

luteus Latin adjective, yellowish + *in* noun suffix denoting an organic chemical compound
Lutein is a fat-soluble, yellow pigment found in fat cells and in the corpus luteum (Latin, yellow body), the medical name for a burst ovarian follicle that fills with yellow fat and secretes hormones that prevent menstruation if an egg has been fertilized. Lutein also helps prepare the uterus to receive a fertilized egg.

luteinizing hormone (LH)

LH is secreted in the pituitary gland and travels to the ovaries where it causes the egg-bearing follicle to burst, releasing the egg during ovulation. Also isolated is LHRH (luteinizing hormone-releasing hormone), made in the hypothalamus of the brain but acting on the pituitary gland to induce release of LH.

lymph, lympho-

lympha Latin, clear water; cognate with or derived from Greek *nympha*, any of several minor water goddesses

Lymph is a thin, watery, extracellular fluid that bathes most body tissues. Lymph collects in and is circulated by lymphatic vessels, and is filtered at the lymphatic nodes. Excess lymph is emptied into the blood stream through the thoracic duct located where the subclavian and jugular veins join.

lympho-cyte

lympha + *kytos* cell

A lymphocyte is a modified white blood cell involved in immunity, a cell produced by lymphoid tissue in the lymph nodes. Lymphocyte B cells recognize antigens and produce antibodies against them. Lymphocyte T cells secrete immunological biochemicals and help B cells. Lymphocytes circulate from the blood to the lymph system and then back into the bloodstream.

lympho-granul-oma venereum

lympha + *granulum* Latin, a small grain kernel + *oma* tumor; *venereus* Latin, of Venus, Roman goddess of sexual love; hence the medical adjective, venereal: caused by genital contact or sexual intercourse

Lymphogranuloma venereum is a sexually transmitted disease, or venereal disease, caused by a *Chlamydia* bacterium. Symptoms include ulcers on the genitals, swollen lymph nodes in the groin, fever, headache and general malaise. Ulcers on the walls of the rectum are less common. A herpes-like sore begins the infection a week or two after contact. Later buboes appear. A lymphogranulomatous bubo is an enlarged, tender lymph node in the groin. Although the buboes heal, they may leave scar tissue that blocks smaller lymph vessels. Treatment with tetracyclines may cure the acute clinical signs but cannot, of course, alter old scars.

lymph-oma

lympha + *oma* tumor
Non-Hodgkin's lymphomata or lymphomas are a group of malignant, hard
tumors found in lymphoid tissue, mostly in the lymph nodes.

-lysis

lysis Greek, a loosening, a breaking down, a weakening

ana-lysis

ana up + *lysis* Greek, loosening, breaking up
The basic meaning of analysis is breaking something up to determine its
component parts. The noun is widespread in all branches of science, and the
'something' broken up may be a chemical, a belief, an emotion, etc.

cata-lysis

kata Greek, down + *lysis* a breaking, so that *katalysis* =
dissolving, breakdown
A catalyst is a substance that speeds up a chemical reaction, or is necessary for
that reaction to occur, but is not itself altered in the reaction it assists. Such a
catalytic process is called catalysis.

dia-lysis

dia through + *lysis* Greek, loosening, dissolving, breaking up
Dialysis is filtering waste materials in the blood through a semi-permeable
membrane as a replacement for natural kidney function. Hemodialysis filters
blood using an artificial kidney machine.

para-lysis

para beside; but ancient Greek used the prefix and preposition
to sometimes mean 'abnormal' + *lysis* Greek, loosening or
weakening of the limbs
Paralysis is a loss of motor and/or sensory function in a part.

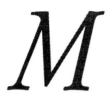

macro-

makros Greek, large, of abnormal size

Many terms denoting congenital enlargement of a body part begin with this prefix, for example macrocephaly (*kephale* Greek, head), a head and brain abnormally large in relation to the rest of the body, resulting in mental and growth retardation. Macroglossia (*glossa* Greek, tongue) is a congenital enlargement of the tongue, often seen in Down's syndrome. The opposite of macro- is micro-, small. Microcephaly is abnormal smallness of the head and brain in relation to the rest of the body.

macro-cyte

makros abnormally large + *kytos* cell

A macrophage is an abnormally big red blood cell, symptomatic in macrocytic anemia due to vitamin B_{12} deficiency. Macrocytosis is the proliferation of such cells in peripheral blood.

macro-drip

makros large

A macrodrip is a device for delivering intravenous solutions where the size of the droplets of the fluid being infused into the patient is controlled by the diameter of the plastic delivery tube. Droplets via macrodrip are bigger than droplets via microdrip (*mikros* Greek, small).

macro-phage

makros large + *phagos* Greek, eater, glutton

A macrophage is any large, mononuclear white blood cell that engulfs and digests foreign micro-organisms and cell debris, as an important part of the immune response to inflammation. Fixed macrophages do not circulate. Free macrophages circulate in the bloodstream. Chemical attractors like MAF (macrophage activating factor), prepare these cells to attack certain antigens. Macrophage migration-inhibiting factor stops the movement of a macrophage after it has come into contact with a specific antigen.

macro-scopic

makros large + *skopikos* Greek, pertaining to viewing or examining

Something macroscopic is large enough to see with the naked eye, or simply very large. Its opposite is microscopic.

macula

macula Latin, spot, blemish; *maculatus* spotted

A macula or macule is a flat, pigmented skin blemish like a freckle, or like a mole that is not above the surface of the epidermis.

macula lutea retinae

macula Latin, spot; *luteus* Latin, yellow; *lutea* is feminine to agree with *macula*. All nouns in Latin have gender and are feminine, masculine, or neuter. The neuter singular form is *luteum; retinae* Latin, of the retina.

The macula lutea is the yellow spot of most acute vision at the center of the retina. It contains the fovea centralis (Latin, center pit) where concentrated cone cells permit what is termed central vision, the most focused and detailed sight.

macular degeneration

Macular degeneration is the most common impairment of vision after the age of 50 years. If it is due to excess blood vessel growth under the retinal layer, laser therapy can destroy these vessels and loss of central vision can be stopped or significantly lessened.

maculate

maculatus Latin, stained, spotted

Maculate or maculated skin is spotted with small discolored patches that are flush with the surface of the skin. Note the Christian belief concerning the immaculate conception. An immaculate conception (*in* > *im* not + *maculatus* stained, spotted) is one not blemished or spotted by earthly sin.

malacia

malakos Greek, soft, weak > *malakia* softness

Malacia is abnormal, degenerative softness of a tissue or an organ. The word is usually suffixed to a root denoting the part so affected. See below. Malacosis is a synonym.

chondro-malacia patellae or runner's knee

chondros cartilage + *malakia* Greek, softening + *patellae* Latin, of the kneecap

Athletes who strain a knee by the constant pounding shocks of running may suffer chondromalacia patellae, in which articular cartilage degenerates.

cranio-malacia

cranium Latin, skull < *kranion* Greek, skull + *malakia* softness

Craniomalacia is softening of the bones of the skull.

osteo-malacia

osteon Greek, bone + *malakia* softness

Osteomalacia is an adult form of rickets, in which bones become so soft that their flexibility and brittleness cause deformities. The two Greek roots are reversed in the rarer, less apt, but synonymous word, malacosteon.

mal-

male Latin adverb and prefix, bad

This is a frequent prefix in English words derived from Latin, like malevolent (*malevolens* Latin, ill-wishing), malefactor, malicious, malignant, maladjusted, malcontent, malodorous, malnutrition, malpractice and maltreat. *Mal* is also seen in English words derived from French: maladroit, malady, malaise, *mal de mer* (seasickness) and malinger. The root has ultimate position in dismal, from *dis mal*, Old French, from *dies mali* Latin, days of evil.

mal-absorption syndrome

male bad + *ab* away from + *sorbere* to suck up > *absorptio, absorptionis* a sucking away from; *syn* together + *dromos* a running > syndrome, a running together of symptoms that indicate a particular disease

To absorb is to uptake substances into or across tissues. A familiar medical example is intestinal absorption, in which food fluids, solutes, proteins, fats and other nutrients are taken from the lumen of the small intestine up into the epithelial cells lining the intestine and thence into the blood and lymph systems. Malabsorption syndrome is a group of symptoms produced by the impairment of the way nutrients are taken into the digestive tract and absorbed. Symptoms include loss of appetite, weight loss, abdominal bloating, cramps, irritable bowel, undigested fat in stools and then anemia and fatigue. It is caused by infections and disorders of the intestinal mucosa, and may be seen postoperatively after surgeries like stomach resection or ileal bypass.

malaise

malaise French, discomfort

Malaise is a word for general feelings of bodily discomfort and weakness that accompany the onset of an illness.

mal-aria

mala aria Italian, bad air

Francisco Torti, an Italian physician, coined the term in 1718 to name a fever he believed was contracted from the noxious fumes of the Pontine marshes near Rome, which even the ancient Romans tried to drain. In 1717, another Italian physician had suggested that the transmitting agent might be a mosquito.

Malaria is a serious infectious disease, often recurrent, whose symptoms include chills, fever, and sweats, in that order as primary symptoms; then follow headache, anemia, muscle ache, and an enlarged spleen. It is caused by a protozoon parasitic in the blood of the Anopheles mosquito. Certain asexual reproductive stages of the protozoon occur in human red blood cells. Prevention includes draining swamps where the mosquito breeds, avoiding bites by use of insecticides and mosquito netting, and taking antimalarial drugs like chlorquine, quinine, and pyrimethamine, if travel to malarial areas is planned.

malignant

malignans, malignantis Late Latin, growing worse

Malignant is said of cancerous growth that may be fatal and highly virulent. Thus a malignancy is the cancerous tumor itself, or, sometimes, a synonym for any carcinoma (see entry). The opposite is benign (*benignus* Latin, mild, with the root *bene*, well, good), said of a tumor that is not cancerous.

malleus

malleus Latin, hammer

English words from this Latin word include mallet, malleable (able to be hammered thin), and even shopping mall: from the Pall Mall in London, originally the site of an imported ball game like croquet called palemail, from Italian *pallamaglio* (*palla* ball + *maglia* mallet < *malleus* hammer).

In medicine, the malleus is a hammer-like little bone of the middle ear, one of the three ossicles (little bones) that act like an amplifier to transmit vibrations of the eardrum to the inner ear.

malle-olus

malleus hammer + -*oleus* diminutive noun suffix,
little > *malleolus* little hammer

A malleolus is a bony knob on each side of the ankle. The lower knob of the fibula is the lateral or external malleolus and the lower knob of the tibia is the medial or internal malleolus.

mamma

mamma Latin, breast

Mamma is a reduplication of the much older Proto-Indo-European root *ma*, breast or mother. This is not only the first sound uttered by many human infants, it may also be the most widespread word root in the world. It forms the word for mother in most of the Indo-European languages : Latin *mater,* Greek *meter,* French *mère*, German *Mutter*, Russian *mate*, Icelandic *modher*, Sanskrit *mata*, Irish *mathair*, Welsh *mam*. The Arabic is *oum*; the Hebrew *em*. In Swahili, it's *mama*. The Chinese word for mother is *ma*. The Hawaian word for mother is *makuahine* (*maka* first, beloved < *ma-k* Proto-Polynesian, the mother (?) + *wahine* female, woman). It appears in many, many language families of the world seemingly unrelated to Indo-European. Why? The sounds of *m* and *a* are among the easiest to make and among the first sounds acquired by a human infant. The first noise in life associated with deep pleasure may be the sound made by the infant's mouth sucking milk from the mother's breast. This sound is frequently some variant of *ma-ma*. The movement of the lips made in uttering an *m*-sound is similar to the movement required to suck a nipple.

mammary gland

The distinguishing feature responsible for the name *Mammalia*, the zoological class of animals to which humans belong, is the possession of breasts that secrete milk to feed the young. The mammary glands are found in the breasts. The glands are made up of fatty tissue in which lobular alveoli secrete milk and then ducts permit passage of milk to the exterior by way of the nipple.

mammo-gram

mamma breast + *gram* something written or recorded, like an X-ray
A mammogram is an X-ray film record of the soft tissues of the breast. Periodic mammography is useful in the early detection of breast cancer and benign tumors. Mammothermography (*thermos* Greek, heat) uses infrared sensors to detect temperature differences in breast tissue which can indicate the presence of malignant tumors.

mammo-plasty

mamma breast + *plastia* new scientific Greek, a surgical shaping, a forming
Mammoplasty may be cosmetic surgery to improve the lift or size of breasts or to reconstruct breasts reduced by surgery to remove cancerous tissue. Reductive mammoplasty is that performed to make large breasts smaller.

mandible

mandibulum Late Latin, the lower jaw, literally 'the little chewer' < *mandare* to chew
The mandible is the lower jawbone, the only bone of the skull that moves. It has a round projection at each end called a condyle (*kondylos* Greek, knuckle, joint) that fits into a hollow area called a fossa (Latin, ditch, trench, pit) in the temporal bones at each side of the face. This is the temperomandibular joint, and its articulation allows the chewing motion in which the mandible with its cargo of lower teeth is moved up and down against the maxillary bones (*maxilla* Latin, upper jaw) that form most of the upper jaw and hold the upper teeth.

masseter

masseter Greek, thing that or one who chews, a chewer
The masseter muscle is the thick, rectangular cheek muscle that closes the mouth, the main muscle involved in chewing food.

mast-

mastos Greek, breast

mast-algia

mastos breast + *algia* Greek, feeling pain < *algos* pain
Mastalgia is any pain in a breast.

mast-ec-tomy

mastos breast + *ek* out + *tome* a surgical cutting + *y* noun
ending
Mastectomy is partial or complete removal of a breast or the breasts usually as
treatment of breast cancer. A radical mastectomy involves excision of not only
the breast but also the pectoral muscles, skin, lymph nodes of the armpit and
some subcutaneous fat. Simple mastectomy is sometimes termed lumpectomy, in
which only the tumorous mass is removed and other tissues and structures are
left intact.

mastitis

mastos breast + *itis* inflammation of
Mastitis is inflammation of the breast, most frequent when a woman is lactating.
Micro-organisms often enter through an abrasion in the skin of the nipple. The
chief symptom of cystic mastitis is found on breast examination while feeling
tiny nodes during palpation.

mastoid bone

mastos breast + *eides* Greek, form, hence -*oid* means 'formed
like'
Mastoid means 'shaped like a breast'. It usually refers to the mastoid process of
the temporal bone, felt as the main bump behind the ear. It serves as the point of
attachment for several muscles, as do most processes on a bone.

mastoid-itis

mastoid bone + *itis* inflammation of
Mastoiditis is infection of the mastoid bones, due to middle ear infections in
children, sometimes with small residual hearing losses. This painful
inflammation is treated by antibiotics, or, if they are not effective, by a partial
removal of the infected bone called mastoidectomy.

masturbate

mas, maris Latin adjective, male + *turbare* to agitate, to disturb
Originally the verb referred only to a male's stimulating his own genitals to achieve orgasm. Both sexes and most people use this form of sexual release at some time in their lives. It is a perfectly healthy practice.

mater

mater Latin, mother

dura mater

dura mater Latin, tough mother (layer)
Dura mater is a translation into Late Latin from the Arabic term *oum al-dimagh*, tough mother. Arabic uses *oum*, mother, to mean the greatest of, the most important of. Compare Saddam Hussein's 'the mother of all wars'.

Three meninges or membranes wrap around and protect the brain and spinal cord. The tough outer meninx, singular of meninges, is the dura mater, the tough mother.

pia mater

pia mater Latin, literally, pious mother
Latin *pia*, pious, because a monk mistranslated an Arabic word that means thin as pious. Very unscientific, yet we owe the preservation of many medical texts to the diligence of medieval monks who copied and translated Arabic versions of Greek medical texts that had been destroyed in the West during the fall of the Roman Empire and during the Dark Ages. Thus we can abide *pia*.

Pia mater is the third layer of the three meninges. Nearest the brain, it is rich in blood vessels.

maxilla

mala Latin, jaw + *illa* diminutive suffix of feminine nouns, little > *maxilla*; plural maxillae
A maxilla is one of the two large bones that form the upper jaw.

meatus

meare Latin, to go, to pass > *meatus* a passageway, a channel, a hole

The external auditory meatus or acoustic meatus is the hole in an ear, the short passage that leads to the tympanum (Latin, skin of a drum, ear drum). The urinary meatus is, in the language of the nursery, the pee-hole, the external opening of the urethra in the male and the female.

medicine

The root of this noun is a Latin verb *mederi*, to attend to a person. From that verb came the Roman occupation name, *medicus*, an attendent who ministered to the sick bed, then the developed meaning, later in Roman history, of a physician. After that is found the phrase *ars medicina*, the art of the doctor, from which after a trip through Old French, the word *medicine* entered Middle English.

medi-

medialis Latin, of the middle > *medium* the middle

Medial as an anatomical direction means located toward the center of a body or body part, for example, the medial phalanx of a finger is the bone between the proximal and the distal phalanges, the middle of the three finger bones.

median

medianus Late Latin, in the middle

Median in anatomy means exactly in the middle, e.g. the median nerve of the brachial plexus, a tangle of nerves in the upper back from which stem the main nerves of the shoulder, chest and arms. The median nerve innervates ultimately the forearm flexor muscles, some thumb muscles, the elbow and hand joints.

medulla

medulla Latin, the marrow of a bone, but, literally, the little part in the middle of something; plural medullae, adjective medullary

A medulla is the innermost part of an organ or structure. The adrenal medulla is the inner portion of the adrenal gland that sits atop each kidney, as part of the sympathetic nervous system. When stimulated, it pours adrenaline (also called epinephrine) into the bloodstream. Epinephrine's basic effect is to get organs ready for exertion. Blood is diverted to muscles, the heart pumps more blood and glucose for fuel is released from the liver into the bloodstream.

medulla oblongata

oblongata Latin feminine adjective, rather long

The medulla oblongata is the innermost and lowest part of the brainstem. This medulla is an enlarged bulbous part of the upper spinal column just inside the foramen magnum, the hole in the bottom of the skull through which the spinal cord enters the brain. In evolution, it is the oldest part of the mammalian brain, and the one most vital to life. For in the medulla oblongata are the control centers for breathing, heart and blood functions, and all the neural pathways that send and receive vital impulses. Trauma to the medulla oblongata is fatal.

mega-

megas, megalos Greek, big, large

Mega- and *megalo-* are frequently used in medical words to indicate an abnormal enlargement, for example, megacardia: abnormal enlargement of the heart, also seen with the Greek roots reversed in cardiomegaly (see below) and as megalocardia, all three synonymous terms denoting a cardiac hypertrophy(see entry). Megabladder, megacolon, megarectum and megaureter denote abnormal distension of those structures and organs.

Mega- is also prefixed to words indicating amounts in excess of normal, as in megadose and megavitamin therapy. This usage reflects the prefix's popularity in journalese: megadeal, megadeath, megahit, megaproject, megastar.

megalo-, -megaly

megas, megalos Greek, big, large > *megale* Greek noun, enlargement

acro-megaly

acro- extremities + *megale* abnormal enlargement

Acromegaly is a growth defect after maturity in which the pituitary gland secretes extra growth hormone, causing gross enlargement of the skeletal extremities: fingers, toes, nose, jaw.

hepato-megaly

hepar, hepatos Greek, the liver + *megale* enlargement

Hepatomegaly is abnormal enlargement of the liver. It may be part of cirrhosis, a group of chronic liver diseases in which hepatic functions and structures degenerate.

megalo-cephal-y

megas, megalos large + *kephale* Greek, the head + *y* noun ending
Megalocephaly is abnormal size of the head, a synonym of macrocephaly
(*makros* Greek, big, wide), a head and brain abnormally large in relation to the
rest of the body, often resulting in mental and growth retardation.

megalo-cyte

megas, megalos large + *kytos* cell
A megalocyte is an abnormally large red blood cell.

megalo-mania

megas, megalos large + *mania* Greek, madness
Megalomania is a symptom seen in many psychoses, a delusional
self-importance, in which the patient imagines he or she has power or
importance far beyond what is realistic.

megalo-syn-dactyly

megas, megalos large + *syn* together + *daktylos* Greek, digit,
finger, toe + *y* noun ending
Megalosyndactyly is a congenital enlargement of fingers and/or toes in which
the digits are webbed together.

melano-

melas, melanos Greek, black in color

melan-chol-ia and melan-chol-y

melas, melanos black + *chole* bile + *ia* medical condition (or + *y*
noun ending)
Melancholia and melancholy refer to a clinical depression with physical and
mental effects, or a general sadness and brooding. Early Greek physicians,
believing in the now discredited theory of humors, thought black bile made one
sad. As well, the word *choler* means bile or anger, because later medieval doctors
still believed excess bile made a person of angry temperament.

melan-in

melas, melanos black + *in* noun ending for organic chemical compound

Melanin is a dark skin pigment made and held in special cells in the basal layer of the epidermis. These cells are called melanocytes (*kytos* cell). The more melanin present, the darker the skin. Sun exposure increases melanin to produce a tan.

melan-oma

melas, melanos black + *oma* tumor

A melanoma is any tumor made up of melanocytes. A melanocyte is a cell whose chief function is the formation of melanin. The malignant form of melanoma, chiefly due to overexposure to sunlight, especially in those with light skin color, metastasizes or spreads very quickly. The ultraviolet radiation delivered in tanning salons may also be a factor. Warning signs include any change in the size and appearance of a mole such as bleeding, oozing, or scaliness of local skin.

mela-ton-in

melas black + *tonos* Greek, the action of stretching + *in* noun ending for organic chemical

Melatonin is a hormone produced by the pineal gland in the mammalian brain. In humans, it may help regulate the production of melanin, and sleep, seasonal mood changes, puberty and reproductive patterns like the ovarian cycle. Its use in pseudomedical therapies by health quacks is unwise, until more is known about this hormone.

membrane

membrana Latin, any tissue that covers a body part, skin, sheet of parchment < *membrum* limb of the body, penis, a part of something

English borrowed its modern medical meaning from French, where membrane was used extensively in the work of the great 18th Century French pioneer of histology, M.F.X. Bichat, the Parisian anatomist who first attempted a classification of the tissues of the human body.

A membrane is a thin, soft layer of tissue covering an organ or structure, lining a body cavity, or separating one body space from another. Fibrous membranes, like the fascia, are made of connective tissue. Also fibrous is the interosseous (*inter* between + *osseus* of bones) membrane in the arm that connects the ulna to the radius. Another interosseous membrane in the leg connects the tibia to the fibula. Kinds of membranes include mucous, serous, synovial and cutaneous. See various entries.

membranous labyrinth

membrana Latin, tissue that covers a body part; *labyrinthos* Greek, a maze

The word *labyrinthos* was first applied to royal palaces on the island of Crete, with many interconnecting halls and passageways. A *labrys* was a kind of axe with two blades in ancient Greece and Egypt, so that the word *labyrinthos* means literally 'the place of the double-axe'. Ruins of such a palace bearing emblems of the double-axe have been found at Knossos on Crete. Part of the legend of the minotaur and its maze built by the mythical Daedalus arose as a folktale about this great palace.

In anatomy, the membranous labyrinth is a network of three little ducts filled with fluid which hang down inside the semicircular canals of the inner ear. These ducts sway gently and touch one another as the human body and head move. Part of our sense of balance is created and fine-tuned as the membranous labyrinth sways.

permeable membrane

per Latin, through + *meare* to go + *-abilis* adjectival suffix, able to, capable of

One common scientific apparatus used in medical devices is a permeable membrane, one that allows the passage of fluids like water and certain solutes, but does not permit larger solid particulates to pass through it. Some membranes are semi-permeable, others are specifically selectively permeable. Also referenced in medical literature are phrases like capillary permeability and magnetic permeability.

meninges (singular *meninx*, adjective *meningeal*)

meninx, meningis Latin from *menigx* Greek, membrane. Hippocrates used the word to refer to the dura mater.

Three meninges or membranes wrap around and protect the brain and spinal cord. The tough outer meninx, singular of meninges, is the dura mater. The middle meninx is the arachnoid (*arachn-oides* Greek, netted like a spider's web). The pia mater is the innermost layer of the three meninges. Nearest the brain, it is rich in blood vessels. Inflammation of these vital membranes as seen in meningitis must prompt immediate therapy.

meningo-cele

meninx, meningis brain and spinal membrane + *kele* Greek, hernia, swelling
Meningocele is a congenital hernia in which the meninges push through an opening in the skull or spinal cord, as sometimes seen in spina bifida (see entry). Corrective surgery is effective.

meno-

men, menos Greek, a month, hence English phrases like 'the monthlies' and Latin terms like *menstrualis*
Meno- is prefixed to words related to the monthly female period of normal and abnormal menstrual bleeding.

cata-men-ia

kata Greek, down from + *men, menos* a month, menstruation + *ia* condition
Catamenia refers to the normal cycle of processes associated with the monthly flow of menstrual blood from the uterus during a female's reproductive years.

dys-meno-rrhea

dys painful + *men, menos* Greek, month + *rrhoia* Greek, a discharge
Dysmenorrhea is a monthly period that is painful due to various inflammations or mechanical obstructions or to other symptoms like menstrual cramping.

meno-rrhea

men, menos Greek, month + *rrhoia* Greek, a discharge
Menorrhea refers to a normal, healthy monthly period.

meno-pause

men, menos a month, hence, referring to menstruation + *pausa* Latin, a stopping
Menopause is the cessation of the monthly female period of normal menstrual bleeding, happening at between 35 and 50 years in most women. Sexual desire does not cease. Stressful menopausal symptoms are real – although some symptomatic distress is psychosomatic and picked up from the particular culture

and society in which the female has lived. Hormone replacement using estrogen alone or in combination with other hormones is not a panacea for menopausal symptoms. For many patients, there are too many harmful side-effects. These risks should be made clear to women who choose hormone replacement therapy.

menstruation

menstruatio, menstruationis Late Latin, the monthly
flow < *menses* Latin, literally, the months

Menstruation is the monthly flow of menstrual blood from the uterus during a female's reproductive years. Each month the endometrium (see entry), the lining of the uterus, thickens and proliferates to prepare for a possible pregnancy. If a pregnancy does not occur, the endometrial excess is shed, and this debris along with an average blood loss of 30 milliliters, a thimbleful, is discharged through the vagina. The average menstrual cycle is 28 days, but may vary greatly.

meso-

mesos Greek, middle

mes-entery

mesos middle + *enteron* Greek, gut, intestines < *entos* within, inside

The mesentery is the peritoneal fold that keeps the stomach, spleen, and parts of the small intestine in their position toward the posterior wall of the abdomen.

meso-colon

mesos middle + *kolon* Greek, the large intestine

The mesocolon is the peritoneal fold that keeps the lower colon loosely against the inside abdominal wall.

meso-morph

mesos middle + *morphe* Greek, form, shape

A mesomorph is a person of the middle body type, with good muscular and skeletal development, the type between ectomorph and endomorph.

meta-

This Greek preposition and prefix means 'along with, with, across in space, after in time or position'. *Meta* has the developed meaning of 'change' (something that happens afterward). The root is akin to the German *mit* 'with' and to the *med* in Latin *medium*, and to the *me-* in Greek *mesos*, 'middle'. It appears in ordinary English words like metaphor, meteor and method.

meta-bol-ism

meta across, with changes + *bole* throwing + *ismos* Greek noun suffix, process of

Metabolism comprises all the physical and chemical processes the body uses to maintain itself, including the conversion of food into energy.

meta-carpal

meta after + *carpalis* pertaining to the wrist < *carpus* Latin, wrist

The metacarpals are the five bones of the middle part of the hand that come after the carpals; they form the palm of the hand.

meta-morph-osis

meta after, changed + *morphe* Greek, form, shape + *osis* condition; *morphosis* Greek, formation

The action of biological units changing from one stage to another in their form or structure. In pathology, a metamorphosis is usually a change for the worse, a degeneration. Previously the Latin-derived *transformation* was used. Transformation is a direct translation of each Greek root part into its Latin equivalent.

meta-stasis

meta after + *stasis* Greek, a standing, a state

Although the literal meaning of metastasis is a changing of position, a removal, its normal use in medicine is to describe the movement of malignant cells to a further, new site of cancer in the body. For example, a cancer may metastasize from its initial site in the breast to the lymph nodes in both armpits.

meta-tarsal

meta across + *tarsos* Greek, the flat of the foot between heel and toe

In anatomy, a tarsus is one of the seven bones of the ankle, permitting articulation between the foot and the leg. These bones are also called the tarsals. The metatarsals are the bones of the foot that come after the tarsals and before the phalanges (bones of the toes).

metatarsal arches

Each foot has two arches or areas of curved outline: the transverse arch across the foot, and the longitudinal arch along the length of the foot. In the biophysics of walking upright, arches support and add spring to the step.

metri-

metra Greek, literally mother-thing, mother-essence, hence the womb, the uterus

endo-metrium

endon Greek, inside + *metrium* Latin form of *metra* Greek, uterus

The endometrium is the inner lining of the uterus consisting of epithelial mucosa. The superficial layers, called decidua, are shed during menstruation if pregnancy does not occur.

peri-metrium

peri Greek, around + *metrium* Latin form of *metra* Greek, uterus

The perimetrium is the outer, serous membrane around the uterus.

myo-metrium

mys, myos Greek, muscle + *metrium* Latin form of *metra* Greek, uterus

The myometrium is the smooth-muscle layer of the uterus that surrounds the endometrium. It contracts the uterus during menstrual cycles and during birth.

micro-

mikros Greek, small

micro-scope

mikros small + *skopos* Greek, watcher, viewer, examiner

A microscope is an instrument to enlarge the image of a small object not clearly visible to the naked eye. Lenses, prisms and mirrors were used first and are still used, but now television microscopy and the scanning electron microscope use beams of electrons to form the image instead of light, for viewing on fluorescent monitor screens or cathode-ray tubes.

micro-organism

mikros small + organism

A microscopic organism, such as a virus, bacterium, or protozoon, is one clearly visible only under a microscope.

micro-surgery

mikros small + surgery

Microsurgery is the dissection and repair of minute body structures under microscopic enlargement, and so permitting previously impossible surgery on certain parts of the eye and brain, and allowing the reattachment of severed limbs by the suturing of tiny nerves and blood vessels.

micturate

micturire Latin, to need urgently to urinate < *mingere* to pee + *urire* a desiderative verb suffix which adds the sense of intense desire or need to the basic verbal root

Micturate is a sometimes useful medical euphemism for 'urinate'. The noun is micturition.

milia

milium Latin, millet seed; plural milia

Milia are whiteheads, very small, whitish cysts, especially of facial skin, caused by blockage of sweat glands and hair follicles. Their minuteness and large number caused them to be named after millet, a cereal grain called *milium* by the Romans because it produces abundant tiny seeds in the thousands (Latin *mille*, a thousand). Milia neonatorum, milia of newborns, is a common rash that usually clears up a week or two after birth. Miliaria is prickly heat rash, with plentiful milia or sudamina. Sudamen, a technical term for sweat blister, is the singular of sudamina.

miso-

misos Greek, hatred

miso-gyny

misos Greek, hatred + *gyne* female

Misogyny is a pathological hatred of women. Hatred of males is misandry (*misos* hatred + *andreia* Greek, masculinity).

mitral valve

mitralis Late Latin, having two points like a *mitra* Latin, bishop's hat

The mitral valve has another name, the bicuspid valve (Latin, with two cusps or points). The mitral valve is in the heart between the left atrium and the left ventricle. It permits blood flow from the left atrium into the left ventricle, and prevents backflow or reflux by closing. The mitral or bicuspid valve is the only heart valve with two, rather than three, cusps. Many terms in cardiopathology use the adjective. A mitral murmur is a heart sound caused by a defective bicuspid valve. In mitral valve stenosis, the little leaves of the valve acquire adhesions which block effective closure of the valve, leading to an enlarged left atrium and possible failure of the right side of the heart. In mitral valve prolapse (Latin, a falling in front of) one or both cusps fall back into the left atrium causing incomplete closure and a backflow of blood. This mitral regurgitation can lead to abnormal enlargement of the left side of the heart, and possibly, eventual congestive heart failure.

mono-

monos Greek, single, of one unit or one form

mono-clonal

monos one + *klon* Greek, graft, ancient Greek botanical term, twig, slip, plant cutting used to propagate similar plants > *clonal* scientific English

Monoclonal refers to identical cells all derived from a single mother cell. A clone is an individual organism or group of cells grown from a single somatic cell of its parent and thus genetically identical to it. In medical histology, a clone is a group of cells grown from a single mother cell by mitosis so that all the daughter cells are genetically identical. There are many instances where such uniformity is an advantage, for example in the culturing of monoclonal antibodies, where antibodies are exact copies of an antibody-producing cell and so all of them are potent against a specific antigen.

mono-cyte

monos one + *kytos* cell
A monocyte is a kind of white blood cell (leukocyte) formed in the bone marrow. Monocytes protect other body parts by ingesting foreign bacteria, dead cells and other debris; hence they are macrophages (see entry) and phagocytes (*phagos* Greek, eater).

mono-nucle-osis

monos one + *nucleus* Latin, kernel, nutlet, center of a cell + *osis* diseased condition
Mononucleosis is an acute infectious disease triggered by the Epstein–Barr virus. Hematic symptoms include excess of monocytes with one nucleus.

mons pubis

mons pubis Latin, the mount or hill of the genital area, also called *mons Veneris*, the mount of Venus, goddess of love
The mons pubis is a pad of fat and coarse skin that lies over the pubic symphysis in the female. The pubic symphysis or symphysis pubis (*syn* > *sym* Greek, together + *physis* a growing) is the line of jointure of the two pubic bones. They are separated by a disk of tough fiber and cartilage connected by two ligaments. Thus the symphysis is slightly movable, especially to assist in accommodation of the growth and birth of the fetus. The fat pad of the mons pubis protects this meeting place of the pubic bones. It also acts as a shock absorber to protect the outer female genitalia during intercourse and was a store of fat for our ancient forebears during times of low nutrition.

morph-

morphe Greek, form, shape, structure

a-morph-ous

a not + *morphe* Greek, form, shape + *ous* adjectival suffix
Something amorphous is without definite shape. Certain chemicals and minerals are amorphous, lacking a definite crystalline form or structure.

morph-ine

Morpheys the Greek god of dreams, literally, the shaper < *morphe* Greek, form, shape
Morphine is the chief alkaloid of opium; the hydrochloride and sulfate are narcotic analgesics. In 1803, Adolf Sertürner, a German chemist, named this powerfully addictive hypnotic after the Greco-Roman god of dreams, Morpheus. Dreams to the ancients were forms or shapes brought to the mind by sleep.

bone morphogenic proteins (BMPs)

morphe form + *gen-* Greek, making, producing + *ic* adjective ending
BMPs are a family of large molecules made when an injury to bone tissue occurs. BMPs hone in on certain immature or unspecialized cells in the area of the injury, and send chemical signals that incite these unspecialized cells to become specialized cells like those in bone and cartilage. The BMPs send an inciting chemical that turns on the immature cells' growth factors. Then these immature cells pick up other chemical signals from the tissue near them that tell the immature cells what kind of cell to become. This understanding of the self-healing power of bone, that Hippocrates recognized but could not explain more than 2400 years ago, is one of the most promising discoveries of modern tissue engineering, perhaps heralding treatments in which the body can be induced to grow new bone tissue wherever it is needed.

Morphogenesis is the noun to describe the development in an organism or organ of its essential form and structure.

muco-

mucus Latin, slime, phlegm, mucus

mucus

mucus phlegm, mucus
Mucus is a viscid secretion of dead cells, mucin, salts and water. Mucus acts as a protective coating on membranes that line certain body parts.

muc-osa

mucus slime, mucus + *osus, osa, osum* Latin adjectival suffix
denoting 'an abundance of'
Mucosa is any membranous body tissue that secretes mucus and covers or lines
many interior parts of the body, e.g. the oral mucosa lining the mouth. It is also
called a mucous membrane. A descriptive adjective is mucomembranous, but
mucosal is commoner.

muc-in

mucus slime
Mucin is a sticky glycoprotein in connective tissue that is also the mucilage-like
cementing biochemical in mucus.

muco-purulent

mucus slime, mucus + *purulens, purulentis* containing pus < *pus,
puris* Latin, pus
Mucopurulent discharges, that follow many infections, are composed of mucus
and pus.

muscle

musculus Latin, a little mouse < *mus* mouse + *-culus* diminutive
noun suffix, little, small
The Romans thought that muscles rippling under the skin looked like *musculi*,
little mice. The same metaphor occurred to ancient Greeks, from whom the
Romans may have borrowed it. Greek *mys, myos* meant mouse, then muscle, and
appears in numerous medical terms like myalgia, muscle pain.

A muscle is a long-celled body tissue that contracts to produce movement.
Striated muscle fibers are divided by transverse bands. They are voluntary
muscles normally under the control of one's will, e.g. arm and hand muscles
moved to pick up an object. Smooth muscles with long, spindle-shaped cells are
involuntary, performing their function without conscious thought, e.g. muscles
of the stomach and intestines that work even during sleep. Heart muscle is a
special class of muscular tissue because it is striated and involuntary muscle.

muscular dys-trophy

dys Greek, bad, abnormal: indicates disordered function +
trophe Greek, nourishment
Dystrophy is any disease due to faulty nutrition in a body part. The many
muscular dystrophies are serious degenerative diseases.

mut-

mutare Latin, to alter, to change
A mutant is an individual some of whose genes have undergone alteration in the
way they are expressed. This mutation is often transmitted to the offspring of
the mutant and to future generations. A muton is the smallest DNA segment
whose alteration results in an expressed mutation.

muta-gen

mutare change + *gen* Greek, producing
A mutagen is any chemical agent that induces a genetic alteration or increases
the rate at which mutations occur in specific organisms.

myco-, myceto-

mykes, myketos Greek, mushroom, fungus
Mycology is the study of diseases caused by fungi. Mycosis is any disease caused
by a fungus, for example, athlete's foot and candidiasis (see entry).
Mycotoxicosis is the poisoning caused by toxins made by certain fungal
organisms. A mycotic aneurysm (see *aneurysm* entry) is the abnormal widening
of a blood vessel in the heart tissues caused by bacterial endocarditis.

Myco-bacterium

mykes fungus + bacterium
Mycobacterium is a genus of rod-shaped bacteria, two species of which are serious
disease-producers in humans. Leprosy is caused by *Mycobacterium leprosae*, and
tuberculosis by *Mycobacterium tuberculosis.*

my-, mye-, myo-

mys, myos Greek, muscle

myo-ton-ia

mys, myos muscle + *tonos* Greek, stretching quality, tone + *ia* medical condition

In myotonia, a muscle or muscle group has a very long period of contraction and does not relax fully after contraction. Myotonus is tonic spasm of a muscle or group of muscles.

my-oma

mys, myos muscle + *oma* tumor

A myoma is a benign tumor of muscle tissue. Plural: myomata.

myo-cardium

mys, myos muscle + *kardia* Greek, heart

Myocardium is heart muscle, cardiac muscle that surrounds the heart in a tough, thick layer. A myocardial infarction is a heart attack due to closing off of a coronary artery that causes an infarct of heart muscle. Part of the muscle dies from lack of oxygen.

myelo-

myelos Greek, spinal cord, confusingly *myelo-* also means bone marrow

myel-in

myelos spinal cord + *in* noun ending for organic chemical compound

The myelin sheath is a white, greasy cover that protects most nerve cells and fibers. Myelin also covers parts of the spinal cord and the white matter of the brain. Neural tissue that is not myelinated, or not covered with myelin, is gray. Hence the term 'gray matter' of the brain and spinal cord.

de-myelin-ation

de Latin, apart, undoing + *myelos* spinal cord + *ation* noun suffix

Demyelination occurs in certain diseaes of the nervous system when the myelin sheath disintegrates and nerve cells fail to transmit impulses well. Multiple sclerosis is an example.

myel-oma

myelos bone marrow + *oma* tumor
Myeloma is a rare tumor of bone marrow cells.

myelo-graphy

myelos spinal cord + *grapheia* Greek, a writing, a recording
Myelography is an X-ray of the spinal cord.

polio-myel-itis

myelos Greek, spinal cord + *polios* Greek, gray in color + *itis* inflammation of
Polio or poliomyelitis is a severe viral infection of the gray matter of the spinal cord that may cause paralysis, because it affects nerve cells at the front of the spinal cord responsible for signalling muscle contraction. The Salk and Sabin vaccines offer methods of prevention.

myxo-

myxa Greek, mucus, and akin to the Latin *mucus*

myxo-virus

myxa Greek, mucus + *virus* (see entry)
Myxovirus is any of certain RNA viruses including the ones that cause influenza and mumps, characterized by red blood cells forming mucus-like aggregrations.

myx-oma

myxa Greek, mucus + *oma* tumor
Myxoma is a usually benign tumor of connective tissue that has a jelly-like, mucus-like character. Myxomatosis is a disease characterized by many myxomata.

myx-aden-itis

myxa Greek, mucus + *aden* Greek, gland + *itis* inflammation of
Myxadenitis is inflammation of any mucous gland.

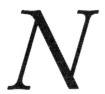

N

nano-

nanos Greek, dwarf

In addition to its use to describe anatomical anomalies as shown below, *nano-* is one of the numerical prefixes of metric measurement used widely in scientific calibration to mean 'one-billionth of'. A nanogram is one billionth of a gram in weight. A nanocurie is a unit of radiation, one billionth of a curie. A nanosecond is one billionth of a second.

nan-ism

nanos dwarf + *ismos* Greek noun suffix indicating a condition

Nanism is dwarfism, an abnormal smallness of the body. Types include pituitary nanism, renal nanism, and senile nanism. Nanous is the adjective. A medical synonym and useful euphemism for dwarf is nanus or nanosomus (*soma* Greek, body). Dwarfism is also called nanosomia or nanosoma. Nanoid is dwarf-like.

nano-cephal-y

nanos dwarf + *kephale* Greek, the head + *y* noun ending

Nanocephaly or nanocephalism is having an abnormally small head.

nano-corm-ia

nanos dwarf + *kormos* Greek, the trunk of the human body + *ia* condition

Nanocormia is dwarfism with the trunk of the body abnormally small in comparison to the head and the limbs.

nano-mel-ia

nanos dwarf + *melos* Greek, limb, extremity + *ia* medical condition

Nanomelia is dwarfism with the arms and legs abnormally small in comparison to the head and the trunk of the body.

narco-

narke Greek, originally, numbness of an extremity, then, a stupor, a torpor

narco-hypnosis

narke stupor + *hypnos* Greek, sleep + *osis* abnormal kind of
Hypnosis is an artificially induced sleep-like state, where the hypnotized subject is often responsive to suggestion. In narcohypnosis, the hypnotic state is produced by the administration of a powerful narcotic drug like sodium pentothal or sodium amobarbital.

narco-lepsy

narke stupor + *lepsis* Greek, a seizure, a sudden onset of
Narcolepsy is a sleep disorder in which the patient falls asleep suddenly during normal daytime activity. It runs in families and may be controlled by one faulty gene. Slightly less than half of narcoleptics also suffer sudden loss of muscle tone and may fall to the ground during an attack but will remain conscious. If they are sitting down, their knees may buckle and their heads fall forward.

narc-osis

narke stupor + *osis* abnormal condition; Hippocrates used the word *narcosis* to mean the artificial numbing of a painful part or injury
Narcosis now means an unconscious state induced by any drug that depresses the central nervous system when given in appropriate, small, medical doses.

narco-tic

narkotikos Greek, of a substance that numbs pain
A narcotic depresses central nervous system activity, and so relieves pain. All powerful narcotics are deeply addictive. A narcotic also produces sleep, but in excess causes depression, slow heart rate, decreased breathing rate, deep sleep, unconsciousness, and possibly coma and death. Dangerous narcotic subtances include codeine, opium, morphine, heroin, crack cocaine and newer synthetic drugs.

naris

naris Latin, nostril

Naris is the anatomical name for the nostril. The English word *nostril* has an interesting derivation, being a compound of Old English *nosu* nose + *thyrel* hole, and thus having the literal and apt meaning of 'nose-hole'. Plural: nares.

nasal, naso-

nasalis of the nose < *nasum* Latin, nose

nasal septum

nasalis of the nose; *septum* Latin, plural *septa*, partition, wall < *saepire* to fence in

The nasal septum is the partition of cartilage dividing the two nasal cavities.

nasal speculum

nasalis of the nose; *speculum* Latin, a looking glass, a mirror < *specere* to observe, to see

A speculum is an instrument to examine a body cavity that opens on the surface, such as the nose, throat, rectum or vagina. A nasal speculum helps dilate a nasal passage and often provides light to make inspection of interior nasal tissues easier.

naso-pharynx

nasum Latin, nose + *pharygx* Greek, throat

The pharynx or throat may be divided into three areas. The nasopharynx is the muscular back wall of the nose, just above the soft palate. When one swallows, the nasopharynx is closed off by a reflexive raising of the soft palate. The cavity of the middle ear joins the nasopharynx by the Eustachian tube, which keeps pressure inside the eardrum equal to pressure outside. The other two areas of the throat are the oropharynx (*os, oris* Latin, mouth), the mouth part of the throat for passage of food and air; and there is the laryngopharynx, the part of the throat near the voice box or larynx.

natal

natalis Latin, relating to birth; compare *Buon Natale*, Italian, Merry Christmas, literally 'Good Birthday' (of Christ)

Natal means pertaining to birth or the day of birth. From the different root *nates*, Latin, buttocks, natal also means pertaining to the buttocks. Natality is the birth rate of a population.

neo-natal

neos Greek, new, young + *natalis* Latin, relating to birth
Neonatal is relating to a newborn baby, precisely the first six weeks after birth. A neonate is a newborn infant up to the age of six weeks, and neonatology is the care and treatment of such newborns.

peri-natal

peri Greek, around + *natalis* relating to birth
Perinatal relates to the period just before and just after birth.

post-natal

post Latin, after + *natalis* Latin, relating to birth
Postnatal pertains to the period after birth.

pre-natal

prae Latin, before, in front of + *natalis* Latin, relating to birth
Prenatal relates to the period before birth, as in prenatal care, clinics, diagnosis, etc.

nausea

nausia Greek, original meaning as used by Hippocrates: seasickness < *naus* Greek, ship
Nausea later came to refer to the uneasy feeling just before one vomits. The technical term for true seasickness is nausea navalis.

nausea gravidarum

gravidarum Latin, of pregnant women < *gravida* pregnant
Nausea gravidarum is the morning sickness of pregnant women. Gravid is a somewhat rare synonym in medical English for pregnant. A nulligravida is a female who has never been pregnant. A primigravida is a female with her first pregnancy.

necro-

nekros Greek, dead

necro-philia

nekros dead + *philia* Greek, fondness, liking for

Necrophilia is a sexual perversion and a psychiatric disorder in which (usually) men want to have sexual intercourse with a female corpse. But the adjective necrophilic can refer to certain bacteria that feed on and prefer dead tissue.

necr-osis

nekros dead + *osis* diseased condition

Necrosis is limited tissue death with areas of healthy living tissue near it. Necrotic tissue describes limited bone destruction or small areas of tissue. Necrosis is often seen in advanced stages of syphilis and tuberculosis. Gangrene (see entry) refers to larger areas or whole organs. A disease which produces necrosis as a major symptom is referred to as necrotizing. Necrotizing enteritis is an acute bowel inflammation caused by a *Clostridium* bacterium. Other diseases include necrotizing fasciitis, popularly termed 'the flesh-eating disease', and necrotizing vasculitis.

neo-

neos Greek, new

neo-log-ism

neos new + *logos* word + *-ismos* state, condition

In psychiatry, neologism is a private vocabulary, new words coined by and used only by the patient, and sometimes not understandable by others. Some neologism presents as the patient giving new and private definitions to common words. It is a symptom in some schizophrenic disorders. However, a neology is a legitimate new word, freshly coined and not yet in a dictionary.

neo-plasm

neos new + *plasma* Greek, a thing formed < *plassein* to mould, to form

A neoplasm is a new formation of tissue as in a tumor. Neoplasm implies malignant growth in most of its modern medical uses. A neoplasm has no biotic function and proliferates at the expense of normal tissue and a healthy organism. Neoplasm is a frequent medical euphemism for cancer. Neoplastic is the adjective, not to be confused with neoplasty, which is the surgical formation or restoration of body structures.

nephro-

nephros Greek, kidney

The Latin word for kidney is *ren, renis* and is also used extensively in medical vocabulary, e.g. renal artery. Sometimes the two different roots produce synonyms, for example, a kidney stone may be a nephrolith (*lithos* Greek, stone) or a renal calculus (*calculus* Latin, stone, pebble).

nephron

nephros Greek, kidney

The nephron may be termed the basic unit of the kidney. The nephron is one of about a million tiny filters in the inner layer of the two kidneys where urine is made by filtering blood in a coil of blood vessels called a glomerulus (Latin, little ball), which empties into a tubule carrying urine to the renal pelvis, to the ureters, and then to the bladder.

nephr-osis

nephros kidney + *osis* diseased condition

Nephrosis is degenerative changes in the renal tubules of the kidney caused by inflammation. Nephrotic syndrome includes symptoms like low protein in the blood, high protein in the urine and edema. There are many causes, some outside the kidneys themselves.

nephro-stomy

nephros Greek, kidney + *stoma* Greek, mouth, making a mouth-like opening + *y* noun ending

Nephrostomy is the insertion of a draining catheter into an obstructed kidney. Carried out by making an incision to insert a catheter through the skin, it is termed a percutaneous nephrostomy (see *percutaneous* entry).

pyelo-nephr-itis

pyelos Greek, basin, pelvis, renal pelvis + *nephros* kidney + *itis* inflammation of

Pyelonephritis is inflammation of the renal pelvis and the other essential structures of the kidney. *Pyelo* (see entry) indicates the renal pelvis, as in pyelogram, an X-ray of the renal pelvis and ureter. The renal pelvis is the expanded end of the ureter nearest the kidney. The renal pelvis lies inside the kidney and receives urine before it enters the ureter. An intravenous pyelography (IVP) involves making an X-ray of the renal pelvis and other structures of the kidney.

neuro-

neuron Greek, nerve, akin to Latin *nervus*

neuron

neuron nerve

A nerve is a bundle of fibers that conduct impulses. A neuron is a nerve cell, the basic cell of the nervous system. There are three kinds of neurons. Motor or efferent neurons conduct impulses *from* the brain and spinal cord (*efferens* Latin, leading from, and *motor* Latin, thing that moves). Sensory or afferent neurons lead impulses *to* the brain or spinal cord (*afferens* leading to, and *sensor* thing that senses). Connecting or associative neurons conduct impulses from one neuron to another.

neuro-transmitter

neuron nerve + *trans* Latin, across + *mittere* Latin, to send

When an electrochemical nerve impulse reaches the end of one nerve fiber, it passes on to the next fiber by means of a neurotransmitter, a chemical transmitter that lets the impulse leap across the gap between two neurons. This gap or meeting place between the thread-like projections of neurons is called a synapse, from a Greek word that means 'clasping together'. One common neurotransmitter is acetylcholine, to which muscle fibers respond.

neur-itis

neuron nerve + *itis* inflammation of

Neuritis is inflammation of a nerve or nerves, but also a general term for any nerve pain, sometimes used as a synonym for neuralgia.

neur-algia

neuron nerve + *algos* Greek, pain

Neuralgia is a general term for any nerve pain, but since all pain ultimately is transferred by nerves, its generality makes it not terribly useful. It lacks specific reference and is redundant.

neuro-logy

neuron nerve + *logos* Greek, word, reason, study of
Neurology is the branch of medical science that deals with the structure and diseases of the nervous system, as neurosurgery is any surgery of the nervous system.

nil per os (NPO)

nil per os Latin, nothing by mouth
NPO is a frequent nursing order given several hours before some surgeries or tests.

nodule

nodulus Latin, a little knot, diminutive of *nodus*, a knot
A nodule is a small, firm swelling or node of tissue, larger than a papule, and detectable by touch. Nodular is pertaining to a nodule. Milker's nodules are hard bumps on the unprotected hands of those who milk cows infected with cowpox. Surfer's nodules are fibrous granulomas over the bony parts of the feet and legs, due to chronic inflammation and repeated trauma from kneeling on surfboards.

noxious

noxiosus Late Latin, poisonous, full of harm, *noxa* Latin, harm, injury < *nocere* to injure + *osus* Latin adjectival suffix, full of, abounding in. English words like innocent and innocuous derive from the same root
Noxious substances are destructive to life, or morally harmful.

per-nic-ious anemia

per Latin, through, thoroughly + *noxiosus* full of harm (the *o* alters to an *i*) + *anemia* disease of the blood
In pernicious anemia, the body fails to absorb vitamin B_{12}. Symptoms include low red blood cell count, pallor and weight loss. Treatment includes supplementary vitamin B_{12}, folic acid and iron.

nucha

nukha Arabic, spinal marrow

In Medieval Latin, the Arabic word acquired the same meaning it has in modern medical English, where the nucha is the nape or back of the neck. Compare the French *nuque*. In the birth distress called nuchal cord, the umbilical cord may get wrapped around the neck of a baby as it is born. It is easily slipped off or cut. Even within the uterus, fetal nuchal cord is correctable. The nuchal ligament is a thick, elastic, triangular fiber band that helps support and separate the muscles which attach at the back of the skull.

nucleus

nucleus, a contracted form of *nuculeus* Latin, kernel, nutmeat, literally, little nut < *nux, nucis* nut, literally, the part that nourishes. English *nut* and German *Nuss* are akin to *nux*.

The *nu* root, whose basic meaning is 'feed, nourish', appears in many words like nurse, nourish, and nutritious. The equivalent Greek word for kernel or nut is *karyon* and gives medical words like the synonym for nucleus, karyon, and a term for abnormal enlargement of the cell nucleus, karyomegaly. Several terms in cytology have the root too: karyogenesis, the development of a cell nucleus, and karyokinesis, the dividing in two of nuclear substance that occurs in cell division.

Nucleus has several meanings in scientific English. A nucleus is the control structure inside a living cell. Spherical, surrounded by a nuclear membrane, the nucleus contains genetic instructions for growth, reproduction and maintenance of life systems of the cell. For clarity, this is often referred to as the cell nucleus. A nucleus is also a group of cells in the central nervous system, chiefly in the brain, that together control a major body function like smell, hearing, or sight. A nucleus is also the center of an atom around which electrons rotate.

nucleus pulposus

pulposus Late Latin, full of pulp

The nucleus pulposus is the pulp-filled center of each pad-like disc between vertebrae.

e-nucle-ation

e, ex Latin, out of + *nucleus* nut-shaped object + *atio, ationis* Latin noun suffix, act of

In surgery, enucleation is the removal of an organ or tumor in one piece. Enucleation can refer specifically to surgical excision of the eyeball, due to carcinoma, obliterative injury, and other causes.

mono-nucle-osis

monos one + *nucleus* center of a cell + *osis* diseased condition
Mononucleosis is an acute infectious disease triggered by the Epstein–Barr virus. Hematic symptoms include excess of monocytes with one nucleus.

nuclear magnetic resonance (NMR)

Nuclear magnetic resonance imaging provides more accurate images of soft tissue than X-rays. An electromagnetic field stimulates the nuclei of atoms, making them release energy that can be recorded. NMR is particularly useful in obtaining images of heart tissue, large blood vessels, and the brain. Of course, it cannot be performed on persons with metallic insertions in their bodies, such as heart pacemakers or the aneurysm clips that work by means of magnetized iron.

nulli-para

nullus Latin, not + *para* scientific Latin, female parent < *parere* to bear children
A nullipara is a woman who has never borne a viable child. A unipara is a woman who has given birth to one viable offpsring. Viable here means able to live outside the mother's body. Thus primipara is also a term for a woman who has borne one viable child. A secundipara has borne two viable children. A multipara has borne two or more. Clinical abbreviations include primip and multip.

O

O.B.

abbreviation for obstetrics or obstetrician, see *obstetrics* entry below

ob

a Latin preposition and prefix, its complex, basic meanings include: facing towards, at the back of, behind (obverse), against (object as a verb, to throw against), upon (obfuscate, to cast darkness upon), completely (obdurate, thoroughly hardened, stubborn). Etymologically, *ob* is akin to Greek *epi* and English *up*.

oblique

ob towards + *liquis* Latin adjective, indirect, oblique < *liqu* Latin root, flowing, liquid

The modern English meanings of oblique are inclined, 'at a side angle', not straightforward, indirect, hence devious. In anatomy, an oblique or obliquus muscle may be situated obliquely, that is, neither perpendicular to a body plane nor parallel to it. Similarly, in birth, an oblique presentation sees the long axis of the fetus oblique to the long axis of the mother. An oblique bandage is wrapped around a limb in slanting spirals.

obliquus

obliquus Latin, oblique

The thin, flat muscles that form the middle and outer layers of the side walls of the abdomen. The outermost is the obliquus externus abdominis (Latin, of the abdomen), one on each side of the abdomen. The obliqui externi act to squeeze abdominal contents and so assist in urination, defecation, birth and forcing

251

breath out of the lungs. Both obliqui externi flex the vertebrae, and each obliquus externus itself helps bend and rotate the spinal column.

The obliquus internus abdominis is one of two muscles that lie immediately under the obliqui externi. These internals perform functions similar to the externals.

obstetrics

ob in front of + *stetrix* one who stands, therefore originally, a midwife who stands in front of the birthing mother. *Stetrix* = Latin feminine form of *stator* one who stands < *stare* to stand.
Obstetrics, or O.B., is the branch of medicine devoted to pregnancy, birth and postpartum care. It derives from a Latin phrase for the art of the midwife, *ars obstetricia*.

obstetric forceps

Those designed to facilitate delivery of the fetal head are named after the gynecologists who invented them: Barton, Elliot, Kielland and Simpson forceps.

ob-tur-ator

ob up + *turare* to close, akin to English *door* + *-ator* agent noun suffix, thus obturator is literally a thing that stops up or closes off something
The obturators are thigh muscles. The obturator externus covers the front wall of the pelvis and helps to flex and to turn the thigh to the side. The obturator internus covers a large area of the lower portion of the hip bone. It surrounds the large opening on each side of the lower portion of the hip bone called the obturator foramen (Latin, hole).

An obturator is also a prosthetic device used to block or fill a space left by surgical excision of diseased tissue or by a congenitally absent body structure. In some forms of cleft palate, an obturator is implanted to cover such a gap in the palate.

obturator sign

This classic clinical sign is diagnostic for acute appendicitis. The examining physician gently rotates the hip inward, tightening the patient's obturator internus muscle, and frequently abdominal pain and discomfort help confirm a severely inflamed appendix.

oc-ciput

ob > oc Latin, behind, at the back of + *caput, capitis* Latin, head
Occiput is a general term for the back of the head or skull. *Bregma*, the Greek
word for the top front of the head, is used in medical vocabulary. Thus, an
adjective that refers to the top front and the back of the skull is
occipitobregmatic.

occipital bone

ob > oc at the back of + *capitalis* of the head
The occipital bone forms the saucer-shaped back of the skull and part of the
skull base and contains the large opening where the spinal cord enters the brain,
the foramen magnum.

occipito-frontalis

frontalis Late Latin, of the forehead < *frons, frontis* Latin,
forehead; origin of the English word 'front'
The occipitofrontales are the scalp muscles, a pair of broad muscles covering the
top of the skull. They permit scalp tissue to be pulled back over the skull bones,
thus raising the eyebrows and contributing to other facial movements.

oc-clusal

ob > oc up + *cludere* Latin, to close
Occlusal is a frequent adjective in dentistry to refer to the closing contact
between teeth of the upper and lower jaws. Occlusion or occlusal harmony is
the natural relationship between teeth that meet in this way. Malocclusion (*male*
Latin, badly) is any abnormal contact between upper and lower teeth. But in
anatomy, an occlusion is a blockage of any passageway in the body. Blood
vessels can be variously occluded.

oc-cult

ob > oc very, thoroughly + *cultus* Latin past participle, hidden
Occult blood is hidden from ordinary view. Traces of occult blood in the stool
are diagnostic of bleeding in the digestive tract. During birth, an occult prolapse
of the umbilical cord, in which the cord sticks out beside or ahead of the
presenting part of the fetus, must be corrected.

oculus

oculus Latin, eye

oculus dexter (OD)

dexter Latin, right, on the right side, right-handed. Thus, dexterity, with its general meaning of using both hands well

Oculus dexter is medical chart shorthand for the right eye.

oculus sinister (OS)

sinister Latin, left, on the left side, left-handed

In the ancient Roman magic practice of augury, foretelling the future by a variety of preposterous means, the left hand was not used because it was considered unlucky and of evil omen, hence sinister acquired its later meanings of unlucky and evil. *Oculus sinister* for the Romans was the evil eye, a concept still alive today in the rural Italian term, *malocchio*, the evil eye (*occhio* < *oculus*).

Oculus sinister is the left eye.

in-ocul-ate

in Latin, in + *oculus* eye + *ate* common verb ending. Inoculate is, literally, to make an eye, but *oculus* here means bud, and the English verb came from Medieval Latin *inoculare*, to graft, a term in medieval horticulture.

To inoculate is to inject a substance into the body to force an immune response to disease. The substance injected, the inoculum, may be a toxin, a live or killed virus or bacterium, or an immune serum.

odonto-

odous, odontos Greek, tooth, akin to Latin *dens, dentis*, and to English *tooth*. Thus, odontology is the scientific study of the teeth and other structures of the oral cavity.

odonto-genic

odous, odontos tooth + *genikos* Greek, making, producing

Odontogenic means 'developing in tissues that make teeth'.

odontogenic fibro-sarc-oma

fibra Latin, thread; the *fibro-* prefix denotes fibers or fibrous tissues + *sarx, sarkos* Greek, flesh + *oma* tumor

Odontogenic fibrosarcoma is an invasive cancer of the jaw made up of malignant connective tissue that begins in tooth germ or another inner tissue of a tooth.

odont-oid process

odous, odontos tooth + *eides* Greek, form, hence *-oid* means 'shaped like'

The tooth-like odontoid process sticks out from the upper surface of the second cervical vertebra. It is the pivot on which the first cervical vertebra or atlas rotates, permitting the head to turn.

olfactory

olfacere, olefacere- Latin, to cause to smell, to apply a perfume or scent; *olere* Latin, to smell, akin to Latin noun for smell, *odor* + *factor* Latin, maker of + *y* adjectival suffix

The olfactory center is a complex of neurons in the brain that amass stimuli and create the sense of smell. The olfactory nerves in the upper mucous membranes of the nose carry electrochemical impulses that can be decoded in the olfactory center and olfactory cortex as smells. In the nasal epithelium are bipolar nerve cells called olfactory receptors. Their neural axons eventually turn into olfactory nerve fibers.

oligo-

oligos Greek adjective, few, not many, a small quantity of, fewer than normal

oligo-dactyly

oligos fewer than normal + *dactylos* Greek, finger, toe + *y* noun ending

Oligodactyly is a congenital absence of one or more fingers or toes.

oligo-spermia

oligos fewer than normal + *sperma* Greek, seed, semen

Oligospermia is too few spermtazoa in semen, insuffucient to insure a normal chance of fertilizing an ovum.

-oid

eidos Greek, form, shape, so the suffix oid = similar to, shaped like

chondr-oid

chondros Greek, cartilage + oid

Chondroid means ' like cartilage' or cartilaginous. For example, a chondrolipoma is a tumor made up of fatty tissue (*lipos* Greek, fat) and chondroid tissue.

delt-oid

delta fourth letter of the Greek alphabet, equivalent to *d* + oid

Deltoid means shaped like the Greek capital letter delta, which is Δ, in other words, triangular. For example, the deltoid, the triangular muscle of each shoulder cap. Bodybuilders work on their 'delts'.

hy-oid

hu colloquial Greek name for upsilon, a letter of the Greek alphabet that resembles a U + oid

Hyoid means shaped like the Greek letter upsilon, U-shaped. The hyoid is a U-shaped bone at the root of the tongue.

lambd-oid

lambda, the letter *l* in the Greek alphabet + oid

Lambdoid is L-shaped like the Greek letter lambda, e.g. the lambdoid suture, the line of juncture between the occipital and parietal bones of the skull, vaguely L-shaped.

-oma

-oma, -omatos Greek noun suffix, has medical meaning of benign or malignant tumor, or swelling

hemat-oma

haima, haimatos Greek, blood + *oma* tumor, swelling
A hematoma is clotted blood that has escaped from its vessels and collected in an organ, tissue or space. A bruise is a hematoma.

circum-orbital hematoma

circum Latin, around + *orbitalis* Late Latin, pertaining to the orbis < *orbis* Latin, the spherical cavity holding the eyeball and its nerves, vessels and muscles < *orbs* Latin, sphere, globe
A circumorbital hematoma is bruising of tissue in a circular pattern around the eye, often from a blow or punch; a black eye, a shiner.

carcin-oma

karkinos Greek, crab, cancer
Carcinoma is a cancerous or malignant tumor. The adjectival form is carcinomatous. A synonym of carcinoma is cancer.

omentum

omentum Latin, fat, bowels, plural *omenta*; origin obscure but possibly a contraction of a putative form like *abdomen-tum*. The Greek equivalent was *epi-ploon* 'over-fold' and appears as the synonym for omentum, epiploon, and for the adjective 'omental' in anatomical phrases like the epiploic foramen, the opening between the greater and the lesser peritoneal cavities.
An omentum is a fold of the peritoneum, like a large purse of tissue that partially encloses, attaches, and supports the stomach and nearby viscera. The greater omentum hangs down from a curvature of the stomach and drapes over the intestines like an apron. The tissue is fat-filled and insulatory, acting to keep heat inside it. Its mucosa make it slippery, so that it prevents friction between abdominal organs. The lesser omentum below covers the front and sides of the stomach and part of the upper duodenum. Sometimes, as in omentoplasty, small swatches of tissue from the greater omentum are used as grafting material in rejoining other body tissues.

omphalo-

omphalos Greek, navel, belly button, akin to Latin *umbilicus*

omphalo-tomy

omphalos navel + *tome* Greek, a surgical cutting + *y* noun ending

Omphalotomy is the necessary division of the umbilical cord at birth.

omphalo-cele

omphalos navel + *kele* Greek, hernia

Omphalocele is a birth defect, a congenital hernia of the navel. Portions of internal abdominal muscles or bowels protrude through a weakness at or near the navel. Surgical repair is effective.

onco-

ogkos Greek, mass, bulk, tumor

onco-logy

ogkos tumor + *logos* study of

Oncology is the study of tumors including cancerous or malignant tumors, and an oncologist is in popular speech a cancer specialist.

onco-genic

ogkos tumor + *genikos* Greek, making, producing

Oncogenic is an adjective applied to certain viruses. It means 'causing tumors'. Oncogenesis is the production, induction, or formation of tumors (*genesis* Greek, birth, start).

onco-RNA-virus

An onco-RNA-virus is one that contains ribonucleic acid (RNA) and produces tumors.

onycho-

onyx, onychos Greek, claw, talon, fingernail, toenail

onycho-gryph-osis (also spelled onychogryposis)

onyx, onychos fingernail, toenail + *grypos* Greek, curved, hooked + *osis* diseased condition

Onychogryphosis is hypertrophy (overgrowth) of the fingernails or toenails, with thickened, inwardly curving nails that resemble claws. The root *gryph-* from *gryp* is influenced by the mythical bird, the griffin, or gryphon, with its large gripping talons.

onycho-lysis

onyx, onychos fingernail, toenail + *lysis* Greek, a loosening of

In onycholysis, nails become detached from their nail beds, due to injury, fungal and bacterial infections, and as a symptom of some skin disorders like psoriasis and severe dermatitis of the hands.

onycho-phagy

onyx, onychos fingernail, toenail + *phagos* Greek, eater, glutton + *y* noun ending

Onychophagy is the neurotic habit of biting (sometimes eating) the fingernails.

oo-

oon Greek, egg, a synonym and akin to the Latin *ovum*. In English medical words with this root, both *o*'s are pronounced.

oo-cyte

oon ovum + *kytos* cell

An oocyte is an early form of the ovum, not completely developed. Oocytin is a biochemical instigator in the spermatozoon that is released after the sperm has penetrated the ovum, to trigger formation of the fertilization membrane. An oogonium (*gone* Greek, seed) is the precursor cell, the primitive cell which develops into a mature ovum. An ootid is a ripe ovum after the first of its two stages of maturation.

oophor-

oon ovum + *phoros* Greek, carrying, bearing = *oophoron* Greek, egg-bearer, hence ovary

oophoro-cyst-ec-tomy

oophoron ovary + *kystis* Greek, cyst + *ek* out + *tome* a surgical cutting + *y* noun ending

An oophorocystectomy is the surgical excision of ovarian cysts.

oophoro-salping-ec-tomy

oophoron ovary + *salpinx, salpingos* Greek, trumpet, trumpet-shaped object, hence Fallopian tube, oviduct + *ek* out + *tome* a surgical cutting + *y* noun ending

An oophorosalpingectomy is surgical excision of a Fallopian tube and an ovary. If both tubes and ovaries are removed, the female becomes sterile, and menopausal symptoms begin. Hormone therapies lessen the menopausal symptoms. The surgery is performed to remove cancers, abscesses, cysts and highly inflamed local tissues.

ophthalmo-

ophthalmos Greek, eye

ophthalm-ia neonatorum

ophthalmos eye + *ia* medical condition; *neonatorum* Latin, genitive plural of *neo-natus* newborn = of newborn babies

Ophthalmia neonatorum is a common type of inflammation of the conjunctiva of the eye in newborns who contract the disorder from the mother while passing through the birth canal. Gonococcal ophthalmia is a serious form contracted from a mother infected with gonorrhea. The regular practice of placing a few drops of a silver nitrate solution in the eyes of newborns kills the offending micro-organisms. So do many topical antibiotics.

ophthalmo-log-ist

ophthalmos eye + *logos* study of + *-istes* Greek agent noun suffix, equivalent to English *-er*, one who performs an act

An ophthalmologist is a doctor who specializes in diseases of the eye and eye surgery. An ophthalmoscope is a medical instrument for viewing interior structures of the eyeball.

-opia

-opia scientific Latin and Greek, disordered condition of sight < *ops, opos* Greek, eye

ambly-opia

amblys Greek, dull, dim + *opia* disordered condition of sight
Amblyopia is a dimness of vision with no eye lesion.

my-opia

myein Greek, to squint + *opia* disordered condition of sight
Myopia is nearsightedness, when vision is better for objects nearer the eye than for those farther away. A sufferer is a myope.

nyct-al-opia

nyx, nyktos Greek, night + *alaos* Greek, blind + *opia* disordered condition of sight
Nyctalopia is night blindness as a disease. This reduced-from-normal ability to see in faint light is symptomatic in diseases like retinitis pigmentosa and vitamin A deficiency. Tobacco-smokers often exhibit nyctalopia.

presby-opia

presbys Greek, old + *opia* disordered condition of sight
In presbyopia, old age makes the crystalline lens of the eye less elastic, less able to focus light rays, hence the eye loses some of its power of accommodation when a person tries to see objects at a distance.

optic

optikos Greek, pertaining to sight
Optics is the scientific study of light and vision. An optician is a technician who fits eyeglasses, grinds lenses and sells frames. An optometrist (*metristes* Greek, measurer) holds a doctor of optometry degree, measures vision, and determines if non-drug therapies may help vision, i.e. lenses and prisms.

optic chiasm, chiasma

optikos Greek, pertaining to sight; *chiasma* Greek, making an X, an X-like junction, anything resembling the Greek letter chi, written χ

At the optic chiasm in the brain, the optic nerve fibers cross to make an X-shape.

optic glioma

optikos Greek, pertaining to sight; *glia* Medieval Greek, glue + *oma* tumor

A glioma is any tumor made of glial cells, sticky neural cells that support connective tissue. Sites of optic glioma include anywhere on an optic nerve, but especially at the optic chiasm in the brain. Among the symptoms may be severe squinting, cross-eyedness, a pop-eyed stare and even paralysis of eye muscles.

orchi-, orchio-, orchid-

orchidion Greek, single testicle, diminutive form of *orchis*, *orchios* testicles

The orchid plant was named by an early Greek botanist who thought the pseudobulbs or the underground roots of one Mediterranean species of orchid looked like human testicles.

crypt-orchid-ism

kryptos Greek, hidden + *orchidion* testicle + *ismos* noun suffix, a condition

Cryptorchidism is also called undescended testicle(s), when one or both testes do not descend into the scrotum. The testes are formed in the abdominal cavity and do not migrate down until late in fetal life, into the inguinal canal and then down into their carrying bag of skin, the scrotum.

They operate efficiently at a lower temperature than other organs and so are carried outside the body. About ten percent of boys are born with one or both testes not yet descended. Most testes descend within the first few weeks after birth. If they do not, pituitary hormone supplements induce descent. If that fails, surgical means are effective.

orchido-pexy, orchiopexy

orchidion testicle + *pexis* Greek, a fastening to, a fixation + *y* noun ending

Orchidopexy is the usual surgical solution to cryptorchidism, the fixing in the scrotal sac of an undescended testis, or both testes. The testicle is transferred from its site of undescent to the scrotal sac and sutured in place there.

orch-itis

orchis, orchios testicles + *itis* inflammation of

Orchitis is inflammation of the testes, often before or during the mumps, but many other less frequent causes include cancer, gonorrhea and syphilis.

orexia

orexis Greek, appetite

Orexia is a rare synonym for appetite. Its compounds are more common in medical literature.

an-orexia

an not + *orexis* appetite + *ia* medical condition

Anorexia is loss of appetite. When it leads to emaciation and is caused by emotional problems, the disorder may be called anorexia nervosa.

orexi-genic

orexis appetite + *genikos* making, producing

An orexigenic agent stimulates the appetite. Many so-called *digestives* of folk medicine act in this manner, some most effectively.

par-orex-ia

para Greek, outside of, beside, beyond what is normal, hence, often, with a sense of abnormal + *orexis* appetite + *ia* medical condition

Parorexia is a technical term in psychiatry for a perversion of the appetite, either wanting to eat only one kind of food, or wanting to eat items not fit to eat such as paper or wood.

organ

organum Latin, engine < *organon* Greek, engine, thing that does work < *ergon* work

An organ is a structural unit of the body, often with several kinds of tissue, designed for one or two chief functions, such as the lungs, the kidneys, the liver, or the eye. In biochemistry, organic refers to compounds that contain carbon, and often participate in life processes. Organic disease refers to a disorder whose symptoms include detectable changes in an organ or organs.

organelle

organ + *elle* French diminutive suffix indicating extreme smallness

In histology and molecular biochemistry, organelles are tiny particles of living substance found in cells, for example mitochondria, lysosomes and centrioles.

org-asm

orgasmos Greek, literally of the male, swelling with lust, having an erect penis < *orge* lust, passion

Orgasm is sexual climax, strong involuntary contractions of the muscles of the genitals; in the male, ejaculation of semen accompanies orgasm.

oral, ori-

oralis Late Latin, of the mouth < *os, oris* mouth. The Greek equivalent is *stoma, stomatos*, also widely used in medical terms. Oral is of, for, or by the mouth.

orbicularis oris

orbicularis Latin adjective, pertaining to a little circle < *orbiculum* Latin, a little circle < *orbis* a circle; *oris* Latin, of the mouth

The orbicularis oris muscle is the complex sphincter muscle surrounding the mouth. It helps close the lips, permits puckering and protruding the lips. When one says, 'Hoot' the contraction is obvious.

ori-fice

orificium Latin, making a mouth or a mouth-like
opening <*facere* to make
An orifice is a mouth-like opening, an aperture, an entrance, an exit. The oral
orifice is the opening into the mouth. The external urethral orifice is the
opening through which urine is voided, and in the male, semen, also called the
urethral meatus.

ortho-

orthos Greek, straight, correct, upright, erect

orth-odont-ist

orthos straight + *odous, odontos* Greek, tooth + *istes* one who
performs an action
An orthodontist is literally a straight-tooth-ist, a dentist who specializes in
correcting poorly positioned teeth, malocclusions etc.

ortho-ped-ics

orthos straight + *paidikos* Greek, pertaining to children <*pais,
paidos* child
Orthopedic surgery treats deformities of the musculo-skeletal system, originally
in children, now in all patients.

ortho-pnea

orthos standing upright or straight + *pnoe* Greek, breathing
Orthopnea is difficulty in breathing except when standing upright or sitting up
in bed at night, often seen in patients with congestive heart failure or some lung
disorders. Acute symptoms include cyanosis (see entry), and the patient bracing
himself or herself against a solid object to make their respiratory exertions less
of a struggle.

os

os, oris Latin, mouth, plural *ora*
Os is a formal anatomical name for a mouth-like opening. Thus, os uteri is the
mouth of the uterus.

os

os, ossis Latin, bone, plural *ossa*
Os confusingly is also the formal anatomical name for a bone. This ought to be changed. Of the long list of formal anatomical names for bones, a few are: os calcis, the heel bone, and os pubis, the pubic bone.

os-culate

osculum Latin, little mouth < *os, oris* mouth + *ate* common verb ending
To osculate is literally to make a little mouth, hence to kiss.

os-cill-ate

oscillum Latin, a little mouth < *os, oris* mouth + *ate* common verb ending
An *oscillum* was a little mouth, then came to mean a little face, in particular a little mask of the wine god Bacchus. Romans hung *oscilla* on branches in orchards and vineyards to ensure the god of wine granted a bountiful harvest. These *oscilla* moved in the wind; they oscillated. Thus the word oscilloscope, in which oscillating lines display data variations on a cathode ray tube.

osmo-

osme Greek, odor, smell

osmesis

osmesis Greek, act of smelling
Osmesis is the sense of smell, equivalent to its Latin-based synonym, olfaction. Another related term is osmesthesia, to denote the power to perceive and distinguish various odors.

osmo-receptor

osme Greek, odor + *receptor* Latin, thing that receives
An osmoreceptor is a group of cells in the brain receptive to odor stimuli. Osmoreceptors for sensitivity to osmotic pressure in the serum of the brain lie in the hypothalamus. Note that osmosis derives from *osmos* Greek, push, impulse. Osmosis is the passage of solvent molecules through membranes, from

solutions of low concentration to those of higher concentration of a particular solute. In biochemistry, the solvent is water.

osseo-, ossi-

osseus Latin, bony < *os, ossis* a bone
Osseous is bony.

ossi-fication

os, ossis a bone + *-ficatio, ficationis* Latin, a making into < *facere* to make, to do
Ossification occurs when cartilage turns into bone in early childhood. Certain later ossifications of softer tissue are pathological.

ossicle

ossiculum Latin, little bone < *os, ossis* a bone
An ossicle is literally a little bone, but specifically, one of the three little bones of the middle ear. These auditory ossicles are the malleus (Latin, hammer), the incus (Latin, anvil), and the stapes (Latin, stirrup of a saddle). In conjunction, these three ossicles act like a tiny amplifier to conduct sound waves through the middle to the inner ear.

osteo-

osteon Greek, a bone

end-osteum

endon Greek, within, inside + *osteon* a bone
Endosteum is the tissue that lines the bone marrow cavity inside a bone.

osteo-malacia

osteon Greek, bone + *malakia* softness
Osteomalacia is an adult form of rickets, in which bones become so soft that their flexibility and brittleness cause deformities.

osteo-por-osis

osteon a bone + *poros* Greek, a passage, a pore + *osis* diseased condition

In osteoporosis, bones lose calcium, become less dense, more brittle, more porous and more subject to fracture. Calcium supplements may counter this tendency.

osteo-tome

osteon a bone + *tomos* Greek, knife, slicer, cutter

An osteotome is a surgical knife used to cut, divide, or section bone tissue.

peri-osteum

peri Greek, around, surrounding + *osteon* a bone

Periosteum is the hard, fibrous outer tissue covering bones.

oto-

ous, otos Greek, ear

ot-itis

ous, otos ear + *itis* inflammation of

Otitis is inflammation of the ear, labeled to indicate which portion of the ear is inflamed. Otitis externa is any inflammation in the structures of the external auditory canal. Otitis interna is inflammation of the labyrinth of the ear. Otitis media, common in childhood, is a possibly more serious inflammation of the inner ear, caused frequently by bacteria or viruses, with accumulation of serous fluid which does not drain away because the Eustachian tube is blocked. Sometimes a tympanostomy (making a small opening in the eardrum to insert a draining catheter) is carried out; sometimes more invasive surgical means are necessary. Otitis media is commonly preceded by infections of the upper respiratory tract.

oto-rhino-laryngo-logy

ous, otos ear + *rhis, rhinos* Greek, nose + *larynx, laryngos* Greek, throat + *logos* study of

Otorhinolaryngology is the scientific study of functions, diseases and treatments of the ear, nose and throat.

par-otid

para Greek, beside + *-otid* combining form of *ous, otos* Greek, ear

The parotid glands are beside the ear; the largest salivary glands are compressed when one chews, and saliva pours through the parotid duct into the mouth.

ovum

ovum Latin, egg, plural *ova*

A human ovum is the female reproductive cell that is fertilized by a spermatozoon to create a new human embryo. Oval is egg-shaped. The ovary is one of two glands in the female that produce ova. Ovarian is pertaining to an ovary. To ovulate is to discharge a mature egg from an ovary.

ovi-duct

ovum Latin, egg + *ductus* New Latin, canal to conduct fluids

An oviduct is one of the two Fallopian tubes which conduct an egg from an ovary to the uterus.

ovule

ovulum Latin, little egg

An ovule is a young egg forming in its follicle in the ovary (*folliculus* Latin, little bag).

pachy-

pachys Greek, thick; thus a pachyderm is an animal with thick skin, like an elephant

pachy-derma vesicae

pachys thick + *derma* skin; *vesicae* Latin, of the bladder

Pachyderma vesicae is a pathological thickening of the mucous membrane lining the urinary bladder.

pachy-lepto-meningitis

pachys thick + *leptos* thin + *meninx, meningis* Latin from *menigx* Greek, brain membrane + *itis* inflammation of

Three meninges or membranes wrap around and protect the brain and spinal cord. The tough outer meninx, singular of meninges, is the dura mater, the thickest, prompting the *pachy* root in pachyleptomeningitis. The middle meninx is the arachnoid (*arachn-oides* Greek, netted like a spider's web). The pia mater is the innermost layer of the three meninges. Nearest the brain, it is rich in blood vessels and thin. It prompts the *lepto* root in pachyleptomeningitis, or 'thick-and-thin-layer meningitis'. Inflammation of these vital membranes is seen in various forms of meningitis.

pachy-onych-ia con-genita

pachys thick + *onyx, onychis* Greek, fingernail, toenail + *ia* medical condition; *con-genita* Latin = *con* < *cum* with + *genitus* born

Pachyonychia congenita is an inborn abnormality of the genes that regulate the formation of keratin, the hard, fibrous protein in nails, hair and horny tissue. Pachyonychia presents as grossly thickened finger- and toenails, thick skin on the palms of the hands and feet, hyperkeratosis (excess production of keratin) at the knees and elbows, and leukoplakia of mucous membranes. Leukoplakia is hard, white spots and patches that may split and may become malignant.

palat-, palato-

palatum Latin, derivation obscure, the palate

The palate or roof of the mouth separates the mouth from the nasal cavity. It is a horizontal structure made of muscles, membranes, and supported by bones. The palate has two parts, the hard and the soft palate. The hard palate in front is formed by the floor of the upper jawbone. The soft palate behind the back teeth is a fibrous span of tissue whose muscles draw it up to close the back of the nose when one swallows. Palatine bones are small bones that form part of the floor of the nose. When palate means a discriminating sense of taste, it is, anatomically, a misnomer. Only a very few taste buds are on the soft palate. Most are on the tongue.

cheilo-gnatho-palato-schisis

cheilos Greek, lip + *gnathos* jaw + *palatum* palate + *schisis* a splitting of

Cheilognathopalatoschisis is a congenital irregularity in which there is a cleft or split in the lips, in the upper jaw, and in the hard and soft palates.

cleft palate, palato-plasty, palato-rrhaphy, palato-schisis

Cleft palate or palatoschisis (*schisis* Greek, abnormal splitting) is a congenital defect. The two halves of the palate fail to fuse properly. Results range from a tiny groove at the edge of the lip, to total midline separation of the palate. Plastic surgery corrects this. Often palatoplasty (*plastia* a forming by means of surgery) is an operation in two parts, each years apart. In severe cases, where the baby cannot suck milk easily, an early palatorrhaphy (*rrhaphe* surgical suturing) permits palate and lip function. Later, further plastic surgery of a cosmetic nature improves appearance.

palpate

palpare Latin, to stroke with the palm of the hand < *palpus* palm of the hand

To palpate is to examine medically with the hands external parts of the patient's body, feeling for size, firmness and general consistency of parts as part of initial diagnosis of certain diseases or abnormalities. Thus palpable is detectable by touch, and palpation is the noun. In light-touch palpation, the outline of organs of the abdomen may be determined by gently palpating the abdominal wall with the fingers. Palpatory percussion is tapping the body's exterior and detecting vibrations against the palm of the examiner's hand.

palpebra

palpebra Latin, eyelid, literally 'the part that flutters'. See next entry.

In anatomy, the palpebra inferior is the lower eyelid and the palpebra superior is the upper eyelid. Palpebral cartilages are flat, slender plates of cartilage-like tissue that form the supporting framework of the eyelid. To palpebrate is to wink.

palpitate

palpitare Latin, to throb, to flutter; frequentative verb from *palpare* to stroke, to pet

When the heart beats rapidly, it is said to palpitate. Cardiac palpitations are usually detected by the patient during strong emotional arousal. Palpitations also accompany some cardiac abnormalities.

pan-

pas, pasa, pan Greek adjective, all. Shown here are the masculine, feminine, and neuter singular; the genitive is *pantos*

Panchromatic film registers all the colors. Pandemonium may include all the devils. A panoroma includes all the view. A pantomime performance is all mime.

pan-acea

pan all + *akea* Greek, cures, plural of *akos* cure

A panacea is an all-cure or a cure-all, an imaginary universal remedy.

pancreas

pan all + *kreas* Greek, meat. To early Greek hunters, the pancreas was 'all meat', thus edible as sweetbreads.

The pancreas is a compound gland located behind the stomach. It secretes pancreatic juice containing important digestive enzymes like trypsin (see entry) which enter the pancreatic duct, then the common bile duct, and empty into the duodenum. The pancreas is also an endocrine gland that secretes hormones like insulin and glucagon.

papill-oma

papilla Latin, nipple, teat, pap + *oma* tumor

In anatomy, a papilla can be anything vaguely nipple-shaped. A papilloma is a benign, epithelial tumor with many nipple-shaped branches or lobules.

papule

papula Latin, pimple

A papule is a skin lesion that is small, hard and raised up; for example, an acne pimple with no pus. The classic skin spots of chickenpox are papules. A weal is a large papule, usually a single, itchy skin lesion with a red margin and a paler center. It is smooth, raised, swollen and is often seen in allergic reactions.

para-

para Greek, alongside of, beside

The prefix can also mean 'abnormal' as in paranoia (*nous* Greek, mind) and can mean 'closely resembling' as in paratyphoid and parainfluenza virus.

para-lysis

para abnormal + *lysis* Greek, a loosening, a weakening

The Greeks used the word *paralysis* to mean any abnormal weakening of the limbs. Paralysis is loss of motor or sensory function in a part.

para-medic

para beside + *medicus* Latin, physician

Paramedical personnel trained in supportive emergency medical procedures work beside or along with medical personnel like doctors and nurses. Paramedic is the agent noun. Paramedics may include, for example, X-ray technicians and audiologists.

para-plegia

para beside, on one side + *plegia* suffering a stroke

A paraplegic patient is paralyzed in the lower body including the legs.

par-otid

para beside + *ous, otos* Greek, ear

Parotid means beside the ear, e.g. the parotid glands.

-para

para scientific Latin, female parent < *parere* to bear children

A para is a woman who has given birth to one or more viable offpsring. Viable here means able to live outside the mother's body. Other words using this suffix include nullipara (*nullus* Latin, not), a woman who has never borne a viable child. A unipara is a woman who has given birth to one viable offsring. Primipara is also a term for a woman who has borne one viable child. A secundipara has borne two viable children. A multipara has borne two or more.

parietal

parietalis Late Latin, of a wall < *paries* wall, plural *parietes*

Parietal means pertaining to the inner walls of a body cavity, as opposed to visceral, pertaining to the viscera or contents of a body cavity (*viscera* Latin, guts, intestines). The parietal bones of the cranium are the two bones that form the top and the upper sides of the skull. The cranium is the part of the skull that encloses the brain. The parietal lobes of the cerebral cortex are protected by the parietal bones of the skull. These lobes are involved in recording sensory messages.

patella

patella Latin, saucer, small pan

In anatomy, the patella is the kneecap. The human kneecap does *not* look like a small pan, but the Latin name is 600 years old. The kneecap bone is actually an irregular rectangle in shape.

chondro-malacia patellae or runner's knee

chondros cartilage + *malakia* Greek, softening + *patellae* Latin, of the kneecap

Athletes who strain a knee by the constant pounding shocks of running may suffer chondromalacia patellae, in which articular cartilage degenerates.

patellar reflex

patellaris New Latin, of the kneecap

Patellar reflex is a medical term for knee jerk. Tapping lightly on the tendon below the patella with a rubber mallet produces a contraction of the quadriceps

274

muscle and a slight kicking outward of the lower leg. The response is a very general indication of neural function.

patency, patent

patens Latin, standing wide open, clear, unobstructed (of passages)

In many diagnostic procedures, the physician checks the patency of airways, tubes, and other passageways. In severe constipation, is the anus patent? In paroxysmal choking, which airways are patent?

patent medicine

In the phrase 'patent medicine', patent is the same adjective as in the above entry, but it derives from a British legal term, where letters patent were legal documents open to be read by the public, and later referred to patents by which owners and inventors secured exclusive legal right to make and sell inventions. Patent medicines are those able to be trademarked and sold without a prescription, also called proprietary drugs.

patho-

pathos Greek, feeling, disease; the noun suffix is *-pathy*. This is one of the most frequently occurring roots in medical words.

angio-pathy

angio vessel + *pathos* disease + *y* noun ending

Angiopathy is any disease of the arteries, veins or lymph vessels.

a-pathy

a no + *pathos* feeling + *y* noun ending

Apathy means 'lack of emotion, listless indifference to ordinary concerns of living'. *Pathos* in Greek first meant 'deep feeling' then 'disease'.

cardio-myo-pathy

kardia heart + *mys, myos* Greek, muscle + *pathos* disease + *y* noun ending

A cardiomyopathy is any disease of heart muscle.

encephalo-myelo-pathy

enkephalos the brain + *myelos* spinal cord + *pathos* disease + *y*
noun ending

An encephalomyelopathy is any disease of the brain and spinal cord.

myo-pathy

mys, myos Greek, muscle + *pathos* disease + *y* noun ending

Myopathy is any disease of muscle tissue.

osteopath

osteon Greek, a bone + *pathos* disease

An osteopath is a physician who specializes in the relationship of organs and the
musculoskeletal system, although osteopathy uses all the other recognized forms
of medical therapy and diagnosis. Some structural defects are correctable by
osteopathic manipulation.

patho-gen

pathos disease + *gen-* Greek root, making, producing

A pathogen is any micro-organism, like a bacterium, capable of producing
disease. The development of a disease from such a specific cause is pathogenesis.

patho-logy

pathos disease + *logos* study of + *y* noun ending

Pathology is the study of diseases, particularly of the causes and effects of disease
on the tissues of the human body. Pathologists work in laboratories analysing
diseased cells and tissues. Pathologists can specialize in autopsy or forensic
pathology (*forensis* Latin, of the forum, of the law court, hence related to legal
matters). Clinical and surgical pathology are also specializations. Pathology has a
looser, secondary meaning as well, referring to the condition produced by a
disease, or, in even looser medical parlance, pathology can be a synonym for
disease.

sym-pathy

sym Greek, assimilated form of *syn* with, together + *pathos*
feeling, disease + *y* noun ending

Sympathy in its prime meaning is feeling with another person or persons. For that division of the autonomous nervous system called sympathetic, see the *sympathetic* entry. Sympathetic irritation is common in those body parts that are paired. Infection in one eye may lead to sympathetic symptoms in the other eye.

pector-

pectus, pectoris Latin, chest, thorax

pectoral muscles

pectoralis New Latin adjective, of the chest
The major or greater pectoral muscle fans out across the chest. It pulls the arm in toward the body, helps pull the arm down when one does the breast stroke while swimming, and also pulls the arm up when one climbs by hand. The pectoralis minor or smaller pectoral muscle draws the shoulder forward and down, and helps raise the ribs when one breathes in quickly.

angina pectoris

angina Latin, a squeezing pain + *pectoris* of the chest
Angina pectoris is a severe chest pain due to reduced oxygen supply to heart muscle. The pain typically radiates down the left arm and is accompanied by a choking feeling. It is often due to fatty plaque coating the walls of the coronary arteries and thus narrowing the lumen of those arteries, hence denying blood to the heart during times of high cardiac activity such as exercise, cold, or stress. Rest from such exertions and vasodilator drugs may bring relief, before therapy for the underlying causes is begun.

pelvis

pelvis Latin, washbasin, wide bowl
The pelvis looks like a bowl of bone. It includes the lower part of the backbone and the two hipbones. This pelvic girdle encloses and protects the lower intestines and most reproductive organs, and supports, as a bowl might, the weight of innards that occupy the thoracic and abdominal cavities.

pelvi-metry

pelvis + *metron* Greek, device that measures + *y* noun ending
Pelvimetry is measuring the diameter and hence the capacity of the pelvis. A pelvimeter may determine if a small pelvis will cause difficulty to a woman during childbirth.

-penia

penia Greek, poverty, need, lack of
This suffix is common in blood work and pathology reports.

cyto-penia

kytos Greek, cell, blood cell + *penia* lack of
Cytopenia is a lack of a sufficient number of blood cells, a deficiency in cell quantity.

leuko-cyto-penia, leukopenia

leukos Greek, white + *kytos* blood cell + *penia* lack of
Leukopenia is an abnormal decrease in the number of white blood cells. It is seen in several pathologic conditions, including leukopenic leukemia.

thrombo-cyto-penia

thrombos Greek, lump, blood clot + *kytos* blood cell + *penia* lack of
Thrombocytes are blood platelets, the smallest of the blood cells, disk-shaped, and necessary for blood coagulation. Thrombocytopenia, often due to bone marrow diseases, is a frequent cause of abnormal bleeding and hemorrhagic disorders.

penis

penis Latin, tail, male sex organ
The Indo-European and very widespread root is *pe* as seen in Greek *peos* penis, Sanskrit *pasas* penis, and even the English nursery term for urine, pee (not, as many dictionaries suppose, a Victorian contraction of *piss*, but in fact of much older origin). Since the word meant the tail of an animal in early Latin, as well as the human sex organ, penis is often described in dictionaries as derived from Latin *pendere*, to hang down. It is not. There is better linguistic evidence that the Latin reflex of the Indo-European root has been influenced by or blended with another Latin root, *pene*, inside, seen in our verb 'to penetrate', to go inside. Thus penis is *pene* + *s*, *s* being the common male nominative suffix in Latin. Therefore the true etymological meaning of penis is best stated as the part that goes inside, that is, inside the vagina. Penile is the adjective pertaining to the penis.

A Greek synonym, *phallos*, produces many medical terms relating to the penis, like ithyphallic, phallic and phalloplasty. The Latin form *phallus* is a synonym in medical terminology. The Greek *phallos* was probably in origin an affectionate diminutive of the Indo-European root, that is *pe*, with the root aspirated to *ph*, originally not an *f*-sound in Greek but a *p* followed by a breath + *ll* diminutive marker in many Indo-European languages like Latin, Greek and English + *os* masculine noun ending.

peps-in

pepsis Greek, digestion + *in* noun ending for organic chemical compound

Pepsin is the main enzyme of protein digestion, secreted by gastric glands in the mucosa of parts of the stomach.

peptic ulcer

peptikos Greek adjective, of digestion

Peptic ulcers occur in the digestive tract, anywhere from the lower end of the esophagus to the stomach to the duodenum, where damaged mucosa succumb to gastric acids. Some damage may be caused by bacteria. Drugs that reduce gastric acid levels often provide symptomatic relief.

per

per Latin preposition and prefix, through, in excess, intense

Seen in Latin phrases used in medical vocabulary, like *nil per os*, nothing through the mouth, an order given several hours before some operations and tests, or necessary in some disorders. Per anum, per rectum and per vaginam are used also as euphemisms for 'through the anus', 'through the rectum', and 'through the vagina'. Rarer is per vias naturales, 'using natural ways and methods'.

per-meate

per through + *meare* Latin, to go, to pass. Compare the noun *meatus* used in anatomy to describe a passageway, an entrance, an exit.

A permeable membrane might permit gas to pass through, to permeate, its pores, but not water.

per-fusion

per through + *fusio, fusionis* Latin, a pouring

Perfusion is pouring fluid through the vessels of an organ. For example, a perfusionist operates a heart–lung machine that oxygenates blood outside the body. Such blood is perfused with oxygen.

peri

peri Greek, around, near, surrounding, similar to Latin *circum*. Loan translations from Greek to Latin sometimes show up in English borrowings, e.g. circumlocution for periphrasis.

peri-cardium

peri surrounding + *kardia* Greek, the heart + *ium* Latin neuter suffix for nouns

The pericardium is a protective fibrous sac around the heart and large heart vessels. The outside layer is tough fiber, the inside serous, that is, it secretes a liquid that lubricates the beating muscles of the heart and prevents friction. Pericarditis is inflammation of this heart sac.

peri-meter

peri around + *metron* Greek, device that measures

A perimeter is a line bounding an area, a measurement around a thing. A perimeter is also a device used by an eye doctor to measure peripheral vision.

peri-toneum

peritonaion Greek, wrapped or stretched around < *peri* around + *tonaion* stretched

The peritoneum is a membrane that lines the abdominal cavity. It is a closed, empty bag. The stomach, intestines, liver, spleen and other viscera are *not* inside it. They are behind it and grow out, so that the peritoneum enfolds the organs and holds them in place. Two layers of the peritoneum join behind the intestines, and the intestines hang down in this fold, kept in place by it. The peritoneum secretes a serous fluid that coats and lubricates the visceral organs so that they can move or be moved without friction. Injury often makes this membrane self-adhering.

periton-itis

peritoneum + *itis* inflammation of

Peritonitis is inflammation of the peritoneum. Although it has great healing powers, this membrane becomes vulnerable if punctured, for example, from the intestine by a burst appendix. The peritoneal cavity incubates bacteria quickly. Women suffer peritonitis more than men, since the Fallopian tubes open directly into the cavity, and infection may spread from the female reproductive organs to the peritoneum. A perforated gastric ulcer may leak acid on the membrane, inflaming the tissue. Peritonitis, when it heals, may lead to adhesions and a bowel obstruction.

-pexy

pexis Greek, a fastening to, a fixation

nephro-pexy

nephros Greek, kidney + *pexis* a fastening + *y* noun ending
Nephropexy is the rare procedure of fixing a floating kidney by surgically fastening it in place.

retino-pexy

retina + *pexis* a fastening + *y* noun ending
The retina is a mesh of nerve fibers and their light-sensitive endings lining the back of the eye. For the retina to function, it must be evenly, smoothly attached to the underlying choroid layer. A detached retina, often due to injury, may be fixed back in place by use of a laser beam to make tiny injuries that, as they heal, cause adhesions, which stick the retina back to the choroid layer from which it was detached.

phag-

phagos Greek, eater < *phagein*, to eat

eso-phagus

oiso- Greek dialectic variant of *es* or *eis* which means 'to, toward, into' + *phagos* eater
The esophagus is the muscular gullet tube, about 9 inches long in an adult, that connects the pharynx to the stomach. Peristaltic contractions of encircling muscles help pass food through the esophagus.

phago-cyte

phagos eater + *kytos* cell

A phagocyte is a scavenger cell that ingests foreign cells, debris and disease micro-organisms. Some phagocytes are fixed in liver, spleen and bone marrow. Others, such as leucocytes, circulate in the blood. They play a significant defensive role in immune reactions.

phalang-

phalagx, phalangos Greek, a line of battle; plural *phalanges*

Aristotle first named the bones of the toes and fingers *phalanges* because they were arranged in rows like an ancient Greek infantry battalion.

Each digit (finger or toe) except the thumb and great toe has three phalanges. The proximal phalanx is nearest the hand (*proximus* Latin, nearest). The middle or median phalanx is in the middle. The distal phalanx is at the tip of the finger or toe, most remote from the midline of the body (*distalis* New Latin, remote). The great toe and the thumb have two phalanges.

pharyngo-

pharygx, pharyngos Greek, throat

The pharynx or throat may be divided into three areas. The nasopharynx is the muscular back wall of the nose. When one swallows, the nasopharynx is closed off by a reflexive raising of the soft palate. The cavity of the middle ear joins the nasopharynx by the Eustachian tube, which keeps pressure inside the eardrum equal to pressure outside. The oropharynx is the 'mouth' part of the throat for passage of food and air (*os, oris* Latin, mouth). The laryngopharynx is the part of the throat near the voice box or larynx.

phleb-

phleps, phlebos Greek, a vein

phleb-itis

phleps, phlebos a vein + *itis* inflammation of

Phlebitis is inflammation of a vein, often resulting in blood clots in the vessels that may cause pulmonary embolism or blood clots in the arteries of the lungs (*pulmonarius* Latin, of the lungs and *embolos* Greek, plug, clot).

phlebo-tomy

phleps, phlebos a vein + *tome* a surgical cutting + *y* noun ending
Phlebotomy is cutting into a vein to permit blood-letting, the discredited,
abandoned practice of bleeding a patient to drain off 'the vile humors'.
Phlebotomy is used today, but rarely, in polycythemia (too much blood) to
reduce volume.

photo-

phos, photos Greek, light

photic epilepsy

photikos Greek, pertaining to light; *epi* on + *lepsis* a seizing =
epilepsis a seizure. Aristotle used the form *epilepsia* for any
convulsive seizure.
Photic epilepsy is neural seizure induced by exposure to flickering lights.

photo-refractive kerat-ec-tomy

phos, photos light; *re* Latin, back, up + *fractus* Latin, broken,
bent, deflected; *keras, keratos* Greek, horny substance, the
cornea of the eye + *ek* out + *tome* a surgical cutting
Refraction in the human eye is the bending or deflecting of light rays which
enter the eye straight and are changed from that direction slightly as they pass
through various tissues of the eye, such as the cornea, lens and the aqueous and
vitreous humors. Photorefractive keratectomy can lessen or eliminate certain
kinds of myopia caused by thickening of the cornea. A precisely timed laser
beam removes thin layers of cells from the corneal surface to improve the focus
of entering light rays as they converge on the fovea (see entry).

photo-retin-itis

phos, photos light + retina + *itis* inflammation of
Photoretinitis is inflammation caused by damage to the retina of the eye by
excess exposure to strong sunlight without the protection of effective sunglasses.

photo-taxis

phos, photos light + *taxis* Greek, an arrangement, a putting in order, an ordering, but with the further sense of motion toward or away from

Taxis is an organism's movement in response to a stimulus, either away from or toward the source of the stimulus. Thus phototaxis is movement toward light, as displayed, for example, by moths.

photo-trop-ism

phos, photos light + *tropos* Greek, a turn, a change + *ismos* noun suffix

Phototropism is the growth response toward light of most plants, including certain lower plant forms responsible for some human diseases.

phren-

phren Greek, abdominal diaphragm; it also meant 'the human mind'

phrenic nerve

The phrenic is a general sensory and motor nerve innervating the pericardium, the peritoneum and diaphragm. The diaphragm is a flexible wall of muscle and membrane that separates the abdominal cavity from the chest cavity, and assists breathing.

phren-ology

phren the mind + *logos* Greek, study of

Phrenology is a pseudoscience, the quackery in which bumps on the skull are read as indicators of psychological traits, a diagnostic procedure of charlatans. The English word *frenzy* derives from *phren* as well.

physic-, physio-

physikos Greek, natural, but with the implication of human nature < *physis* nature

Physical is pertaining to the body and to material things; also, related to physics.

physician

physikos Greek, pertaining to nature

Physikoi were early Greek philosophers who thought about nature rather than studying it firsthand. But they did teach medicine, and eventually their name was applied to doctors, first in French, then in Middle English.

physio-logy

physis living nature + *logos* study of

In medicine, physiology is the study of the function of cells, tissues and organs that goes hand-in-hand with anatomy, the study of their structure.

physio-therapy

physis living nature + *therapeia* Greek, literally, the serving and tending of the sick, then 'healing'

Physiotherapy is treating disease by physical methods like massage and exercise. A physiotherapist in a hospital may give patients exercises for stiff joints, breathing routines for the bed-ridden to prevent pneumonia, and flexing tips for muscles after a stroke.

physique

The French adjective became a noun meaning the form of a human body. In the late 20th Century it also signified the unnatural, hypertrophied monstrosity of certain bodybuilders.

pili-, pilo-

pilus Latin, hair

pilar cyst

pilaris New Latin, pertaining to hair; *kystis* Greek, sac, bladder

In medicine, a pathologic cyst is an abnormal sac or pouch, with a wall lined with epithelial cells, and usually distended by liquid or semi-solid material. A pilar cyst springs from the middle epithelium of a hair follicle and presents in the epidermis of the scalp.

pilo-motor reflex

pilus hair + *motor* Latin, mover

The hairs on the surface of the skin erect when stimulated by cold, by emotions like fear and awe and by certain irritants. The operation together of the tiny muscles that erect the hair is the pilomotor reflex.

pilo-nidal cyst

pilus hair + *nidus* bird's nest + cyst

These cysts resemble microscopically little bird's nests filled with hair. They occur most frequently at the midline of the back just above the tailbone. To the naked eye, a pilonidal cyst may look like a hairy dimple. This hair in an enclosing structure is seen in pilonidal sinus, often in the armpit or navel, where a hair has lodged in a fold of skin.

pineal

pinealis Latin, shaped like a *pinea* pine cone < *pinus* a pine tree

The pineal gland is a small, cone-shaped gland anchored to the side of the third ventricle in the center of the brain where it secretes two hormones, melatonin and serotonin, whose functions are just beginning to be understood. Serotonin is produced by many tissues. It is a vasoconstrictor important in control of bleeding. In the brain, serotonin may assist the transmission of nerve impulses between nerves. Melatonin seems to be an endocrine inhibitor. A pinealoma is a tumor of the pineal gland.

plantar wart

planta pedis Latin, the flat part of the foot, the sole. This is the origin of the verb *plantare* which has the prime meaning of putting seeds or seedlings in the ground and firming them into the soil with the sole of the foot; *wearte* Old English, bump, knob, wart, outgrowth.

A wart is a hard, benign tumor of the epidermis caused by a virus. Some warts disappear, others can be removed. The Latin synonym, *verruca*, is used in medical literature. A plantar wart is one on the planta pedis, the sole of the foot. Because of the pressure exerted on it during walking, this wart develops a hard ring, a callus, around its soft central part, and is painful. Cryosurgery and cautery are two therapies.

plasia

plasis Greek, a forming, so in medicine the development and growth of tissue and cells. The adjectival form is *-plastic*.

ana-plasia

ana Greek, without + *plasis* development

In many tumor tissues which are very malignant, the cells are not differentiated and not aligned as they would be normally, and do not function normally. This anaplasia is common to most cancerous tissue.

a-plasia

a not + *plasis* development

Aplasia is lack of development of an organ or tissue, e.g. aplastic anemia.

dys-plasia

dys Greek, negative prefix indicates difficult or disordered function + *plasis* development

Dysplasia is abnormal cell growth, usually pre-malignant, for example in cervical dysplasia, where abnormalities occur in the tissue covering the neck of the uterus. Alloplasia or heteroplasia (*allos* Greek, other, another; *heteros* different) is the growth of tissue in a place where that kind of tissue does not normally occur, for example, bone can be replaced by vascular fibrous tissue in certain disorders.

hyper-plasia

hyper Greek, over, above normal, akin to Latin *super* + *plasis* development

Hyperplasia is excess growth of tissue due to increase in the number of cells.

plastic surgery

plastikos Greek, molding, forming < *plassein* to mold, to form

Plastic surgery is the restoration of visible body defects using tissue from the patient or inert materials.

-plasty

plastia new scientific Greek, a shaping, a forming, with later implication of 'forming by means of surgery'

angio-plasty

angio blood vessel + *plastia* forming by means of surgery
Angioplasty is any surgery of the blood vessels.

glosso-plasty

glossa tongue + *plastia* a shaping, a forming by means of surgery
Glossoplasty is plastic surgery of the tongue, often to repair cleft tongue.

mammo-plasty

mamma breast + *plastia* a surgical shaping
Mammoplasty may be cosmetic surgery to improve the lift or size of breasts or to reconstruct breasts reduced by surgery to remove cancerous tissue.

plexus

plexus Latin, a braid, a plait; plural *plexus*
A plexus is a tangle or intermingling of blood vessels or nerves or lymph vessels, for example, the solar plexus. We've all heard of a boxer getting a hard back slam, or getting punched in the solar plexus. It is also called the celiac plexus (*coeliacus* Latin, abdominal), a network of nerve fibers and ganglia at the upper back of the abdomen. It is named solar after the Latin word *solaris*, of the sun, because sympathetic and parasympathetic nerves radiate out from this plexus like rays from the shining sun.

pleura

pleuron Greek, rib, but its plural *pleura* referred to the membrane covering the lungs; medicine uses the Latin plural, *pleurae*
The visceral pleura is a serous membrane covering the lungs; the parietal pleura lines the chest wall and covers the diaphragm. The pleural cavity is the lung-containing space. The pleural space between the visceral and parietal pleurae holds a lubricating fluid. Pleurisy or pleuritis is inflammation of the

parietal pleura, with severe pain when breathing in. Its causes may be viral, pneumonic, tubercular or malignant.

pneum-

pneumon Greek, the lungs < *pneuma* air, gas, spirit < *pnein* to breathe

pneumon-ia

pneumon the lungs + *ia* medical condition

Hippocrates, the early Greek father of medicine, used pneumonia as the term for any acute inflammation of the lungs, now known to involve fluid and cellular debris exuding through the walls of vessels into surrounding tissue. Pneumonitis is the more apt medical term. Bronchopneumonia starts in the bronchioles. Double pneumonia affects both lungs. Aspiration pneumonia is often due to breathing gastric acid into the lungs during severe vomiting. Viral pneumonia may be due to influenza virus.

poly-

polys Greek, many; Latin equivalent is *multi-*

poly-cystic

polys many + *kystis* Greek, sac + *ikos* adjectival suffix

Polycystic is having many pathological cysts, for example, an ovary with many ovarian cysts is a polycystic ovary.

poly-dactyl-ism

polys many + *daktylos* Greek, digit, finger, toe + *ismos* noun suffix indicating a condition

Polydactylism is a minor birth defect in which the baby has extra fingers or toes.

poly-odont-ia

polys many + *odous, odontos* Greek, tooth + *ia* medical condition

In dentistry, polyodontia is the presence of supernumerary or extra teeth.

post

post Latin, after, behind

The Latin preposition is used directly in several Latin phrases of medicine. Post partum is after birth, e.g. a post partum depression. Post mortem is after death, for example, a coroner's post mortem examination of a corpse. Postoperative is after an operation, after surgery.

post cibum (p.c.)

post after + *cibum* Latin, food, a meal

P.c. means to be taken after meals, as seen on prescriptions for medication, as opposed to a.c., ante cibum, before meals (*ante* Latin, beforehand).

pre-

prae Latin, before, in front of, abnormally early

The prefix is common in medical words, such as precancerous, said of a growth that is not but may become malignant, and precursor, in biochemistry a chemical substance that precedes the production of another later substance whose appearance is chemically linked with its precursor (*cursor* Latin, runner). Prenatal care is that given before birth.

pre-coc-ious

praecox Latin, premature, abnormally early in development

Precocious dentition in children is an abnormally early eruption of permanent teeth. Precocious puberty is sexual maturity in girls before the age of eight, in boys before the age of ten. Dementia praecox is an obsolete term for various forms of schizophrenia, based on the mistaken early belief that it was a kind of premature senility.

pre-puce

prae in front of + *putium* Latin root, penis

The prepuce, or in formal anatomical description the preputium, is the foreskin of the penis, a fold that covers the glans. In the female, a clitoral prepuce, a fold of the labia minora, covers the clitoris. Preputial glands circle the corona of the penis and secrete a lubricating sebum. See *circumcision* entry.

presby-

presbys Greek, old

Presbyterians named their Christian denomination from their use of governing bodies or presbyteries that consisted of clergy and various councils of elders. The comparative of *presbys* in Greek is *presbyteros* 'older, elder' and this word was used by early Christians to name 'elders' and also to refer to orders of priests.

presby-opia

presbys old + *opia* disordered condition of sight

In presbyopia, old age makes the crystalline lens of the eye less elastic, less able to focus light rays, hence the eye loses some of its power of accommodation when a person tries to see objects at a distance. One so affected is a presbyope. Progressive hearing loss due to the normal aging process is presbyacousia (*akousis* Greek, sense of hearing).

pro-

pro Latin and Greek preposition and prefix, in front of, in favor of, on behalf of, on account of, before in time

pro-cess

pro Latin, in front of + *cessus* a going

Process has a special meaning in anatomy. A process is an outgrowth of bone or tissue, a bump or projection out from the surface. For example, the tooth-like odontoid process sticks out from the upper surface of the second cervical vertebra. It is the pivot on which the first cervical vertebra or atlas rotates, permitting the head to turn. Ciliary processes (*cilium* Latin, eyelash, slender hair) are little hair-like ridges on the choroid coat of the eye where the ligaments that help suspend the lens in place are attached to the choroid layer.

pro-geria

pro Greek, before in time + *geras* Greek, old age

Progeria is a rare childhood retardation characterized by premature aging symptoms like wrinkled skin, gray hair, small stature and hardening of the arteries. This progressive and early senility contributes to a shortened life span.

pro-gnosis

pro Greek, beforehand + *gnosis* knowledge, knowing

Prognosis is predicting the course and outcome of a disease.

pro-lapse

pro Latin, in front of + *lapsus* a slipping, a falling, thus collapse 'to fall together' and elapse 'to slip out, to slip past', like elapsed time
Prolapse is a slipping forward or falling of an organ from its normal position, e.g. prolapse of the uterus or prolapse of the rectum, due to muscular laxness in herniation, and other causes.

prostate

pro Greek, in front of + *states* Greek, standing. The prostate stands in front of the bladder.
The prostate gland in the male rings the neck of the bladder just where the vas deferens joins the urethra and adds a secretion to semen that helps sperm movement. As men age, the prostate may enlarge causing urine retention and difficult or even painful urination. Benign enlargement sometimes requires removal of the obstructing tissue, possibly by transurethral resection of the prostate. This transurethral prostatectomy involves removal of the benign growth through the urethra. Resection is partial removal.

procto-

prokton Greek, anus

procto-clysis

prokton anus + *klysis* Greek, a washing, a cleaning. Note the related agent noun in Greek *klyster* which gives a medical synonym for enema, clyster, and the Greek *klysma* which gives a medical word for the act of giving an enema, clysma.
Clysis is the injection of fluid not given by mouth into the human body. In certain medical instances, an intravenous injection is not possible. In proctoclysis, normal saline at body temperature is slowly (40 to 60 drops per minute) delivered by a lubricated rectal catheter, to resupply the body with fluid after hemorrhage, severe vomiting, or diarrhea. Body temperature is sometimes lowered by means of an ice-water proctoclysis.

procto-logy

prokton anus + *logos* Greek, study of
Proctology is treating and studying the diseases of the colon, rectum and anus.

procto-scope

prokton anus + *skopos* viewer, examiner
A proctoscope is an instrument for examining the rectum.

proct-ec-tomy

prokton anus + *ek* out + *tome* a surgical cutting
Proctectomy is surgical removal of the rectum or anus, often necessitating a
colostomy (see entry).

procto-sigmoid-ec-tomy

prokton anus + *sigmo-eides* Greek, S-shaped (colon) + *ek* out +
tome a surgical cutting
Proctosigmoidectomy is surgical removal of the rectum that includes removal of
the sigmoid colon, usually due to cancer or severe ulcerative colitis.

proto-plasm

protos Greek, first, original + *plasma* any formed
thing < *plassein* to form
Protoplasm is, literally, the first thing formed. In cytology, the study of cells,
protoplasm is all the material of a cell.

proximal

proximus Latin, the nearest
Proximal as an anatomical position means nearest the center of the body, or at
the beginning of a structure. The opposite of proximal is distal. The proximal
end of the thigh bone, the femur, forms a joint with the socket of the hip bone.
The distal end of the femur articulates with the tibia and the knee-cap. Each
finger has three bones called phalanges. The proximal phalanx is the finger bone
nearest the body. The distal phalanx is the fingerbone most remote from the
body, at the tip of the finger.

pruri-

pruriens Latin, itching, craving for
Thus, in general English, a prurient interest is one that appeals to unusual,
immoderate sexual desire, an interest that raises an itch for sex.

pruritus vulvae

pruritus Latin, an itching + *vulvae* Latin, of the vulva
Pruritus vulvae is severe itching of the female external genitalia, often due to yeast infection or dermatitis, or it may be a sign of diabetes mellitus.

prurigo

prurigo, pruriginis Latin, itchiness
Prurigo is an itchy skin lesion with vesicles that crust over. It may be due to allergic or drug reaction, or endocrine imbalance. The adjective is pruriginous.

pseudo-

pseudos Greek, false, fake

pseudo-gout

pseudos false + *gout* Old French, a drop of liquid < *gutta* Latin, drop
Pseudogout is false gout, a disorder resembling gout, but, in the synovial fluid in the joints is a build-up of calcium salts, rather than uric acid salts.

pseudo-cyesis

pseudos false + *kyesis* Greek, conception, pregnancy < *kyein* to conceive, to bear in the womb
Pseudocyesis is false pregnancy, the development of many signs of pregnancy but without the presence of an embryo. One form used to be called hysterical pregnancy, now called phantom pregnancy, due chiefly to severe psychological disorders.

psoriasis

psoriasis Greek, itching = *psora* itch < *psen* to rub + *iasis* medical condition
Psoriasis is a chronic skin disease with red patches covered with white scales notably on the scalp, knees, elbows, genitals and sites of injury. The cause is unknown, but genetic predisposition has been noted.

psycho- .

psyche Greek, soul, spirit, the breath of life, mind < *psychein* to breathe, echoic in origin, that is, it imitates the sound of an outward breath

psych-iatry

psyche mind + *iatreia* doctoring < *iatros* physician
Psychiatry is the branch of medicine concerned with the treatment and prevention of mental disorders. A psychiatrist is, first, a medical doctor. Psychoanalysis is one method by which a psychiatrist records a patient's past experiences in seeking to lessen the present expression by the patient of long-repressed unconscious conflicts of childhood, many of these psychoneuroses sexual in origin.

psych-ology

psyche mind + *logos* scientific study of
Psychology is the study of normal and abnormal mental processes. A psychologist is not necessarily a medical doctor.

psych-osis

psyche mind + *osis* diseased condition
A psychosis is a major mental disorder, so disruptive that the patient loses touch with reality and suffers personality disintegration. Delusions and hallucinations often accompany a psychosis, and hospitalization is required.

psycho-somatic

psyche mind + *soma, somatos* Greek, body
Psychosomatic pertains to the relationship between mind and body. Psychosomatic disorders often show more clearly than merely physical diseases the close links between the mind and the body.

ptosis

ptosis Greek, a falling down
Ptosis is the displacement of a body part from its normal position, also called prolapse. The adjective is ptotic or ptosed, both meaning fallen or prolapsed. For

example, blepharoptosis or eyelid droop, involving weakness of the muscles that move the upper eyelid (*blepharos* Greek, eyelid).

nephro-ptosis

nephros Greek, kidney + *ptosis* a falling down

Nephroptosis is floating kidney, with the implication that it needs to be re-attached by a nephropexy, an operation only rarely indicated today (*pexis* a fixing, a fastening).

ptyalo-

ptyalon Greek, saliva, synonym for the Latin *saliva*. *Ptyein*, Greek, to spit, is echoic, imitating the sound of spitting, much like the English spitting interjection, ptui!

ptyal-in

ptyalon saliva + *in* noun ending for organic chemical compound

Ptyalin is an enzyme in saliva that helps begin the digestion of starch and glycogen.

ptyal-ism

ptyalon saliva + *ismos* noun suffix indicating a condition

Ptyalism is the excessive secretion of saliva. Another Greek word for saliva, *sialon*, gives the synonym sialorrhea (*rrhoia* Greek, a flowing of). Ptyalism or sialorrhea may be seen in acute oral inflammations, pregnancy, malnutrition, alcoholism and other conditions.

ptyalo-litho-tomy

ptyalon saliva + *lithos* stone, calculus + *tome* surgical cutting

A ptyalolithotomy is the surgical removal of a salivary calculus, a small stone-like concretion usually found in the submandibular gland that stops the flow of saliva and causes severe pain and swelling, especially during eating.

pubes, pubic

pubes Latin adjective, grown-up, able to reproduce

In medicine it first meant the pubic area, then the pubic bone. Pubes is still used to refer in general to the genital area of the body.

mons pubis, mons Veneris

Latin, the hill of the pubis, the hill of Venus, the Roman goddess of love
The mons pubis is a pad of protective fat over the pubic symphysis in the female.

os pubis

os pubis Latin, bone of the pubis
Os pubis is the pubic bone, the lower front part of the pelvis. Two pubic bones meet in front of the pelvis and fuse at the pubic symphysis (*sym* > *syn* together + *physis* a growing, nature). This juncture of tough, fibrous tissue is rigid in the male, but slightly elastic in the female to allow small pelvic adjustments during childbirth.

pulmo-, pulmono-

pulmo, pulmonis Latin, lung

pulmonary circulation

pulmonarius Late Latin, of the lung
The blood passes from the heart to the lungs by way of the right cardiac ventricle to receive fresh oxygen and then returns to the heart by the left cardiac atrium.

pulmonary edema

pulmonarius Late Latin, of the lung; *oidema, oidematos* Greek, a swelling
Edema results when excess fluids build up in the intercellular spaces and cause swelling. Accumulation of fluid in the lungs, as seen in pulmonary edema, is due to heart failure, usually of the left side of the heart, so that more blood is pumped into the lungs than can be withdrawn.

pulmonary muco-ciliary clearance

pulmonarius Late Latin, of the lung; *mucus* Latin, mucus, slime; *ciliarius* Latin, pertaining to fine hair-like objects < *cilium* eyelash
Pulmonary mucociliary clearance (PMC) is the natural process of removal from the lungs of inhaled particles, cell debris and excess secretions by cells, using fine hair-like projections. These ciliated cells wave and pulse, stirring up the mucoid debris and propelling it out of the bronchi and trachea. PMC is thus the major defense mechanism of the respiratory tract.

punctum

punctum Latin, pin-prick, pointy hole

This anatomical term is seen in such phrases as punctum lacrimale, the tiny tear-hole of each lacrimal duct through which tears flow to the lacrimal sac of each eye. The punctum caecum (Latin, blind) is the blind spot in the body of the eyeball where the optic nerve enters it.

pupil

pupilla Latin, a little doll < *pupa* girl child, puppet

The pupilla or pupil of the eye was so named because a tiny image of a person looking into another's eye is reflected in the pupil and this reflection looks like a little doll. Contraction and dilation of the pupil are useful diagnostic signs in various diseases and drug-induced disorders. Fixed and dilated pupils are one of the signs of death.

pur-, pus

pus, puris Latin, pus. It is akin to *pyon*, the Greek word for pus, with its many medical words containing *pyo-* (see below).

Pus is a yellowish fluid produced by inflammation due to bacteria. Pus contains white blood cells and fluid that has leaked from blood vessels, dead bacteria and cell debris of damaged tissue.

muco-purulent

mucus slime, mucus + *purulens, purulentis* containing pus < *pus, puris* Latin, pus

Mucopurulent discharges, that follow many infections, are composed of mucus and pus.

pus-tule

pustula Latin, pimple < *pus*

A pustule is an infected pimple, a small blister of purulent (pus-containing) material.

sup-pur-ation

sub > *sup* Latin, under + *puratio, purationis* New Latin, a forming of pus

Suppuration is the formation or presence or discharge of pus. The verb is to suppurate. A near synonym is purulence, pus-like matter.

pyelo-

pyelos Greek, basin, pan, a synonym of the Latin *pelvis*. In medical words, pyelo- refers to the renal pelvis.

pyelo-gram

pyelos the pelvis of the kidney + *gram* something written or recorded

A pyelogram is an X-ray made of the renal pelvis and the ureter. An intravenous pyelogram uses a contrast agent, a dye, introduced by a line into a vein. A retrograde pyelogram (*retrogradus* New Latin, walking backwards) is an X-ray of the renal pelvis and the ureter where dye is injected through a catheter placed in the ureter. Pyelitis is inflammation of the renal pelvis.

py-, pyo-

pyon Greek, pus

em-py-ema

en > *em* in + *pyon* pus + *-ema* Greek noun suffix, diseased condition

Empyema is the accumulation of pus in the pleural cavity, often needing surgical drainage.

pyo-nephr-osis

pyon pus + *nephros* Greek, kidney + *osis* diseased condition

Pyonephrosis is the collection of pus in an obstructed kidney.

pyo-rrhea

pyon pus + *rrhoia* Greek, a flowing through, a discharge

Pyorrhea is a great discharge of pus, especially in alveolar pyorrhea, pus formation in the alveoli, or in sockets of the teeth. It may be part of general periodontal disease.

py-uria

pyon pus + *ouron* Greek, urine + *ia* medical condition
Pyuria is the abnormal presence of pus in the urine.

pyr-

pyr Greek, fire, fever; akin to pyre, pyrite, German *Feuer*, and fire

pyro-gen

pyr fire, fever + *gen-* Greek root, making, producing
A pyrogen is a substance that is released by white blood cells during an acute inflammatory response that has the effect of raising the body temperature above normal.

pyro-mania

pyr fire + *mania* Greek, madness
Pyromania is an obsessive compulsion to set fires, and it refers also to the morbid love of fire by a pyromaniac.

pyret-

pyretos Greek, fever (fire in the body, so-to-speak)

anti-pyretic

anti Greek, against, counter to + *pyretikos* Greek, pertaining to a fever
An antipyretic agent reduces body temperature in a patient with fever.

pyrex-ia

pyrexis Greek, feverishness + *ia* medical condition
Pyrexia is fever, when the temperature of the body rises above normal, which is 98.6°F or 37°C. A common clinical acronym seen on charts is P.U.O., or pyrexia of unknown origin.

quadri-ceps femoris

quadri- combining form of *quattuor* Latin, four + *-ceps* suffix
form of *caput* Latin, head; *femoris* of the femur

The quadriceps femoris is a large muscle on the front surface of the thigh that
extends the leg. It is named four-headed because it is made up of four smaller
muscles: the rectus femoris, the vastus lateralis, vastus medius, and vastus
intermedius (*rectus* Latin, straight; *vastus* extensive, broad). The common
knee-jerk response is sometimes called the quadriceps reflex because that muscle
is involved in the movement produced (see *patella* entry).

quadri-plegia

quadri- combining form of *quattuor* Latin, four + *plege* Greek, a
paralyzing stroke

Quadriplegia is paralysis of the arms and legs caused by spinal cord trauma,
often in car and sporting accidents. The trunk of the body below the injured
portion of the spinal cord is also usually paralyzed.

quarantine

quarantina Italian, a period of forty days, from *quaranta giorni*
forty days

The practice of isolating suspected bearers of infectious disease began at Venice
in AD 1374 at the time of a great plague known as the Black Death. The precise
number of days during which strangers were considered contagious was not
based on science, but was chosen as forty, being a semi-legal and semi-mystical
number. Consider the forty days of Lent, the forty days of a medieval truce, the
forty days in medieval law in which a recent widow could live in her dead
husband's house. Most influential may have been Hippocrates' belief that the
fortieth day of a disease was a critical moment on which an attending ancient
physician might predict a patient's recovery or prepare for decline.

rabies

rabies Latin, rage, fury, raving

Rabies is an acute, dangerous viral infection passed to humans by animal bites. The blood, saliva and tissues of a rabid animal carry the virus. Exposed victims need immediate vaccination. French scientist Louis Pasteur invented the first vaccine in 1885. The old name for rabies was hydrophobia, which literally means 'fear of water'. During the crisis of rabies, which can be fatal within a few days, fever, delirium, paralysis and muscle spasms may occur. The patient is thirsty because of the fever, but severe spasm of the throat muscles makes the patient terrified to drink water, hence the 'fear of water'.

rachi-, rachio-, rachis

rhachis Greek, backbone, spine

Rachis is a medical term for the spinal column. A rachiometer measures the curvatures of the spine. Rachischisis (*schisis* Greek, a splitting) is congenital fissure of the spinal column, or spina bifida.

rach-itis, rickets

rhachis spine + *itis* inflammation of

Rachitis is the formal medical term for rickets, a deficiency disease of children. A lack of vitamin D prevents the deposition of calcium and phosphorus in developing cartilage and new bone, producing abnormal, thin and small bones. Bad teeth, humped back, and big knobs on the ends of large bones are typical. Osteomalacia (*osteon* bone + *malakia* softness) is an adult form of rickets, in which bones become so soft that their flexibility and brittleness cause deformities. A classic clinical sign of rickets is 'the rachitic rosary', in which the ends of the rib bones widen and produce a line of rosary bead-like bumps running down either side of the front chest wall.

radial, radius

radius Latin, a rod, a ray of light, the spoke of a wheel
The radius is the shorter forearm bone that early anatomists thought resembled
the spoke of a wheel. The radius goes partly around the ulna. The radius makes a
joint proximally with the upper arm bone, the humerus, and distally with the
ulna and wrist bones. The radial nerve is the largest of the arm nerves. The
radial pulse is the pulse of the radial artery taken at the wrist. Pain may radiate,
or ray out, from one area of the body to another along the course of a nerve.

radical

radicalis Latin, deeply rooted, from the original root of an idea
or movement < *radix* root, from which the vegetable *radish*
derives, being a root
In medicine, radical is directed to the root cause, for example, a radical
mastectomy, total removal of breast tissue designed to rid the site of all vestiges
of malignancy.

radicle

radicula Latin, rootlet, little root, diminutive of *radix*
A radicle is a very small branch of a vessel or nerve. Radiculitis is inflammation
of spinal nerve roots.

radio-

radio- a combining form of *radius*, with the developed meaning
of 'radioactive' or 'of radio waves'
Referring originally to the ray-like waves of a radio signal, the prefix *radio-*
today usually pertains to radioactive substances and their use in medical
diagnosis, in imaging techniques or therapies.

radio-logy

radio- radioactive + *logos* study of
Radiology is the study and application of radioactive substances to medical uses,
including X-rays and radioactive isotopes used in medical imaging and disease
treatment. A radiologist is a medical doctor who diagnoses and treats diseases
using radioactive materials. A radiologic technician operates and maintains X-
ray machines, fluoroscopic diagnostic devices, and other systems designed to
produce images for medical use.

radio-lucent

radio- of radio waves + *lucens* Latin, shining through
Radiolucent objects let X-rays pass through them. Air is radiolucent and shows up on the X-ray as dark gray or black. Uric acid stones in the urinary bladder are radiolucent.

radi-opaque

radio- of radio waves + *opacus* Latin, shaded, dark
Radiopaque objects do not let X-rays pass through them, e.g. the lead sheeting used as a shield around radioactive equipment. A radiopaque dye may be injected as a contrast medium before an X-ray of some internal organ, to help obtain a clear image of the organ's interior. Calcium stones in the urinary system are radiopaque.

rale

rale French, a rattling sound in the lungs
Rale is the moist or dry wheezing sound made by air passing through clogged bronchi and bronchioles. Bronchi congested by secretions, thickened walls and mucus make a variety of squeaks, whistles, pipings, cracklings, bubblings and gurglings. There are many phrases to differentiate these noises, but no universal method of classification that is at all scientific. When a rale sounds like snoring, it is often called a rhoncus (*rhogchos* Greek, a snoring).

raphe

rhaphe Greek, a suture, a seam, a sewn-up wound
In formal anatomical nomenclature, a raphe is a seam, a ridge, a heightened line where two parts have joined naturally. For example, the scrotal raphe is a visible midline external and central on the scrotal sac.

hernio-rrhaphy

hernia Latin, a rupture, a protruding + *rrhaphia* Greek, a sewing, stitching, suturing
Hernia is the abnormal protruding of an organ or body part through a muscular wall that usually contains the organ. Herniorrhaphy is the surgical repair of a hernia with suturing.

episio-rrhaphy

epision Greek, pubic area + *rrhaphia* a sewing
Episiorrhaphy is the suturing of the labia majora or of a lacerated perineum, usually post partum (after birth), often to repair an episiotomy, an incision of the vulva to prevent ripping and tearing of maternal tissue and to protect the emerging baby during a difficult birth.

re-

re Latin prefix, back in space, time, or state; hence again, repeated
Thus, in their original Latin senses, a reflex is a bending back, a reflux is a flowing back, a remission is a sending back (to health when a disease abates). A remedy was originally a *remedium*, from *mederi* to attend medically, that is, a medical tending that brings back health.

recto-, rectum

rectus Latin adjective, straight. The neuter singular is *rectum*.
The rectum is the last four or five inches of the colon, an intestinal passage that is relatively straight and leads to the anus. The rectum is sometimes involved in colitis and dysentery. It is a site of intestinal cancer whose early symptoms include blood or mucus in the stool and changes in bowel habits such as unexplained constipation. Anorectal means 'involving the anus and the rectum'.

renal

renalis Latin, of a kidney < *ren* kidney
The renal cortex is the outer part of a kidney comprised of glomeruli and tubules (*cortex* Latin, outer tree bark). The renal medulla is the inner layer of kidney containing nephrons (*medulla* Latin, little middle part, also means marrow). The renal pelvis (*pelvis* Latin, wide basin, lower part) is the funnel at the upper end of the ureter where urine collects before descent to the bladder. A renal calculus (*calculus* Latin, pebble) is a synonym for a kidney stone.

respiratory

respiratorius New Latin, pertaining to any breathing apparatus, natural or synthetic < *respirare* to breathe
In respiratory distress syndrome of the newborn, acute lung dysfunction is caused by a congenital lack of sufficient pulmonary surfactant. Surfactants in the

lungs are lipoproteins that act to reduce the surface tension of normal lung fluids, thus permitting the necessary exchange of gases across alveolar tissue.

rete

rete Latin, net; plural: *retia*

In anatomy, a rete is any network, like a plexus (see entry) of nerves or blood vessels. For example, two vertebral retia or plexuses of nerves extend from the top of the spinal column right down to the tailbone.

reticular

reticulum Latin, network, little net < *rete* net

Reticular tissue is connective tissue formed of a net-like mesh of fibers and star-like cells with tiny processes that connect them with adjacent cells. Reticular tissue abounds in bone marrow, liver tissue, kidney tissue, lymph nodes and the walls of blood vessels.

reticulo-endothelial system (RES)

reticulo- pertaining to reticular connective tissue + endothelium

Endothelium is tissue composed of flat and scale-like cells that line the internal organs of the body like the heart, as well as the veins and arteries. The RES refers to the phagocytes (see entry) in connective tissue that engulf and remove from circulation cell debris, pathogens and foreign bodies. These phagocytes abound in the spleen, liver, lymph nodes, alveoli, brain, blood vessels and many mucous membranes. They are the chief actors in non-specific immune responses.

retina

Medieval Latin extension of *rete*, net. The word was coined by Gerard of Cremona, a translator of Arabic medical texts into Latin. The word was in English by AD 1400.

The retina is the innermost layer of the eye which receives the image through the lens. Among the many retinal pathologies are actinic retinitis, inflammation of the retina due to intense light or other radiant energies. Diabetic retinitis is seen in protracted diabetes where the blood vessels of the retina dilate abnormally, hemorrhage and exude a fluffy, waxy substance.

retro-

retro Latin adverb used as a prefix meaning 'backwards, behind'

Thus retrobulbar is located behind the eyeball (*bulbus* Latin, onion, ball, bulb).

retro-cecal

retro behind + *caecalis* Medical Latin, of the cecum < *caecum* Latin, blind, because it's the blind part of the gut that ends with the appendix and, in a sense, leads nowhere

Retrocecal is behind the cecum. The cecum is the pouch that is the first part of the large intestine. At the end of the cecum is the appendix. But sometimes the appendix may be located retrocecally, and this may make an appendectomy more difficult to perform than usual.

rhesus factor

First discovered in the red blood cells of the rhesus monkey, hence the label, the rhesus factor appears in the blood of humans as well. It can produce agglutination problems in certain blood transfusions. In pregnancy a mother who is rhesus (Rh) negative, carrying a fetus that is Rh positive, can produce antibodies that may endanger subsequent fetuses.

rheum-, rheumat-

rheuma, rheumatos Greek, a discharge, a flow < *rhein* to flow

Rheum is any watery discharge from mucous membranes of the head and throat.

rheumat-ism

rheuma, rheumatos a discharge + *ismos* noun suffix indicating a condition

Rheumatism is a general term for arthritic inflammations of the joints, and stiff, sore muscles. Rheumatoid arthritis, gout, rheumatic fever, even gonorrhea may be implicated.

rhino-

rhis, rhinos Greek, nose, equivalent to Latin *nasum*

Rhinitis is inflammation of the nasal mucosa, the lining of the nose, due to cold or hay fever. A rhinoplasty is a nose job, plastic surgery to repair the nose, one of the most ancient surgeries.

oto-rhino-laryngo-logy

ous, otos ear + *rhis, rhinos* Greek, nose + *larynx, laryngos* Greek, throat + *logos* study of
Otorhinolaryngology is the scientific study of functions, diseases and treatments of the ear, nose and throat, and the upper respiratory tract in general.

rub-

ruber Latin adjective, red. The Latin noun is *rubor*, redness.
Rubor is the redness of tissue that is inflamed, the redness due to increased blood flow to the site of infection. Rubor is one of the classic signs of inflammation.

rubella

rubellus Latin, reddish, pink
Rubella is German measles, a mild viral infection named from the pink rash, but it may be very serious in pregnant women.

rube-osis

ruber red + *osis* diseased condition
Rubeosis of the iris involves formation of new tissue on the surface of the iris, accompanied by consequent reddening, often a sign of diabetes.

-rrhea

rrhoia Greek, a flowing, a discharge

a-meno-rrhea

a not + *men, menos* Greek, a month, hence English phrases like 'the monthlies' and Latin terms like *menstrualis. Meno-* is prefixed to words related to the monthly female period of normal and abnormal menstrual bleeding + *rrhoia* a flowing.
Amenorrhea is lack of a monthly period, due to dysfunction or pregnancy.

dia-rrhea

dia Greek, through + *rrhoia* Greek, a flowing
Diarrhea is too-frequent bowel movements of watery stools, a flowing through of waste.

dys-meno-rrhea

dys Greek negative prefix indicates difficult or disordered function + *men, menos* a month + *rrhoia* a discharge
Dysmenorrhea is a monthly period that is painful.

pyo-rrhea

pyon Greek, pus + *rrhoia* a discharge
Pyorrhea is a copious flow of pus, as in severe gingivitis (inflammation of gum tissue).

S

sac

saccus Latin, a bag made of rough cloth < *sakkos* Greek, a garment made of coarse hair, a bag made of sackcloth < *saq* Biblical Hebrew, the hair-shirt of penance, a bag < *chaqqu* Assyrian, rough shirt < *shagadu* Sumerian, an under-garment

Thus sac is possibly the oldest word used in medical English, with a long history stretching back as an almost intact lexical unit more than 8000 years. Sac has derivatives and diminutives borrowed into English from French, e.g. sachet and satchel, both from *saccellus,* little bag. To sack a village by plundering it derives from Medieval Latin *saccare* 'to pillage a place by putting the booty in rough bags and making off with it'.

In anatomy, a sac is a pouch or bag-like part of a structure or organ. The pericardium surrounds the heart as a tough, bag-like membrane sometimes called the pericardial sac or the heart sac. The human embryo shows an abdominal sac that later develops into the abdominal cavity. The amniotic sac is a thin membrane filled with serous fluid enclosing the embryo. The air passageway into the lungs terminates at the alveolar sacs. Each pouchlike alveolar sac, also called an air sac, is connected by a small duct to a bronchiole. Sometimes the diminutive form is used and these little pocket-like structures are labeled air saccules (*sacculus* little bag). When an artery weakens and a localized part of its arterial wall protrudes, and when this ballooning outward resembles a little bag on the arterial wall, the abnormality may be called a saccular aneurysm (see *aneurysm* entry).

sacrum, sacral, sacro-

os sacrum Latin, holy bone, a translation of a Greek phrase that meant great bone

The sacrum is the largest bone of the spinal column, a fused triangle at the base of the spine, composed of five vertebrae at birth, which fuse together in the child.

sacro-iliac

sacrum + *ilium* hipbone

Sacroiliac joints occur where each hipbone or ilium meets the sacrum. These joints are capable of a very slight articulation, and this makes them subject to the stress and strain ailments of all joints, and to disorders like rheumatism. Sacroiliac strain is especially common in women.

sagittal

sagitta Latin, arrow

In anatomy, a longitudinal section, like a virtual slice through an axis, is used to locate body parts. This section through an axis is called a plane. One is the sagittal plane, a front-to-back plane parallel to the midline of a body, like an arrow passing through the body. Planes are important in the preparation of many medical imaging devices. The sagittal suture of the human skull runs right down the midline of the cranium at the front. It is the solid fusing between the two parietal bones of the skull, supposedly like an arrow, but in fact serrated, since this tooth-like meshing of projections makes for a firmer juncture.

sal-

sal, salis Latin, salt; adjectival form, *salinus* salty

The bare root was used in pharmacology in old chemical names, still seen occasionally, like sal ammoniac for ammonium chloride and sal soda for sodium carbonate. A saline solution has widespread uses when infused intravenously in medical hydration, reintroducing fluids into body parts that have lost fluid. A saline cathartic (*kathartikos* Greek, cleansing) produces evacuation of the bowel within four hours. A saline enema treats certain worm infestations.

saliva

saliva Latin, spittle; akin to *sialon* Greek, saliva, also used in medical terms (see below)

Saliva is secreted by salivary and mucous glands in the mouth. It wets food as a chewing and swallowing aid, and contains the enzyme ptyalin to begin starch digestion. There are three pairs of salivary glands named by their location, the parotid near the ear, the submandibular under the lower jawbone and the sublingual under the tongue. A stone-like accretion in one of these glands is called a salivary calculus, using Latin roots, or, using Greek roots, a sialolith (*sialon* saliva + *lithos* stone, pebble). An agent that promotes the secretion of saliva is a sialogogue (*agogos* Greek, leading forth).

salpingi-, salpingo-, salpinx

salpigx, salpingos Greek, a trumpet

The salpinx is the Fallopian tube, because the end of the tube flares open like a trumpet where finger-like fimbriae catch the ovum as it leaves the ovary. Confusingly, salpinx is also applied to the tube of the middle ear, the Eustachian tube. To avoid this confusion, formal anatomical labels are: salpinx auditiva for the Eustachian tube, and salpinx uterina for the Fallopian tube.

salping-itis

salpigx, salpingos a trumpet + *itis* inflammation of

Salpingitis is inflammation of the Fallopian tubes. Popularly called 'hot tubes', it may be part of pelvic inflammatory disease.

salpingo-gram

salpigx, salpingos a trumpet + *gram* something written or recorded

A salpingogram is an X-ray of the Fallopian tubes to determine their patency (if they are wide open), used in fertility studies. To restore the opening and permit ova to pass, a salpingostomy (*stoma* Greek, mouth) may be performed by making an artificial, mouth-like opening in a Fallopian tube.

saphena

saphenes Greek, obvious, plain. An early Greek writer, translating the Arabic of Avicenna's medical texts into Greek, mistook the Arabic term *al-safan* 'the hidden one' for a Greek word that meant the opposite 'clear, manifest'

The saphena is either of the two large, superficial veins that pass up the leg. The great saphenous vein runs up from the foot to an opening in the thigh muscles through which it passes. The small saphenous vein runs up the back of the leg to join the popliteal vein at the back of the knee (*poples* Latin, ham of the knee).

sarco-

sarx, sarkos Greek, flesh; Latin equivalent is *carnis*

sarc-oma

sarx, sarkos Greek, flesh + *oma* tumor

A sarcoma is a highly invasive cancer of the soft tissue in fibrous structures, and in fat, muscle, vessels and nerves. It arises chiefly in connective tissue including bone in a malignant osteosarcoma. Common sites are the bladder, kidneys, liver, spleen and lungs.

scalpel

scalpellum Latin, little carving knife < *scalpere* to cut, to carve
One of many designs of a small surgical knife with a convex, very sharp blade.

scapula

scapula Latin, shoulder blade
The scapula is either of the flat, triangular bones that form the back part of the shoulder girdle. It articulates with the collarbone or clavicle, and is a 'hitching post' for the attachment of many muscles and ligaments. A scapulary is a shoulder bandage used to fix a larger body bandage in place. A clinical testing sign is the scapulohumeral reflex, induced by tapping solidly the edge of the scapula near the spinal column. Normally the upper arm is then draw up and rotated outward.

-schisis

schisis Greek, a splitting, an abnormal fissure < *schizein* to split

cheilo-schisis

cheilos Greek, lip + *schisis* abnormal splitting
Cheiloschisis is the anatomical name for harelip.

palato-schisis

palato of the palate + *schisis* abnormal splitting
Palatoschisis or cleft palate is a congenital defect. The two halves of the palate fail to fuse properly. Results range from a tiny groove at the edge of the lip to total midline separation of the palate. Plastic surgery corrects this. In cheilo-gnatho-palato-schisis, the abnormal cleft separates the lip, the upper jaw (*gnathos* Greek, jaw), and the hard and soft palate.

schisto-

schistos Greek, split, cleft, divided

schisto-cyte

schistos split + *kytos* cell

A schistocyte is a red blood cell fragment seen in hemolytic anemia (*haima* blood + *lytikos* pertaining to a breaking up of). Hemolysis is the destruction of red blood cells in which hemoglobin seeps into surrounding tissues and fluids. And schistocytosis is the abnormal condition of having many schistocytes in the blood.

schisto-som-iasis

schistos split + *soma* body + *-iasis* Greek, diseased medical condition

Schistosomiasis is chronic infestation by blood flukes of the genus *Schistosoma* (split-body). A fluke is a trematode or flatworm, common in the tropics and Far East.

schisto-thorax

schistos divided + *thorax* Greek, breastplate in ancient Greek armor, hence, chest

Schistothorax is a rare birth defect with split breastbone or chest fissure.

schizo-

schizein Greek, to split, to divide

schiz-oid

schizein to split, but here implying schizophrenia + *eides* form, thus *-oid* means 'like, similar to'

Schizoid personality disorder begins in early adulthood as withdrawal from normal social interactions. Patients appear cold and aloof from ordinary human interests like friendships and sexual contacts.

schizo-phrenia

schizein to split + *phren* Greek, mind + *ia* medical condition

The word *schizophrenia* was coined by pioneering psychiatrist Eugen Bleuler in 1911. It is a very broad, general label for a very large number of psychotic disorders. Bleuler did not mean *split* to refer to multiple personality disorders, but to the apparent split in these patients between feeling and thought.

Schizophrenia now encompasses so many signs and symptoms of disturbed mental and emotional processes that it is virtually useless as a scientific label; but, of course, it is long established and still widely used – and misused.

sciatica

Low Latin corruption of ischiadikos *Greek, of the* ischion *Greek, hip and loin area*

Sciatica appears twice in the writings of Shakespeare. Sciatica is an inflammation of the sciatic nerve, a long, many-branched nerve that arises in the sacral plexus and innervates the muscles of the thigh, leg and foot. The clinical signs are the pain and tenderness of 'lower back pain', felt down the back of the thighs and legs. Causes of sciatica may include compression of the sciatic nerve by herniated discs between the vertebrae. Rest and, occasionally, surgery are treatments.

sclera, sclero-

skleros Greek, hard and dry

Sclera is the tough, fibrous tissue surrounding the eyeball that helps keep its shape and also protects the softer inner tissues of the eye.

scler-osis

skleros hard + *osis* diseased condition

Sclerosis is disease-produced hardening of nerve tissue or of the blood vessels, e.g. in arteriosclerosis.

a-myo-trophic lateral sclerosis (ALS), Lou Gehrig's disease

a not + *myo* of muscle + *trophe* Greek, nourishment; *lateralis* Latin, at the side of the body

In amyotrophic lateral sclerosis, motor neurons of the brain stem and spinal cord in middle-aged patients degenerate, usually fatally. It produces wasting of the muscles of the arms and legs and spreads to the rest of the body's musculature.

-scope, -scopy

skopia Greek, a watching, a viewing, an examining

315

Many medical terms pertaining to the clinical examination of specific organs and body parts end with this suffix, for example, laparoscope, sigmoidoscopy, proctoscope, otoscopy.

broncho-scopy

brogchos Greek, windpipe + *skopia* an examining
Bronchoscopy is using a bronchoscope to look inside bronchi, the major air-carrying vessels of the lungs.

cysto-scope

kystis Greek, bag, bladder + *skopos* viewer, examiner
A cystoscope is a medical device used to examine visually the urinary bladder.

endo-scopy

endon Greek, inside + *skopia* an examining
Endoscopy is a general term for examining the inside of a body cavity with any of various instruments called endoscopes. A cystoscope is an endoscope.

seb-, sebum

sebum Latin, originally, hog fat, lard, fat < ultimately from Indo-European root *sus* pig, with related words like swine, sow, French *suif* 'tallow, candle fat', suet and the farmer's common pig-call in many languages, *suee-suee*. *Sebum* is not akin to *sapo*, *saponis* Latin, soap.
Sebum is the oily secretion of the sebaceous glands in the dermis layer of the skin. It is emptied through sebaceous ducts into the hair follicle to coat and protect individual hairs, and make the skin supple.

sebaceous cyst

sebaceus Late Latin, oily, greasy + *kystis* Greek, sac
A sebaceous cyst is a tiny sac of often rancid sebum, sometimes involving a hair follicle.

sebo-rrhea

sebo- sebum + *rrhoia* Greek, a discharge of

Seborrhea is an inflamed skin condition due to excess sebum production, also called seborrheic dermatitis.

sepsis, septic

sepsis Greek, rotting, decaying, infection of a wound

In medicine, sepsis is infection of tissue by bacteria and their toxins; it is also contamination introduced by a wound or surface lesion. A wound that is infected is septic.

anti-sepsis

anti Greek, against + *sepsis* infection

Antisepsis is the destruction of bacteria causing infection by an antiseptic agent.

a-sepsis

a not + *sepsis* infection

Asepsis is the state of freedom from infection and germs. Surgical asepsis is the elimination of and protection against infection during surgical procedures by the diligent use of sterile techniques. Aseptic body image is a mental awareness technique used by personnel in an operating room to maintain a sterile surgery even as certain areas become contaminated.

septic-emia

septikos infected + *em* short for *haima*, Greek, blood + *ia* medical condition

Septicemia is blood poisoning by disease-producing bacteria.

sero-, serum

serus Latin, originally, late or coming last, then the neuter form of the adjective, *serum*, came to mean 'whey', the watery portion of milk left over (at the last) during the making of cheese

Serum is the fluid that separates from clotted blood. In other words, serum is the plasma without the clotting agents, such as fibrinogen and prothrombin. In shed blood, fibrinogen converts to fibrin, which is threads of a hard, insoluble protein. Blood cells mesh in fibrin, then the fibrin contracts, squeezing out a clear, yellow fluid called serum. In immunology, an antiserum is a liquid containing antibodies.

ser-ous

serosus scientific Latin, abounding in serum, viscid

Serous means consisting of or producing a liquid like serum; for example, many body membranes secrete a lubricating, serous fluid.

sinoatrial node

See *node* entry

sinus

sinus Latin, anything hollowed out, the fold of a garment, a bay or gulf of water

In anatomy, the paranasal sinuses are cavities inside the bones near the nose. Also called the accessory nasal sinuses, they are lined with epithelial mucosa and act to moisten, warm and filter air, and perhaps they act as resonators for the human voice. A sinus is also a channel for venous blood, for example the aortic sinus is a widened part of the aorta or pulmonary artery opposite a semilunar valve. A draining sinus is a pathological passageway formed to permit the escape of pus from an abscess.

sinus-itis

sinus + *itis* inflammation of

Without proper drainage, a paranasal sinus may become blocked, due to viral or bacterial infection or allergies. In acute suppurative sinusitis (*sub* > *sup* under + *pus, puris* pus), pus, pain, fever, chills and headache must be relieved by bedrest, and possibly antibiotics, extra fluid intake and hot packs. In chronic hyperplastic sinusitis, polyps crowd the lumen of a sinus and surgical remedy may be necessary.

sito-

sitos Greek, grain, food

para-site

para Greek, beside + *sitos* food, literally, a beside-feeder, one who scrounges food, a hanger-on

An ancient Greek *parasitos* was a freeloader who sat beside you at your table, ate your food, but did not pay for it or contribute to its preparation. A biological parasite lives in or on another organism, obtains food from it, and injures the health of its host. Examples of parasites in humans are viruses, worms and some bacteria.

sito-mania

sitos food + *mania* Greek, madness
Sitomania is a morbid craving for food, like the obsessive hunger seen in bulimia, an appetite disorder whose chief symptom is a cycle of eating binge, followed by self-induced vomiting, followed by depressive fasting.

situ-

situs Latin, position, location, site

in situ

Latin, in its (original) position
In situ means in its normal place, or confined to the site of origin. For example, a carcinoma may be *in situ*. It has not yet spread, and is at its original site. In cervix or bladder cancer, *in situ* means confined to the epithelium. A Pap test may detect such a cervical cancer. In medicine, a site is a position or a locus, a place, a location. To situate is a verb, but in anatomical description situate is also an adjective meaning 'located' or 'beside'.

skeleton

skeletos Greek, dried up < *skellein* to dry up
Ancient Greeks used *skeleton* to refer to a mummy, a dried-up body. Not until the 16th Century was the term applied to the framework of bones that support the human body.

The human skeleton consists of 206 bones, not counting the teeth and sesamoid bones other than the patella. The skeleton provides support and protection for internal organs, and permits body movement through the muscles attached to its bones. The bones also make and store red blood cells. The skeleton is usually divided into two parts. The axis of the skeleton includes the bones of the skull, vertebrae, ribs and sternum. Below the axial skeleton is the appendicular skeleton consisting of the bones of the arms and legs, of the pelvic girdle, and of the pectoral girdle.

solar

solaris Latin, of the sun

solar plexus

plexus Latin, a braid, a plait

In medicine, a plexus is a tangled intermingling of blood vessels or nerves or lymph vessels. We've all heard of a boxer getting a hard back slam, or getting punched in the solar plexus. It is also called the *celiac* plexus, a network of nerve fibers and ganglia at the upper back of the abdomen. It is named solar from the Latin word *solaris* 'of the sun', because sympathetic and parasympathetic nerves radiate out from this plexus like rays from the shining sun.

somni, somno

somnus Latin, sleep

h.s.

Abbreviation for *hora somni* Latin, literally, at the hour of sleep

H.s. is a common short form used on charts and prescriptions, a direction that medication be given or taken at bedtime.

in-somnia

in Latin, not + *somnus* sleep, hence *insomnis* sleepless. The Latin negative prefix *in-* is related to the English *un* as in undo.

Insomnia is a general term for inability to get as much sleep as one needs. It is a common, usually temporary symptom, but if chronic, insomnia needs professional attention.

somn-ambul-ism

somnus sleep + *ambulare* Latin, to walk + *ismos* a condition

Somnambulism is walking in one's sleep, during stages three or four of non-REM sleep. The patient usually has no memory of the motor activity involved, such as leaving the bed and walking around for a few minutes.

spadi-

spadon Greek, a rip, gash, tear, abnormal opening

epi-spadias

epi Greek, on + *spadon* abnormal opening

In the male, epispadias (singular) is a birth defect that causes the urinary passage to be on the upper surface of the penis. In female epispadias, the urethral meatus is abnormally near the clitoris. The cause is often congenital absence of the upper wall of the urethra.

hypo-spadias

hypo under + *spadon* abnormal opening

Hypospadias (singular) is a birth defect in which the urethral orifice opens not at the end of the penis but on the underside. Surgery is required for cosmetic reasons and to permit more effective insemination.

speculum

speculum Latin, a looking glass, a mirror < *specere* to see, with hundreds of related words in English, from inspect to spectacle

A speculum is an instrument to examine a body cavity that opens on the surface, such as the nose, throat, rectum or vagina. A nasal speculum helps dilate a nasal passage and often provides light to make inspection of deeper nasal tissues easier. A vaginal speculum has two adjustable duck-billed, spatulate blades to gently dilate the vaginal orifice, as does a rectal speculum, used to dilate the rectum.

sphen-oid

sphen Greek, a wedge + *eides* Greek, form, hence *-oid* means 'formed like'

The sphenoid bone makes up part of the base of the skull, and part of the floor and sides of the eye socket. The sphenoid was so called because it appeared to early anatomists to be wedged in among the other bones of the skull. The sphenoid sinus is one of two recesses or cavities in the sphenoid bone at the base of the nose. They are air sinuses lined with mucous membrane, in effect, extensions of the nasal cavity. Sinuses act to amplify the voice and to warm and moisten nose air.

sphincter

sphigkter Greek, the squeezer

The Sphinx of Giza was a monster with the body of a lion and the head of a pharaoh. It squeezed victims in its lion claws, as did the Greek sphinx of Thebes, with its woman's head and lioness' body. In Latin, the root drops its *s* to give such akin words as *fingere*, to squeeze or mold with the hands, hence to shape, to sculpt, hence ultimately English words like *fiction* and *fictile*. In Germanic reflexes of the root are seen the origin of English words like *finger*, the digits we use to clutch, squeeze, and hold objects.

A sphincter is a ring of contractile muscle that closes an orifice. The anal sphincters, internal and external, are muscle bands that contract to close the anus after defecation. Sphincter muscles also exist in the bile duct, pylorus, urethra and urinary bladder. The pupillary sphincter consists of circular fibers in the iris that constrict the pupil of the eye.

splen-, spleen

splen Greek, spleen

The spleen is a rubbery, purple sac of lymph tissue behind the stomach, under the ribs on the left side. Among other functions, the spleen filters foreign material out of the blood, destroys used red blood cells, and produces lymphocytes and antibodies as part of the immune system.

Splenectomy is the surgical cutting out of the spleen. Because most spleen functions can be carried out by other organs, in an otherwise healthy adult, splenectomy has few bad effects. If injured, splenic tissue is difficult to repair.

-spir-

spirare Latin, to breathe, akin to *spiritus* 'the breath of life', then 'the divine breath'

Many compound words borrowed by English include conspiracy (a breathing, huddling and planning together of evildoers), perspiration and transpire. Expire is literally to breathe out, or to let out one's last breath, hence to die. A respirator is literally a rebreather, an apparatus that assists weakened or disordered breathing.

a-spir-ate

a > ad to, toward, on + *spirare* to breathe. *Aspirare* literally meant 'to breathe upon' but acquired extensions of meaning like 'to breathe in'.

To aspirate is to draw off fluids by suction. One way of choking is to aspirate food into the lungs during the act of vomiting. This is a danger for the semi-conscious trauma patient. Emergency treatment for certain ingested poisons may involve aspiration of the contents of the stomach (having the stomach pumped).

spondyl-

spondylos Greek, bone of the spine. Its Latin translation *vertebra* is widely used in medicine too.

ankylosing spondyl-itis

agkylos Greek, bent at an angle > *agkylosis* a bending + *spondylos* vertebra + *itis* inflammation

Ankylosing spondylitis is a rheumatoid inflammation of certain vertebral joints with ankylosis, that is, with bending and stiffening of the joint. The chief spinal joints involved are the sacroiliac, the intervertebral, and the costovertebral. If allowed to progress, ankylosing spondylitis may cause total spinal rigidity. Spondylosis is bending and stiffening of the spine and the accompanying degenerative spinal change.

squam-

squama Latin, a scale on a fish or a snake

Squamous is consisting of thin, plate-like structures or squamae; for example the squamous epithelial cells that make up the outer layer of the skin. They are flat, scaly, arranged in many layers. They are one of the reasons the skin peels after a sunburn or scratch. One type of skin cancer is squamous cell carcinoma. Desquamation is the scaling off of skin. Usually the epithelial tissue comes off in sheets or scales. This is also sometimes called desquamative exfoliation.

stapes

stapes Latin, stirrup on the saddle of a horse

The stapes is one of the three ossicles (little bones) of the middle ear. It resembles a little stirrup. It transmits sound waves from the incus to the inner ear. A tiny muscle called the stapedius attached to the wall of the tympanic cavity can pull the head of the stapes backward if the sound waves are too strong, thus preventing some injury to the inner ear. The stapedius acts with the muscle that stretches the ear drum, the tensor tympani.

stat

Abbreviation of *statim*, Latin, immediately

Stat is a beloved buzzword of television medical dramas where health professionals are seen in emergency rooms dashing about insanely and screaming 'Stat!' every few moments. In more realistic medical settings, stat is seen on charts and spoken calmly to reinforce the urgency of a clinical order.

-sten-

stenos Greek, narrow

angio-stenosis

angio blood vessel + *stenos* Greek, narrow + *osis* diseased condition

Angiostenosis is the pathological narrowing of blood vessels. Other vessels subject to abnormal narrowing are indicated in aortic stenosis and pyloric stenosis, where the sphincter muscle around the bottom of the stomach (called the pylorus from *pylouros* Greek, gatekeeper) contracts abnormally, blocking passage of food into the duodenum, and inducing projectile vomiting. An ulcer, congenital malformation, or cancer may cause pyloric stenosis which is correctable by surgery.

stereo-

stereos Greek, hard, solid, with the developed meaning of 'especially realistic' or 'three-dimensional'

chole-ster-ol

chole Greek, bile, gall + *stereos* solid, firm + *ol* biochemical suffix indicating an alcohol

Cholesterol is a solid alcohol of animal fats first isolated in gall stones. Early doctors thought it was solidified bile, hence the name.

stereo-taxis

stereos three-dimensional + *taxis* Greek, arrangement, depiction

Stereotaxis is a term in brain surgery. Stereotactic surgery permits the location of a minute area of the brain by detailed CAT scans (see entry), from which a three-dimensional image of the skull is displayed on a computer screen. Then, guided by data files and their screen display, a needle-like electrode is positioned to monitor electrical activity of neural tissue, and to deactivate and destroy tissue, if it is diseased. Stereotaxis as a three-dimensional arrangement is only apparently three-dimensional, for the illusion of depth is created on a two-dimensional screen by false perspective.

ster-oid

Literally, like sterols, a large group of biochemicals that includes cholesterol

Steroids are hormonal substances affecting growth and sexual processes, secreted mainly by the adrenal glands and the gonads. Steroid hormones include estrogen and androgen. One adrenal gland sits atop each kidney. Each adrenal gland consists of two distinct organs. An outer adrenal cortex surrounds an inner adrenal medulla. The adrenal cortex is an endrocrine (ductless) gland that secretes many hormones including the corticosteroids that are important in maintaining a kind of chemical status quo in the changing environment of the body, thus protecting living tissue which does not tolerate extreme chemical ups and downs. These steroid hormones prevent upheaval of body chemistry by forces like illness, injury, mental stress and great exertion. Without this chemical mediation by the hormones of the adrenal cortex, internal chemical fluctuations might prove lethal. Overdosing with steroid growth hormones by bodybuilders later produces many deleterious side-effects, some of them lethal.

sterno-, sternum

sternum Late Latin, breastbone < *sternon* Greek, the human chest. Sternum did not appear in English until the early 1800s.

The sternum is the breastbone at the middle of the thorax, a long, flat bone that articulates with the clavicles and the first seven ribs. Many muscles are attached sternally. Early anatomists thought the sternum resembled the short sword typically carried by an ancient Roman infantryman. The sternum has three parts. The upper part is the manubrium (Latin, handle, hilt of a sword < *manus* hand). The body of the sternum is the gladiolus (Latin, short sword; the gladiolus flower is named because the leaves of some species are also shaped like a short Roman army sword). At the lower end is a blunt, cartilaginous tip called the ensiform or xiphoid process (*ensis* Latin, sword + *forma* shape, form; and *xiphos* Greek, sword + -*oid* shaped like).

sterno-cleido-mast-oid muscle

sternum breastbone + *kleis, kleidos* Greek, key, clavicle + *mastos* breast + -*oid* shaped like

The sternocleidomastoid is a neck muscle with a long but apt name. It attaches to the mastoid process of the temporal bone behind the ear, to the back of the neck, and by separate heads to the clavicle and to the manubrium of the sternum. The sternocleidomastoid muscle flexes the vertebral column and helps rotate the head to an opposite side.

Kleido- is a combining form meaning clavicle because both words refer to a long bolt or key that locked ancient doors. Latin *clavicula* 'little key' is a diminutive of *clavis* 'key'. Clavicula meant literally 'little key', but in Latin it also denoted a long hoopstick, the water-bent wooden branch that Roman children used to trundle a hoop. This hoopstick was *f*-shaped like a human collarbone. It also referred to a long metal window latch quite like a human collarbone in shape. The clavicle is the long, slender, *f*-shaped collarbone that connects the breastbone (sternum) with the shoulder blade (scapula).

stetho-scope

stethos Greek, chest + *skopos* examiner, viewer

Stethoscope is a misnomer, since it means chest viewer. In fact one listens to or auscultates the heart and lungs with a stethoscope. It is a preliminary but useful method of detecting heart noises. Among the most prominent regular heart noises are 'lubb' and 'dupp'. The heart and its major vessels have valves to insure that the blood flows one way, that no backflow occurs. The slamming shut of the tricuspid and mitral valves makes a 'lubb' sound. The semilunar valves of the aorta and pulmonary artery then close with a shorter, higher 'dupp'.

-sthen-

sthenos Greek, strength

a-sthen-ia

a not + *sthenos* strength + *ia* medical condition

Asthenia is a loss of strength, a weakness, especially debility due to muscular or cerebellar diseases. Chronic fatigue syndrome is sometimes called neurocirculatory asthenia. The cause is unknown, but undue stress is implicated.

my-a-sthen-ia

mys, myos Greek, muscle + *a* not + *sthenos* strength + *ia* medical condition

Myasthenia is muscle weakness. Myasthenia gravis (*gravis* Latin, heavy, serious) is a rare disease of the voluntary muscles associated with problems in the thymus gland, whose surgical excision often removes myasthenic symptoms.

cali-sthenics

kalos Greek, beautiful + *sthenikos* pertaining to bodily strength

Calisthenics is, literally, beautiful strength, a system of rhythmic body exercises done without gym apparati.

stoma, -ostomy

stoma Greek, mouth, small opening; plural stomata

A stoma is any mouth-like opening, often surgically incised and kept open for drainage.

chole-cysto-stom-y

chole gall + *kystis* bladder + *stoma* mouth-like opening + *y* noun ending

Cholecystostomy is the surgical making of a mouth-like opening in the gallbladder through the abdominal wall, often for the purpose of inserting a catheter to drain excess fluid accumulation from the gallbladder.

colo-stom-y

colon + *stoma* mouth + *y* noun ending

Colostomy is making a mouth-like opening between the colon and the body surface for the discharge of fecal matter when, for example, the rectum has been removed because it was cancerous.

cysto-stom-y

kystis bag, urinary bladder + *stoma* mouth + *y* noun ending

Cystostomy is making a mouth-like opening in the urinary bladder for drainage.

stratum

stratus Latin, a flat layer. Our English word *street* is ultimately from the Latin phrase *via strata* 'paved roadway'.

Stratum, plural strata, names several layers of epidermal skin. The stratum corneum (*corneus* Latin, horny) is the horny, outer layer of the epidermis, thickest on palms and soles. The stratum germinativum (Latin, growing) or basal layer of the epidermis is where skin cells reproduce or 'germinate'. The stratum granulosum (Latin, full of granules) is an under layer of the epidermis with granules of old skin cells that die and gravitate to the skin surface to be sloughed off. The stratum lucidum (Latin, transparent) is a clear layer of the epidermis under the horny layer.

sub

sub Latin, under, beneath, below. The final *b* can assimilate to following consonants, for example, in words like success, suffix, suffuse, supplant, support, suppress, suspect, suspend and sustain.

Subcutaneous (*cutis* Latin, skin) is under the skin. Subconscious is below conscious apprehension. Subliminal (*limen* Latin, limit) is below the limit of conscious awareness.

sub-clav-ian

sub under + *clavicula* collarbone + *ianus* Latin, common adjectival suffix

Subclavian is under the collarbone. Clavicle is the anatomical name for the collarbone. The subclavian artery brings blood from the heart, passes deep under the clavicle, and continues as the artery carrying blood to the armpit.

sudor

sudor Latin, sweat, perspiration

A sudatorium is a hot-air bath or sweat bath, or the room in which such baths are taken to induce perspiration. Sudor is sweat. Certain nerves are sudomotor, stimulating the secretion of sweat. The sudoriferous glands of the skin secrete sweat. A chemical agent that produces sweating is a sudorific. A sudamen, plural sudamina, is a whitish blister caused by retention of sweat in the corneous layer of the skin. Sudamina appear during certain fevers and after heavy sweating, and are usually absorbed in a short time.

super

super Latin, above, over, excessive, akin to the Greek *hyper*. A prepositional combining form is supra-.

Supernumerary digits are congenitally extra fingers and toes. Superficial wounds are on the surface of a tissue like the skin (*superficies* Latin, surface).

super-ego

super above + *ego* Latin, oneself

In Freudian psychology, the superego is that part of the psyche that acts as a control over the ego. Psyche here is a special use of the Greek word for 'mind'.

supra-renal

supra Latin, adverb used as prefix, above + *ren* Latin, kidney
This is the correction of an established medical term, namely adrenal, attached
to the kidney. It was decided that suprarenal better described where the glands
are – above the kidney. The term, however, is rare.

superior

superior Latin, more above, higher, on top of. In its form,
superior is a comparative adjective from *super*.
Superior is an anatomical descriptive, meaning above, toward the top,
uppermost. It is the opposite of inferior. The eyes are superior to the mouth, but
inferior to the scalp. The two venae cavae are the large veins that bring
deoxygenated venous blood back to the heart. The superior vena cava, above the
heart, more toward the top of the body, returns blood from the upper part of
the body. The inferior vena cava, below the heart, more toward the lower part
of body, returns blood from there.

supine

supinus Latin, facing up
Supine is lying face up on one's back. The opposite is prone, lying face
downwards on one's stomach. Supination is the act of turning the palm upward
or raising the medial margin of the foot. The supinator is a muscle in the arm
that turns the palm upward. Pronation of the hand is turning the palm down.
Pronation of the foot is lowering the medial margin of the foot. A pronator is a
muscle that pronates a body part.

sym-

syn > sym Greek, one of the common assimilating forms of *syn*
with, together

sym-physis

syn > sym together + *physis* Greek, a growing
A symphysis is a joint at which fibrous cartilage joins the two bones firmly but
allows some slight flexing, e.g. the pubic symphysis of the pelvis where the two
pubic bones join.

sym-ptom

syn > sym together + *ptoma* Greek, calamity, disaster, disease
A symptom is any subjective evidence of disease or disorder that the patient
notices, e.g. a headache, a chronic upset stomach, a feeling of dizziness. Signs are
objective symptoms of disease that others including a doctor may observe, e.g. a
skin rash, a palsy, a motor impediment.

syn-

syn Greek, with, together

syn-apse

syn with + *apsos* Greek, joint, juncture
A synapse is a junction of the processes of two neurons where a nerve impulse is
transmitted from one neuron to another.

syn-drome

syn together + *dromos* Greek, a running
A syndrome is a group of symptoms that occur together, e.g. carpal tunnel
syndrome (see *carpal* entry).

syn-thesis

syn together + *thesis* Greek, a putting, a placing, a making
Synthesis is putting together or creating a thing from its elements, e.g. the
artificial chemical creation of a vitamin that also occurs naturally, like synthetic
vitamin C; hence synthetic is artificial, made-up.

syringe

syrigx, syringos Greek, any hollow tube, hence a reed pipe, a
whistle
In 1853 a Scottish doctor, Alexander Wood, made a hollow metal needle to
inject a narcotic under the skin or hypodermically, and called it a syringe.
Earlier claims do exist. The hypodermic syringe (each word has become a
synonym for the other) appeared in an all-glass version in 1896.

syring-itis

syrigx, syringos hollow tube

Syringitis is inflammation of the auditory tube in the ear, also called the syrinx. In zoology, syrinx is the lower trachea of birds where song is produced. Debussy wrote a flute solo entitled Syrinx, imitating the sound of reed pipes or pan-pipes, as played by a lonely shepherd.

systole, systolic

syn > sys together + *stole* Greek, a putting, a drawing

Systole is the contraction of the ventricles of the heart, when blood is pumped out. Diastole (*diastole* a drawing apart of the ventricles of the heart) is the relaxing and expanding of the ventricles, when blood flows into the heart. Blood pressure measures the pressure against the vessel walls. When the ventricles contract, the highest pressure is produced, the systolic. When the ventricles relax, the lowest, the diastolic pressure, is evident.

syn-cope

syn with + *kope* Greek, a cutting, hency *synkope* was 'a cutting short'

A syncope is a fainting spell, due to temporary loss of cellular oxygen in part of the brain. This transient cerebral hypoxia may be ischemic (*ischein* Greek, to block, to check the flow of + *haemia* blood condition). Ischemia is lack of sufficient blood in a body part due to narrowed or blocked blood vessels.

T

tabes

tabes Latin noun, a wasting away, in medicine the wasting away of body tissue during the course of certain chronic diseases
Tabes dorsalis is a wasting of the dorsal columns of the spine in late stages of syphilis, often producing severe flashing pains and a characteristic tabetic gait with very high steps taken to try to avoid the pains. An older name of this syphilitic wasting was locomotor ataxia, literally, disorder of movement required to get from place to place.

tachy-

tachys Greek, swift, quick

tachy-cardia

tachys quick + *kardos* heart + *ia* medical condition
Tachycardia is a high rate of contraction of heart muscle, to increase oxygen supply to body cells by quickening the circulation of the blood. It occurs naturally during exercise, excitement, even when one laughs. Pathological tachycardia in adults is more than 100 heart beats per minute, seen in some high fevers, hemorrhages and cardiac diseases, and as a reaction to drugs like atropine and nicotine.

tali-pes

talus Latin, ankle + *pes, pedis* Latin, foot; in combination talipes means 'clubfoot'
Talipes is a usually congenital deformity of the foot. In talipes calcaneus (Latin, of the heel), the toes point up and the patient walks on his heels. In talipes equinus (Latin, like a horse), the toes point down and the patient walks on his toes. See also *valgus* and *varus* entries.

tarsus

tarsos podos Greek, Hippocrates' term for the flat of the foot between the heel and the toe
A tarsus is one of the seven bones of the ankle, the tarsi, permitting articulation between the foot and the leg. They are also called the tarsals.

meta-tarsals

meta Greek, after + tarsal
The metatarsals are the bones of the foot that come after the tarsals and before the phalanges (bones of the toes). Each foot has two metatarsal arches or areas of curved outline: the transverse arch across the foot, and the longitudinal arch along the length of the foot. In the biophysics of walking upright, arches support and add spring to the step.

taxis

taxis Greek, arrangement, but with the developed sense of 'motion toward or away from'; combining forms taxi-, taxo-
Taxis is an organism's movement in response to a stimulus, either away from or toward the source of the stimulus.

a-taxia

a not + *taxis* ordinary motion, arrangement
Ataxia is literally unarrangement, an unco-ordination of the muscle actions involved in a body movement. A late stage of syphilis of the spinal cord was called locomotor ataxia (*locomotor* Latin, moving from place to place). See tabes.

chemo-taxis

chemeia Greek, chemistry (the word passed into Arabic and came back into English as alchemy) + *taxis* ordered movement
Chemotaxis is movement toward or away from a chemical. Leukocyte chemotaxis involves white blood cells being attracted to certain chemicals formed in immune reactions. Leukocytes then cluster near the reaction as part of the healing process. Phototaxis is movement toward light, as displayed by moths.

taxo-nomy

taxis arrangement + *nomos* Greek, law + *y* noun ending
Taxonomy is the science or law of arranging and classifying animals and plants.
Thus the study of the laws of the stars would be astronomy (*aster* Greek, star).

T-cell

A short form of thymus cell or thymocyte
T-cells are lymphoid cells made in bone marrow which migrate to mature in the
thymus gland and then circulate in the blood and the lymph. The many varieties
of T-cells are important parts of the body's immune system.

temporal

temporalis Latin, pertaining to the side of the head < *tempus*
time
It also meant the temple of the head. The temple is the flat area at the side of the
head above each ear. No one knows why this area was named with a word
signifying time, but one ingenious guess has been made: namely, that since the
hair begins to first turn grey over the temporal area, time and the temple are
related. The temporal bone is part of the skull around the ear. The temporal
lobe is part of the brain under the temporal bone, associated with hearing and
memory.

temporo-mandibular joint

tempus, temporis developed meaning of temporal bone +
mandibulum Late Latin, the lower jaw, mandible, literally 'the
little chewer' < *mandare* to chew
The mandible is the lower jaw bone, the only bone of the skull that moves. It
has a round projection at each end called a condyle (*kondylos* Greek, knuckle,
joint) that fits into a hollow area called a fossa (Latin, ditch, trench, pit) in the
temporal bones at each side of the face. This is the temperomandibular joint, and
its articulation allows the chewing motion in which the mandible with its cargo
of lower teeth is moved up and down against the maxillary bones (*maxilla* Latin,
upper jaw) that form most of the upper jaw and hold the upper teeth. In
temporomandibular joint syndrome, chewing produces severe pain and clicking
sounds when the joint is moved. Malocclusion, badly fitting dentures, various
arthritides, or tumors may be causative.

tendon

tendo, tendinis medical Latin, a sinew < *tenon* Greek, a stretched band, a sinew

A tendon is a sinew, a tough, whitish cord made of collagen fibers that attaches muscles to bones. A tendon is not a ligament. The most famous is Achilles' tendon. In Greek mythology, Achilles' mother, to protect him from harm, took her son by the foot and dipped him in the magical waters of the River Styx. But she failed to wet the powerful tendon at the back of the heel, the tendon that attaches the triceps surae to the heelbone, so that Achilles was fatally wounded later in that spot. And ever afterward it was called Achilles' tendon.

A ligament (*ligamentum* Latin, a binding, a wrapping, a bond, a tie < *ligare* to tie up, to pull tight) is not a tendon. A ligament is a fibrous band of connective tissue that joins bones where they articulate with other bones. Ligaments help keep joints together, and they help set the limits of joint movement.

terato-

teras, teratos Greek, a wonder, a marvel, a fetal monster

In gynecology, a teras is a severely deformed fetal monster. A teratism is a congenital or acquired structural abnormality. See the *anomaly* entry. Teratology is the branch of medicine that studies the causes of fetal monstrosity. Certain drugs and medications can be teratogenic, producing fetal anomalies. Maternal tobacco smoking is known to cause underweight babies. Heroin, LSD, thalidomide, mercury, polychlorinated biphenyls (PCBs), and certain sedatives and tranquilizers are fetotoxic and teratogenic.

testis

testis Latin, witness

Compare the verb 'to testify', originally, to act as a witness, to swear an oath. In the Old Testament, and many other records of different ancient cultures, a man had to hold his hand not over his heart as we do, but over his genitals when swearing a solemn oath. Testis meaning 'testicle' may also have developed in Latin with the sense that the testicles (little witnesses) were witness or proof of manhood. Under Roman law, a male could not testify unless his testicles were present. No eunuchs were called to court.

The testis is one of two glands in the scrotum that make spermatozoa and produce the chief androgen or male hormone called testosterone. During the growth of a human male fetus, the testes descend, from the abdominal cavity where they form, down into the scrotum. Undescended testicles can be fixed in place by surgery.

tetanus

tetanos Greek adjective, stretched

An anaerobic bacterium, *Clostridium tetani*, grows at the site of surface lesions to produce this severe infectious disease that leads to often fatal tonic spasms of the voluntary muscles. Indicated is immediate and intensive care with tetanus immune globulin, penicillin and other agents. Tetanus antitoxin can produce passive immunity to prevent the development of the disease and is also sometimes used early in active tetanus.

tetany

tetanos Greek adjective, stretched

The confusingly named tetany describes intermittent and painful muscle spasms of the arms and legs, often in young pregnant females and those lactating. Excessive calcium and changes in blood pH make the nerves and muscles too excitable.

-thel-

thele Greek, nipple

endo-thel-ium

endon inside + *thele* Greek, nipple + *ium* Latin neuter noun suffix

Endothelium is epithelial tissue, composed of flat and scale-like cells that line the internal organs of the body like the heart, as well as the veins and arteries. The name was conceived on the analogy of epithelium, itself first coined in 1700 to refer to the cells just surrounding the nipple. Later, when the use of the narrow term was broadened, the inappropriate Greek root for 'nipple' stayed in the word.

epi-thel-ium

epi Greek, on + *thele* nipple + *ium* Latin neuter noun suffix

Epithelium is the varied, external tissue that covers the body, the outer layer of the skin. Epithelium also forms the surface layer of mucous and serous membranes, and thus it lines hollow organs such as the bladder, and the passages of the respiratory, digestive and urinary tracts. Epithelium as a word was first coined in 1700 to refer only to the cells surrounding the nipple. Later, the meaning was expanded but the specific root was not changed. Related words containing the 'nipple' root are thelitis, meaning sore nipples due to inflammation, and the rarer term thelalgia, or pain in the nipples.

epitheli-oma

epithelio + *oma* tumor
Epithelioma is a malignant tumor, a carcinoma, made up of epithelial cells. The tumor originates in the skin or in a mucous membrane. One form is basal cell epithelioma, in which the tumor derives from cells in the basal layer of the epidermis, also called the stratum germinativum.

thel-arche

thele nipple + *arche* Greek, beginning, onset
Thelarche is the onset of female breast development, usually commencing just before puberty.

therapy

therapeia Greek, a tending of the sick, a healing
Therapy is the treatment of a disease or disordered condition. The branch of medicine concerned with specific remedies and treatments is sometimes called therapeutics.

thermo-

thermos Greek, hot, warm

thermo-meter

thermos hot + *metron* Greek, thing that measures
A clinical thermometer measures the patient's temperature at the bedside, often taken two or three times in a row. One reading is not as useful as knowing the progress of the temperature. The rise and fall over a specified time are as meaningful as the precise level taken once. Many kinds of thermometer are used, including gas, recording, rectal and tympanic.

thermo-taxis

thermos hot + *taxis* arrangement
Thermotaxis is the normal adjustment of body temperature. Thermotaxis may also mean movement of an organism in response to heat rise or fall.

thorax

thorax, thorakis Greek, breastplate of armor, then chest
In anatomy, the thorax is the part of the body from the base of the neck to the diaphragm, in ordinary English, the chest area. The bony thorax comprises the thoracic vertebrae, twelve pairs of ribs and the sternum.

thora-centesis

thorax chest + *kentesis* Greek, a surgical puncturing of < *kensai* to prick, to stab
Thoracentesis, also more fully called thoracocentesis, is inserting a large needle through the chest wall to aspirate excess fluids.

thrombo-

thrombos Greek, lump, clot
A thrombus is a blood clot, a solid mass of blood parts stuck to the wall of a blood vessel. Thus thrombosis is the medical condition in which thrombi occur in arteries and veins.

coronary thrombosis

coronarius Medieval Latin, like a wreath, crowning
The coronary arteries are so named because they encircle the heart like a garland or wreath. Here is the source of the lay term 'coronary' for a kind of heart attack, namely a myocardial infarction or occlusion.

A coronary thrombosis is blockage by blood clots of the arteries of the heart and consequent damage to heart tissue. Thrombotic occlusion describes such arterial blockage.

thymo-

thymos Greek, thyme, the sweet-smelling herb
Galen, the ancient physician and medical writer, thought a dissected thymus gland resembled a bunch of thyme leaves – one of the more far-fetched metaphors in medical nomenclature.

The thymus gland is found at the bottom of the neck in the chest behind the breastbone. The thymus is large in children, and gets smaller in adults. It secretes a hormone called thymosin that helps make antibodies against some diseases. The thymus is full of lymphocytes, and is involved in regulating the body's autoimmune responses to its own tissue.

thyroid

thyreo-eides Greek, like a door-shaped shield

The thyroid cartilage was named first. It shields the vocal cords of the larynx. This cartilage (*cartilago* Latin, gristle) sticks out in front of the neck and is called the Adam's apple. A *thyreos* was an ancient Greek army shield shaped like a door (*thyra*), with a notch at the top for the soldier's chin. Gently feel the top of your Adam's apple. It has a notch. An apt name, isn't it? The last part of the Greek word comes from *eidos* form, likeness. It gives us the very common English suffix *-oid*.

The thyroid gland was named after the thyroid cartilage. This gland has a lobe on each side of the Adam's apple. It makes a hormone called thyroxine that controls the rate of chemical reactions in the body, that is, it helps control the metabolic rate. The thyroid gland needs iodine to make thyroxine. If there is a lack of iodine in the diet, the gland must work overtime and may become huge. This enlarging of the thyroid is simple goiter (*goitron* Old French, throat). Calcitonin is also a thyroid hormone that controls blood calcium.

tibia

tibia Latin, a flute, any musical pipe; plural *tibiae*

The tibia is the larger bone of the lower leg. The tibia forms a socket with the femur proximally, and forms part of the knee joint, and distally articulates with the fibula and ankle bone. The medial malleolus of the tibia forms one of the knobs of the ankle. The Anglo-Saxon term was shin or shin bone. The Latin term came into use because the ancient Romans made panpipes from thin reeds and flutes, and whistles from hollow tubular objects like the shin bones of birds. Tibiofemoral is pertaining to the tibia and femur.

tinea

tinea Latin, moth, bookworm, any gnawing worm < *tondere* to gnaw

Tinea is ringworm, a fungal skin disease of various body parts. Athlete's foot is tinea pedis. Dhobie itch, a skin fungus of the genital area, is tinea cruris.

-toc-

tokos Greek, birth, childbirth

Tocology is a rare synonym for obstetrics or midwifery.

dys-toc-ia

dys Greek bad, abnormal + *tokos* childbirth + *ia* medical condition

Dystocia is a prolonged or difficult labor, due to a large fetus, its abnormal position, or an obstruction or constriction of the birth canal.

eu-toc-ia

eu Greek, well, easy, normal, good + *tokos* childbirth + *ia* condition

Eutocia is normal labor in childbirth.

oxy-toc-in

oxys Greek, sharp, sharpening, quickening · *tokos* childbirth + *in* noun suffix for organic chemical compound

Oxytocin is a hormone made by the pituitary gland that stimulates some processes of birth.

-tomy

tome Greek, a surgical cutting, combining form tomo-

ana-tomy

ana Greek, up + *tome* Greek, a cutting, a dissection; in medicine a surgical incision

The original sense of the word *anatomy* was cutting up a body. Now anatomy means the study of the structure of living organisms.

ap-pend-ec-tomy, ap-pend-ix

ad > ap Latin, to, on + *pendix* Latin, hanging part + *ectomy* surgical cutting out of

In Latin *appendix* meant 'addition or appendage'. In anatomy it is any supplementary part of a main structure, like the vermiform appendix. See *appendicitis* entry.

Appendectomy is surgical excision of the vermiform appendix (*vermiformis* scientific Latin, shaped like a worm).

tomo-graph

tomos Greek, a section + *graphe* Greek, a drawing, a picture, a recording of

In tomography, a machine moves an X-ray tube through an arc, so that the X-ray shows one plane of tissue clearly. In a computerized axial tomography scan, hundreds of X-ray pictures are taken as a machine revolves around, for example, the head. The X-rays of these sectional brain views, compared in a computer to previous X-ray series, help the doctor, with other scanner data files, to assess the size and spread of a brain tumor. Axial refers to an axis, an imaginary line drawn through the center of a body part, around which the body part could be said to revolve. By adjusting the axis of the part being scanned, many different axial views are made.

tone

tonos Greek, the quality of being stretched, like a musical note (tone) or a muscle < *teinein* to stretch

Muscle tone is the stretchiness of a muscle, its flexibility and firmness; the steady, lightly contracted state of a normal skeletal muscle that helps keep a human being standing upright, and aids in the return of blood to the heart. It is also called tonus.

iso-tonic and iso-metric

isos Greek, equal, the same + *tonos* stretchiness or + *metrikos* Greek, pertaining to measurement

In isotonic contraction, the muscle shortens against a pulling resistance, but the muscle tone stays the same. Isometric contraction has the muscle tone increasing, but the muscle does not shorten.

-tonia

tonos Greek, stretchiness

a-ton-ia, a-ton-y

a not + *tonos* stretchiness + *ia* medical condition

Atony is a lack of normal tone in muscle or in a muscular sac like a bladder.

dys-ton-ia

dys bad, abnormal + *tonos* stretchiness + *ia* medical condition

Dystonia is abnormal muscle tone, e.g. a spasm due to a drug reaction or to a rare genetic disorder like dystonia musculorum deformans.

myo-ton-ia

mys, myos Greek, muscle + *tonos* stretchiness + *ia* medical condition

In myotonia, a muscle or muscle group has a very long period of contraction and does not relax fully after contraction. Myotonus is tonic spasm of a muscle or group of muscles.

tort-, torq-, tors-, torsion

torsio, torsionis Latin, an act of twisting

Torsion is the act or state of twisting; in dentistry, torsion is turning a tooth on its long axis.

torti-collis

tortus Latin, twisted + *collum* Latin, neck

Torticollis is wryneck, torsion of the neck due to spasm and contraction of the sternocleidomastoid muscle, with bending of the head toward the affected side. Conservative therapy includes applying heat, stretching exercises, perhaps analgesics. In rare, persistent cases, partial myectomy (muscle-cutting) of the sternocleidomastoid muscle may be involved.

toxic, toxin

toxikon Greek, arrow poison

Toxic means poisonous in medicine. A toxin is the poisonous substance itself. Toxicology is the branch of medical biochemistry that deals with the detection of poison, studying its chemical action in the body, preparing antidotes, and preventing exposure to toxins. Toxicosis is the pathological condition that obtains after poisoning has occurred.

trachea

tracheia Greek, rough

The trachea is the windpipe, a tube of elastic membrane held open by cartilage hoops, that extends from the voice box to just above the lungs where it divides into the two main bronchi, one to each lung. Ancient Greeks called it the rough air-carrier or *arteria tracheia*, whence its medical name in modern English.

tracheo-tomy

trachea + *tome* Greek, a surgical incision

If the larynx is blocked, an emergency passage to get air to the lungs can be made by cutting into the trachea through the neck and then inserting a tube to keep the tracheotomy open.

trans-

trans Latin, across, through

trans-fusion

trans across + *fusio, fusionis* the pouring out of a liquid

Tranfusion is introducing whole blood or blood parts into the blood stream.

trans-plant

trans across + *plantare* Latin, originally, to stamp one's feet on the ground; then, since farmers and gardeners do this when planting crops, it came to mean to seed, to make cuttings and to graft plant parts. Late Latin *implantare* = to graft

Transplant as a noun means grafted tissue; as a verb, to transfer tissue from one part to another.

trauma

trauma Greek, wound, plural traumas, traumata

A trauma is a physical injury or wound. Sometimes trauma refers to a psychological shock. Chief kinds of trauma are car accidents, suicide, homicide, falls, burns and drowning. Birth trauma is injury to a fetus as it is being born. In dentistry, toothbrush trauma is caused by too-vigorous brushing with a stiff brush, producing visible grooves in the teeth and injury to the gums.

343

tri-ceps

tris in threes < *tres* three + *ceps* < *caput* Latin, head, hence, with three heads

Triceps is a muscle of the upper arm with three points of origin called the long head, lateral head and medial head. The triceps helps extend the arm and forearm. The biceps (*bis* Latin, twice) is an arm muscle with two heads, that is, two points of origin or two divisions, a long head and a short head. The biceps helps flex the forearm and turn it up or down.

tricho-

thrix, trichos Greek, a hair

trich-iasis

thrix, trichos a hair, a hair-like object + *iasis* Greek, disordered condition

Trichiasis is turning in of the eyelashes, that then abrade the surface of the cornea and irritate the eyeball. It is usually associated with entropion (Greek, a turning inward), a turning in of the edge of the lower eyelid. Trichiasis can also be labeled trichoma.

tricho-tillo-mania

thrix, trichos a hair + *tillein* Greek, to pull + *mania* madness

Trichotillomania is obsessive pulling out of one's hair, far beyond any nervous gesture of brief duration.

trocar

trois quarts French, three-quarters

A trocar is a medical instrument with a sharp, three-sided point that fits inside a cannula. It is used to pierce the wall of a body cavity. The trocar is then withdrawn, and the cannula or tube is left in place to maintain the patency of the incised hole, usually to permit fluid to drain out of an infected body cavity.

trochanter

trochanter Greek noun, a roller, a runner < *trochos* wheel

Two of the bony processes below the neck of the femur are called trochanters. Both the greater and the lesser trochanter serve as places of attachment for leg muscles.

trop-

tropos Greek, a turn, a turning

hyper-trop-ia

hyper Greek, above + *tropos* Greek, a turning + *ia* medical condition
Hypertropia is a turning upward of the visual axis of the eye, a form of strabismus or eye deviation.

neuro-trop-ism

neuron Greek, nerve + *tropos* Greek, a turning + *ismos* noun suffix indicating a condition
Neurotropism is a tendency of vascular tissues to grow toward certain areas of nerve tissue.

photo-trop-ism

phos, photos Greek, light + *tropos* Greek, a turning + *ismos* noun suffix indicating a condition
Phototropism is the growth response toward light of most plants, including some parasitic to man.

tropo-mys-in

tropos a turning + *mys, myos* Greek, muscle + *in* noun ending for organic chemical compound
Tropomysin is a muscle protein that inhibits contraction.

troph-

trophe Greek, food, nourishment

a-trophy

a not + *trophe* nourishment
Atrophy literally is not feeding, hence any wasting away of bodily tissue with shrinkage in size of the tissue. For example, disuse atrophy, typically muscle atrophy due to lack of normal exercise; 'use it or lose it'.

dys-trophy

dys Greek negative prefix indicating difficult or disordered function + *trophe* nourishment
Dystrophy is any disease due to faulty nutrition in a body part. Note the many muscular dystrophies which are serious degenerative diseases.

hyper-trophy

hyper Greek, over + *trophe* feeding
Hypertrophy is excess tissue growth due to increase in cell size.

tumor

tumor Latin, swelling, neoplasm, cancer
Tumor in its original meaning of swelling is one of the four classic medical signs of inflammation, namely, tumor, rubor, dolor and calor: swelling, redness, pain and heat.

A tumor that is an uncontrolled growth of new tissue may be benign or malignant.

tympanum

tympanon Greek, a broad drum made of skin, then eardrum
Tympanum can refer to the tympanic membrane, the eardrum, or to the tympanic cavity within that is also called the middle ear.

typh-oid fever

Typhoid is an English coinage that means 'resembling typhus'. See next entry
Typhoid fever is a severe, sometimes fatal bacterial infection caused by *Salmonella typhi*. The symptoms include high fevers, diarrhea, delirium, enlarged spleen, coughing and rosy spots on the abdomen. Antibiotics help, and short-term prevention is possible by means of a typhoid vaccine.

typhus

typhos Greek, high fever

Typhus refers to a number of infectious diseases caused by *Rickettsia* micro-organisms, parasitic on certain fleas and lice. Epidemic typhus is thus common where humans are packed together in unsanitary conditions: refugee camps, badly run ships, and so on. Broad-spectrum antibiotics given early in the course of typhus, and rigid cleanliness of the patient's physical site are necessary for effective treatment. Fatalities are high in epidemic typhus.

ulcer

ulcus Latin, a sore, an ulcer, akin to *elkos* Greek, a sore
An ulcer is a limited lesion of the skin or mucous membranes that line many organs and body parts, an open sore with dead tissue due to infection, inflammation, or malignancy.

de-cubitus ulcer

de down + *cubitus* Latin, lying in bed
A decubitus ulcer is a bedsore, an ulceration of tissue lacking blood supply because blood vessels are pressed against bones, common in immobile, elderly, bed-ridden patients. Bedsore sites include elbow, hip, buttocks and shoulder.

ulcerative col-itis

ulcerativus scientific Latin, with ulcers, accompanied by ulcerations; *kolon* Greek, Aristotle's word for part of the large intestine + *itis* inflammation of
Ulcerative colitis is a serious, chronic, episodic inflammatory disease of the large intestine and rectum, whose symptoms include cramping pain, watery diarrhea with blood, mucus and pus in the stools, fever, chills, anemia and weight loss. In children it may disrupt normal growth. Treatments include anti-inflammatory drugs and possibly intestinal surgery.

ulna

ulna Latin, elbow
The word contains a very ancient pre-Indo-European root *el* that seems to have referred to a small measuring rod of specific length, namely, the length of a human forearm. The root gives the name and the shape of the letter *l* in many languages. Our Roman letter *l* derives from the Greek letter *lambda*, itself from Phoenician *lamed* 'goad, stick used as a cattle or sheep prod'. Many Indo-European words for elbow contain this root: *olene* Greek, *Ellenbogen* German, *lokat* Russian. And there was a common European measure of distance called an ell.

The ulna is the larger of the two main bones of the forearm; the smaller is the radius. At the elbow joint, the ulna articulates with the humerus; at the wrist, with the radius. The adjective is ulnar.

ultra-

ultra Latin, beyond, above normal

ultra-violet (UV)

Ultraviolet denotes wavelengths of light beyond violet in the color spectrum, and not visible. Ultraviolet radiation is one therapy used to treat skin disorders like severe acne and psoriasis. Natural ultraviolet radiation in sunlight can harm skin if received in excess.

ultra-sonic

ultra beyond + *sonicus* Late Latin, pertaining to sound
Ultrasonic sound waves are beyond the range of human hearing, higher than 20 000 cycles per second. Ultrasound imaging techniques permit reflected high-frequency sound waves to form an image of an internal structure like a fetus or a heart.

umbilicus

umbilicus Latin, navel, belly button; akin to Greek *omphalos* (see entry)
The umbilicus is the place on the mid-abdomen where the umbilical cord is connected to the fetus. Sometimes the abdominal wall around the navel has a congenital or acquired weakness and a small portion of intestine and omentum may protrude in an umbilical hernia.

uni-

unus Latin, one, single
Many English words borrowed from Latin contain this root: unit, a single thing, a segment of a whole; unity, a making one, a uniting; unify, to make one.

uni-cellular

unus one + *cellula* Latin, a little cell
Unicellular is made up of one cell, e.g. a bacterium.

uni-lateral

unus one + *lateralis* of a side
Unilateral means affecting one side only, as in a hemiplegia or unilateral paralysis.

uni-para

unus Latin, one + *para* New Latin, a female parent, one who has borne offspring
A unipara is a woman who has borne one child, also called a primipara.

urea

urea scientific Latin, from *ouron* Greek, urine
Urea is a nitrogenous waste compound found in urine, blood and lymph. Urea is one of the significant end products of protein metabolism in the body, and the removal of urea is the major function of the human urinary system.

blood urea nitrogen test

A blood urea nitrogen or B.U.N. test is part of blood work that measures the amount of urea in the blood. The results reflect basic kidney function. Excessive urea in the blood is uremia, indicating possible kidney failure, and possible imminent death, unless dialysis is begun immediately.

ureter

oureter Greek, urine carrier
The ureters are two narrow tubes, one from each kidney, about 10–12 inches long, which carry urine from the kidneys down to the urinary bladder. Urine is propelled through the ureters by peristaltic waves of muscle contraction that average one peristaltic wave every 20 seconds.

uretero-lith

oureter ureter + *lithos* Greek, pebble, stone, calculus
A ureterolith (a somewhat obscure term, to be sure) is a stone or abnormal mineral deposit stuck in one of the ureteral tubes. It is surgically removed during a ureterolithotomy.

ureter-ec-tasis

oureter ureter + *ek* out + *tasis* Greek, a stretching
Ureterectasis is a swelling up or distention of the ureter, possibly due to
blockage by a ureteral calculus.

uretero-sten-osis

oureter ureter + *stenos* narrow + *osis* abnormal condition
Stenosis is an abnormal narrowing of a tube-like structure. Thus ureterostenosis
is a pathological narrowing of the ureter. This stricture may be caused by an
adjacent swelling, a bladder tumor, or other disorder.

urethra

ourethra Greek, literally, urine-door = *ouron* urine + *thyra*
door, passageway
The urethra is the tube from the bladder to the body's exterior for the discharge
of urine. The female urethra is approximately one and a half inches long, and
carries urine from the bladder to the urethral or urinary meatus, which is the
external opening of the urethra. The common English terms for this urethral
orifice are from the nursery: pee hole, pee slit. The male urethra is eight inches
long, and carries both urine and semen to the external opening at the tip of the
penis. Encircling an upper portion of the urethra is the prostate gland which
secretes a fluid that aids the movement of sperm.

urin-, urinary

urina Latin, urine
Urine is a fluid formed in the kidneys by filtering blood. This filtration removes
nitrogenous end products of protein metabolism and other waste from the
bloodstream, and helps maintain a balance of water, salts and acids in body
fluids. To urinate or to micturate is to pass urine through the urethra, to void
water.
   The urinary system consists of blood-filters (the kidneys), tubes to lead
urine to the bladder (the ureters), a muscular storage reservoir (the bladder), and
a tube to lead urine outside the body (the urethra).

uterus

uterus Latin, womb < *uter, utris* big wineskin, water sack made
of leather. And see entry for the Greek equivalent *hystero-* also
widely used in medicine.

The non-pregnant uterus is a hollow, muscular organ, about three inches long and pear-shaped, suspended in the pelvic cavity by ligaments. At its top end the uterus connects to the Fallopian tubes; at its bottom end it narrows into a neck or cervix that opens into the vagina, as part of the birth canal through which the fetus passes during birth. This chief organ of the female reproductive system allows implantation of the fertilized egg, embryonic and fetal growth and nourishment during pregnancy. Three uterine layers envelop the organ. The inner layer of mucous membrane, the endometrium, helps form the placenta in pregnancy. The myometrium is the muscular layer that contracts during labor to help expel the fetus. The outer layer or parametrium is serous connective tissue that extends into the broad ligament. The suffix -*metrium* derives from *metra* Greek, womb, by way of a diminutive form *metrion* Greek, 'little mother object, little womb'.

uvea

uveus Latin, grape-like < *uva* grape. Compare modern Italian *uva* grapes

Uvea is a Latin translation of a phrase used by the Roman medical writer Galen. He wrote in Greek and used a phrase meaning 'grape-like tunic' to refer to the choroid layer and the iris of the eye, because, he wrote, they resemble a grape with the stalk torn out leaving a hole in front, the hole being the pupil of the eye.

The uvea is the pigmented layer of the eye, namely the fibrous tunic under the sclera (see *sclera* entry) which includes the iris, the ciliary body and the choroid coating. Uveitis is inflammation of this ocular tract.

uvula

uvula Medieval Latin, a little bunch of grapes

The uvula is a fleshy mass projecting from the soft palate mid-line at the back of the oral cavity, clearly seen when the mouth is wide open. During human speech the uvula helps shape certain guttural sounds. For example, in Parisian French, one uses the uvula in making the rolled *r* sound in *rouge* and *rue*. In the true Scottish pronunciation of *loch*, one vibrates the uvula to make the guttural *ch* sound. In the film of *The Wizard of Oz*, when Bert Lahr as the cowardly lion makes the sound *nong-nong-nong*, his uvula is vibrating like a struck gong.

vaccine

vaccinus Latin, from cows < *vacca* cow

Vaccina was an old term in English medicine for cowpox. The first vaccination was an inoculation of cowpox virus injected hypodermically to produce a human immunity to smallpox, a procedure whose worldwide use has almost eliminated smallpox as a disease. A vaccine is now any suspension in liquid of killed micro-organisms given by several means to induce an active immunity to an infectious disease.

vagina

vagina Latin, sheath for a sword, hence the human vagina, based on a pun in Latin where *gladius* was a name for a short army sword and was also widely used as a colloquial word for penis

The vagina is a muscular tube or canal lined with mucosa that extends from the neck of the uterus to the outside orifice.

vagin-itis

vagina + *itis* inflammation of

Vaginitis is inflammation of the vagina. Atrophic vaginitis (*atrophikos* Greek, not growing, weakened, not fed) may be seen in the postmenopausal female. The epithelial lining of the vagina becomes thin or ulcerated or with mucosal adhesions, all due to a decline in the level of the hormone estrogen, so that therapy may include taking estrogen.

valve

valva Latin, the leaf of a folding wooden door in a Roman house < *volvere* to fold up, to roll up

A valve is an arrangement of tissue folds in the wall of a tube or canal to permit passage of a fluid in one direction only, and therefore to prevent reflux or flowing back of the fluid. Valvulitis is inflammation of a cardiac valve often due to rheumatic fever.

bi-cuspid valve

bi two + *cuspis, cuspidis* Latin, point, sharp end
Bicuspid means 'having two points'. A bicuspid valve in the heart has two valvular leaves and looks a bit like a bishop's hat or miter, and so it was first called the mitral valve.

mitral valve

mitralis Late Latin, having two points like a *mitra* Latin, bishop's hat
The mitral valve is in the heart between the left atrium and the left ventricle. It permits blood flow from the left atrium into the left ventricle, and prevents backflow or reflux by closing. The mitral or bicuspid valve is the only heart valve with two, rather than three, cusps. Many terms in cardiopathology use the adjective. A mitral murmur is a heart sound caused by a defective bicuspid valve. In mitral valve stenosis, the little leaves of the valve acquire adhesions which block effective closure of the valve, leading to an enlarged left atrium and possible failure of the right side of the heart. In mitral valve prolapse (Latin, a falling in front of), one or both cusps fall back into the left atrium causing incomplete closure and a backflow of blood. This mitral regurgitation can lead to abnormal enlargement of the left side of the heart, and possibly eventual congestive heart failure.

varicose vein

varicosus Medical Latin, full of varices. A varix is a dilated, twisted vein, artery, or lymphatic vessel.
Varicose veins are common, especially in obese women and sometimes during pregnancy. Most often affected are the saphenous veins in the legs (see *saphenous* entry). Varicosis may be caused by congenital defects in the valves of veins and by chronic pressure on the inside lining of the veins from occupations that require long standing on the feet. Pain, muscle cramps and a full feeling in the legs are often symptomatic. Superficial veins are often visibly dilated before real discomfort occurs.

vas deferens

vas Latin, vessel, conduit, duct + *deferens* Latin present participle, carrying away

The vas deferens is also called the ductus deferens or spermatic duct. It carries sperm from the testis to join the excretory duct of the seminal vesicle.

vas-ec-tomy

vas vas deferens + *ek* out + *tome* a surgical cutting
A vasectomy is a method of sterilizing a male for birth control by cutting out a portion of the vas deferens. Technically, it is usually a vasotomy. The tube is cut, but no piece of the vas is removed.

vascular

vasculum Latin, little blood vessel. Note a Late Latin synonym, *vascellum*. In 15th Century French, it became *vaissel*, then was borrowed by English as *vessel*.
Vascular tissue is rich in blood vessels. Hence vascular insufficiency is lack of enough peripheral blood flow caused by blockage of veins and arteries.

vaso-

a combining form of *vas* Latin, blood vessel

vaso-dilator

vas blood vessel + *dilator* widener
A vasodilator is a chemical, natural or synthetic, that acts to expand or dilate blood vessels. Vasodilators are often used to treat angina.

vaso-constrictor

vas blood vessel + *constrictor* Latin, device that squeezes or narrows
A vasoconstrictor is a chemical, natural or synthetic, that narrows or constricts blood vessels, e.g. ephedrine in nose drops for a 'cold' acts to constrict nasal blood vessels in the mucosal lining and so decrease their production of mucus.

vaso-pressor

vas blood vessel + *pressor* New Latin, device or person that presses, puts pressure on something
A vasopressor is a chemical substance that helps contract blood vessels, thus increasing blood pressure, e.g. the adrenal hormone, epinephrine or adrenaline.

Another powerful vasopressor is vasopressin, a hormone stored in the pituitary gland.

vector

vector Latin, carrier (of a disease), transporter < *vehere* to carry. A little carrier, a cart, or a carriage in Latin was *vehiculum* which gives the English word *vehicle*.

A vector is an agent that transmits a disease. A biological vector might be a flea or louse or fly on which or in which a disease-producing virus or bacterium completes part of its life cycle. Vector is also used to label an altered retrovirus, in which the genes that cause disease are removed and replaced by helpful genes. This altered virus may then be injected into a patient suffering a viral disease, be reproduced, and 'cure' the disease.

Vector also means a quantity having direction and magnitude. In a vectorcardiogram, heart electrical activity is traced and made visible on an oscilloscope (see *oscilloscope* entry).

vein, vena, veno-

vena Latin, vein; plural *venae*

A vein is a vessel in which blood that has given up most of its oxygen flows back toward the heart, for re-oxygenation in the lungs. Veins have valves to prevent backflow of blood.

vena cava

vena vein + *cava* Latin, empty, because it was often found to be empty during post mortem examination

The venae cavae are two large veins that enter the heart. The superior vena cava transports blood from the upper body, the inferior vena cava from the lower body.

ventilate

ventilare Latin, to move air as a wind does, to fan < *ventus* wind

To ventilate in ordinary English is to provide a space with fresh air. In medicine, it means to provide the lungs with atmospheric air or to provide air and oxygen to blood across the capillaries in the lung. Ventilation is the process in which gases are moved in and out of the lungs. A ventilator (Latin, wind-machine) is a therapeutic device that assists a patient's labored breathing.

ventral

ventralis Latin, of the stomach < *venter* stomach, belly
Ventral as an anatomical location means: of or to the front of the body, where the belly is. Ventral can be a synonym for abdominal, and is the opposite of dorsal. A ventral hernia may be due to muscle weakness in the midline of the abdomen.

ventr-ad

ad Latin preposition and prefix, to, toward + *venter* stomach
Ventrad is an anatomical direction: toward the stomach, toward the ventral side, toward the ventral aspect of a part.

ventr-icle

ventriculum Latin, little belly or little stomach
A ventricle is a small chamber in the heart or the brain.

verruca

verruca Latin, wart
A verruca is a benign skin lesion with a rough surface caused by a common, contagious papovavirus. But verrucous carcinoma is a malignant squamous-cell cancer found in the lining of the mouth, throat and on genitals. It is slow-growing and does not usually spread. See also *wart* entry.

vertebra

vertebra Latin, a turning place, a pivot, a joint < *vertere* to turn
One of the 33 bones of the spinal column, the back bones or joints that permit flexibility of the vertebral column.

vesica

vesica Latin, bladder, a diminutive form of *vas* bladder, dish, little container
Vesica urinaria is the formal anatomical name of the urinary bladder.

vesicle

vesicula Latin, a little sac, a little bladder-like object, a small bag; another diminutive form of *vas*

A vesicle is a small anatomical sac containing liquid, e.g. the seminal vesicles, a pair of pouches at the back of the urinary bladder in the male that make part of the seminal fluid. Vesical means pertaining to the urinary bladder, for example, vesical stones. A pathological vesicle is a limited, raised area of the skin containing clear fluid or serum. For example, a small blister is a vesicle. The vesicles seen in herpes, herpetic vesicles, are fluid-filled blisters. The adjective for this meaning is vesicular.

virus

virus Latin, a poisonous liquid

Virus first meant venom or poison in Latin, and in the 20th Century came to be applied to microscopic, non-living infectious particles. The viral particle is called a virion (note the Greek diminutive ending *-ion*). A virion is not capable of independent metabolism, and can reproduce only within a host cell, where it takes over from the nucleic acid of the host cell and makes many replica virions (or viria, the formal plural). Eventually the host cell bursts apart, spreading the new virions to adjacent tissue. A large number of human diseases are of viral origin.

viscera

Plural of *viscus* Latin, soft flesh, vital organ, entrails, innards < *viscare* to make sticky, compare the adjective *viscid*. Note the term in fluid mechanics, viscosity, the relative ability of a liquid to flow, its sticky thickness or thinness.

The Romans used the word *viscera* to refer to the fleshy interior of a body, especially the bowels or intestines. In anatomy, the visceral cavity contains the abdominal organs. The visceral skeleton encloses the abdominal organs.

vulva

vulva Latin, a covering, a wrapping < *volvere* to roll, to turn

The vulva is the external female genitalia including the labia, mons pubis, clitoris and the openings of the urethra and vagina. Thus vulvovaginitis is an inflammation that includes the vagina and the external genitalia as well. Vulvitis is a tingling, itching and scratching of the vulva as symptoms of atrophic vaginitis in postmenopausal women. It may cause intercourse to be painful, because of dry, scaly skin. Vulvitis may also be an early symptom of diabetes mellitus.

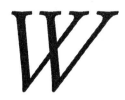

wart

wearte Old English, bump, knob, wart, outgrowth
A wart is a hard, benign tumor of the epidermis caused by a virus. Some warts disappear, others can be removed. The Latin synonym, verruca, is used in medical literature.

plantar wart

plantar Latin, on the sole of the foot < *planta pedis* sole of the foot
A plantar wart is one on the sole of the foot. Because of the pressure exerted on it during walking, this wart develops a hard ring, a callus, around its soft central part, and is painful. Cryosurgery and cautery are two therapies.

venereal wart

venereus Latin, of Venus, goddess of love, hence, associated with the genital area
A venereal wart or a condyloma is a small, pointed, benign growth on the genital skin or anus. A condyloma (*kondylos* knuckle + *oma* tumor) common on the genital or anal skin is a tumor vaguely shaped like a knuckle and called condyloma acuminatum (Latin, tapering to a point).

wen

wenn Old English, a cyst
A wen is a small sebaceous cyst in the epidermis of the scalp, at the back of the neck, or on the forehead. Sometimes called a pilar cyst or hair cyst (*pilaris* Latin, of a hair). The sebaceous glands in the skin secrete a greasy, protective substance called sebum which helps keep the skin lubricated and flexible. When one of these glands is blocked with sebum, a wen occurs. Wens are harmless, but if a patient feels they are embarrassing or unsightly, surgical removal under local anesthetic can be carried out.

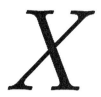

xantho-

xanthos Greek, yellow

xanth-oma

xanthos yellow + *oma* tumor

Xanthoma is a yellow deposit of fat cells in the skin, seen as nodules, papules, or plaque. In some cases, xanthoma is associated with diabetes; in others it may be a hereditary disease in which the body does not store fat properly. Xanthomatosis is a disease of multiple xanthomas or xanthomata caused by disorders of lipid metabolism (how the body uses and stores fat).

xiphoid process

See *sternum* entry

xeno-phobia

xenos Greek, stranger + *phobia* fear

Xenophobia is a morbid, paranoid dread of any person the patient does not already know.

xero-

xeros Greek, dry

xero-derma

xeros dry + *derma* Greek, skin

Xeroderma is a chronic skin condition whose symptoms are dry, scaly, rough, itchy skin. In xeroderma pigmentosa (Latin, colored) a rare congenital intolerance of ultraviolet light produces a wide variety of skin lesions including freckles, keratosis and sometimes skin cancers. Tumors on the eyelids and cornea may produce blindness.

xero-stoma

xeros dry + *stoma* mouth

Xerostoma is dry mouth due to lack of sufficient saliva. Xerostoma is a symptom of diseases like diabetes and many acute infections. The cessation of salivary secretion is sometimes due to facial nerve paralysis.

Z

zona, zone

zona Latin, belt < *zone* Greek, a girdle
An erogenous zone (*eros* Greek, sex + *gen* making, producing) is any body area that stirs sexual desire when stimulated. Such zones vary with the individual.

zona glomerul-osa

zona zone + *glomerulus* cluster + *osus* adjectival suffix, full of, abounding in
The zona glomerulosa is the outer layer of the adrenal cortex with many glomeruli or clusters of small blood vessels. Natural cortisone is secreted by cells in the adrenal cortex.

zonule of Zinn

zonula Latin, a little belt
Johann Gottfried Zinn (1727–1759), a German anatomist, was the author of a classic treatise on the eye. Zinn's zonule or the ciliary zonula is a group of fibers that connect the lens of the eye to the ciliary body.

zoo-

zoon Greek, animal, living thing < *zoe* life

zoo-graft

zoon animal + graft
A zoograft is living animal tissue transplanted by surgery into a human, e.g. a pig's heart valve may replace a damaged one in a human.

zoo-psia

zoon animal + *opsis* Greek, vision
Zoopsia is hallucinations of animals while suffering delirium tremens. Seeing pink elephants is a zooptic instance.

zoo-tox-in

zoon animal + *toxikon* Greek, poison + *in* noun ending for organic chemical compound
A zootoxin is any poisonous substance derived from an animal, for example, a spider's venom.

zygo-

zygon Greek, a yoke for oxen, a pair, a set of twins

a-zygous

a not + *zygon* pair
An azygous structure or organ is one that is not paired, for example the heart or the liver. Note the alternative spelling of the azygos vein, a single vein that arises in the abdomen, branching from the lumbar vein. If the inferior vena cava is ever obstructed, the azygos vein provides a route by which venous blood can return to the heart.

zygomatic bone

zygoma Greek, the cheekbone, literally 'the yoke or pair swelling'
The zygomatic bone forms the hard part of the cheek and the lower rim of each eye socket. By pressing gently on each side of the eye, one may feel the zygomatic arches which protect the eye from lateral injury and form part of the orbit or eye socket. The arches are formed by processes, bony projections, of the zygomatic bone and the temporal bones. If you try to touch your nose with your upper lip, you use the zygomaticus muscle which acts to draw the upper lip upward and outward.

zygote

zygotos Greek, joined, yoked
The zygote is the cell that results from the union of two sex cells, sperm and egg. Zygote is a synonym for fertilized ovum.

Review list of frequent Latin and Greek roots used in medical words

How to use this list to test yourself

1. Read all the entries in the main text of *Dictionary of Medical Derivations* under one letter of the alphabet. After you have read, for example, the medical roots and words beginning with *a*, return to this review list, say aloud each medical root that begins with *a*, then say aloud one or two full English medical words that contain each *a* root. If you prefer, write these words beside the root on these pages, or do so using a separate piece of paper. You may also copy the review list and write in medical words containing the root beside or beneath the root in question.
2. If you are studying medical vocabulary with a fellow student, make a two-person quiz game of testing yourselves. One person reads aloud the medical root, the other answers with a full English medical term containing the root and defines the medical word correctly. Score yourselves, and declare a winner. You might reverse roles for each letter of the alphabet.

A

a	alpha privative indicates a negative, not
ab	*ab* Latin, away from
acantho	*acanthos* Greek, thorn, spine
acet	*acetum* vinegar
acid	*acidus* Latin adjective, sharp, sour-tasting
acro	*akron* Greek, extremity (that is, arm, hand, finger, leg, foot, toe) or *akros* high
ad	*ad* Latin preposition and prefix, to, toward
aden	*aden* Greek, gland
adipo	*adeps, adipis* Latin, lard, hog fat, fat
agog, agogue	*agog* leading, inducing, from *agogia* Greek, a leading, a guiding
alb	*albus* Latin, flat white
algo, algia	*algos* Greek, pain; *algia* feeling pain
allo	*allos* Greek adjective, akin to the Latin *alius*; both have the basic sense of 'another' and the developed sense of foreign, outside the self, other, different, abnormal
alveolus	*alveolus* Latin, little socket, sac
ambul	*ambulare* Latin, to walk
amnio	*amnion* Greek, sac enclosing fetus

amyl	*amilum* Latin, starch < *amylon* Greek, starch
ana[1]	*ana* Greek, up, on, again, against
ana[2]	*ana* Greek, without; a double negative, a combination of alpha privative *an* + another *a* privative
anal, ano	*anus* Latin, rectal opening
andro	*aner, andros* Greek, man, male
aneurysm	*aneurysma* from *ana* through + *eurysma* Greek, a widening
angina	*angina* Latin, a choking pain
angio	*angeion* Greek, a little container, then a vessel that carries a fluid like blood or lymph
ante	*ante* Latin, in front of, before in time
anterior	*anterior* Latin, more in front
anti	*anti* Greek preposition and prefix, against, working against, effective against
aorta	*aorte* Greek, Aristotle's term for the great artery, ultimately from *aeirein* 'to raise'
aperture	*apertura* Latin, an opening, a hole, an orifice in an anatomical space or canal
apex, apical	*apex, apicis* Latin, attachment, the top, summit, the pointed end of a structure
apo	*apo* Greek, from, detached from, opposed to
appendix	*appendix* Latin, *ad* > *ap* Latin, to, on + *pendix* hanging part
ar	adjectival ending
arachno	*arachne* spider, spider's web
artery, arterio	*arteria* Greek, airpipe < *aerterion* air duct < *aer* air + *terein* to carry
arthr	*arthron* Greek, joint
articul	*articulus* Latin, knuckle or any joint of the body
ase	*ase* common ending for name of an enzyme
ate	common verb ending
athero	*athere* Greek, hard, fatty plaque deposits
atri, atria, atrio	*atrium* Latin, hearth, fireplace, with modern medical meaning of the upper chamber of the heart
auris	*auris* Latin, ear; seen in terms like auris sinistra, left ear; auris dexter, right ear
auto	*autos* Greek, self
axilla, axillary	*axilla* Latin, armpit
axis, axial	*axis* Latin, axle, turning point, pivot about which a round object turns

axo, axon	*axon* Greek, axle of a wheel, axis; in medicine, the long extension of a neuron

B

bacill, bacillus	*bacillum* Latin, little iron rod, little stick
bacteria, bacteri	*baktron* Greek, rod, cane, wooden pole + *ion* Greek diminutive ending meaning 'little, small'; a *bakterion* was the small staff of office carried by some officers in ancient Greek armies
bi	*bis* Latin adverb, two times, now a combining form for twice, double, both, two
bili	*bilis* Latin, bile, gall
bio	*bios* Greek, life
blast	*blastos* Greek, a sprout, a bud
blepharo	*blepharos* Greek, eyelid
bol	*bole* Greek, the act of building something
brachi, brachio	*brachion* Greek, upper arm; it came into English from its Latin form *bracchium*
brachy	*brachys* Greek, short
brady	*bradys* Greek, slow
broncho	*brogchos* Greek, windpipe
bucca, buccal	*bucca* Latin, cheek
bulla	*bulla* Latin, bubble
burs, bursa	*bursa* Greek, a leather wine-skin, an oxhide pouch; in medicine, a sac of fluid near joints

C

caecum, ceco	*caecum* Latin, blind thing; in medicine the first part of the large intestine
cal, calor	*calor* Latin, heat
calc	*calx, calcis* Latin, chalk, limestone, stone, heel; acquired scientific meanings 'calcium' and 'heel'
calculus	*calx, calcis* limestone + *ulus* Latin, diminutive suffix indicating smallness, therefore *calculus* = limestone pebble; in medicine a pathologic accretion or stone
cancer	*cancer* Latin, crab, a disease of malignant tumors
candid	*candidus*, shining white; a Roman candidate for office wore a symbolically white toga
cannula	*canna* Latin, hollow reed + *ula* diminutive suffix indicating smallness; now a medical device: a hollow tube that guides a sharp-pointed puncturing instrument

capillary	*capilla* Latin, hair + *arius* adjectival ending
capital, caput	*caput, capitis* Latin, head, adjective *capitalis*, of the head
carcinoma	*karkinos* Greek, crab, cancer + *oma* tumor
cardio, cardium	*kardia* Greek, the heart
carotid	*karotides* Greek, the arteries of the neck < *karos* heavy sleep < *karoun* to choke, to stupefy
carpal, carpo carpus	*carpus* Latin, wrist; *carpalis* adjective, of the wrist
cata	*kata* Greek, down from, lower
catalysis	*kata* Greek, down + *lysis* a breaking, so that *katalysis* = a dissolving, a breakdown
cataract	*kata* Greek, down + *rrhaktes* something that rushes, drops quickly; in medicine, a loss of transparency in the lens of the eye
catarrh	*kata* Greek, down + *rrhoia* Greek, a flowing
catatonia	*kata* Greek, down + *tonos* Greek, stretching + *ia* medical condition
catharsis	*katharos* Greek, pure, clean + *osis* Greek noun ending here indicating process of = *katharsis* a cleansing
catheter	*kath* < *kata* down + *hienai* to send, to cause to go, so *katheter* Greek, thing put in, thing let down into, thing inserted
caud	*cauda* Latin, tail, tail-like anatomical structure
cele	*kele* Greek tumor, swelling
celio	*koilia* Greek, belly, abdomen
cell	*cella* Latin, a small room, from *celare* to hide, to conceal
centesis	*kentesis* Greek, the act of puncturing
cephalo	*kephale* Greek, the head
cer	*cera* Latin, wax; akin to *keros* Greek, wax, beeswax; in medicine the combining form means 'wax' or 'waxy'
cerebellum	*cerebrum* Latin, brain + *ellum* diminutive suffix meaning 'small, little'
cerebra, cerebri, cerebro	*cerebrum* Latin, brain
cervica, cervix, cervico	*cervix, cervicis* Latin, neck, any neck-like structure
cheilo	*cheilos* Greek, lip, combining form meaning 'lip of the mouth'
chiasma	*chiasma* Greek, marking an X, an X-like junction, anything resembling the Greek letter chi, written χ

chlor	*chloros* Greek, green; combining form in chemical names: with a chlorine-containing radical; in medicine, pertaining to chlorides
chole	*chole* Greek, bile, gall
chondro	*chondros* Greek, gristle, cartilage
chrom, chromato	*chroma, chromatos* Greek, color of the skin, then any color; combining form signifying 'color'
chronic, chrono	*chronikos* Greek, of time, persisting through time
chrono, chronic	*chronos* Greek, time
chyle	*chylos* Greek, digestive juice
chyme	*chymos* Greek, fluid, juice
cide	*caedere* Latin, to slay, to cut down with a sword; in medicine the suffix means 'killing, or causing a reduction in pathogenic quantity of'
cilia, cilium	*cilium* Latin, eyelash, small hair; in medicine the plural, cilia, refers to hair-like projections on cells, or, the eyelashes
cine, kine, kinesis, kinet	*kinesis* Greek, movement of
circum	*circum* Latin, around, circling
cirrh	*kirrhos* Greek color adjective, orange-yellow
clasis	*klasis* Greek, a fracturing, a breaking into pieces
clavicle, clavicul	*clavicula* Latin, twig, little stick, hoopstick, human collarbone
clinic, clinical	*kline* Greek, a bed
clitoris, clitorid	*kleitoris, kleitoridis* Greek, clitoris < *kleis, kleidos* Greek, key + *oris* Greek agent noun suffix
clonal, clone	*klon* ancient Greek botanical term, twig, slip, plant cutting used to propagate similar plants
clonus	*klonos* Greek, tumult, convulsion
co	*co* Latin, shortened form of *cum* with, together
cocco, coccus	*kokkos* berry, berry-shaped bacterium
coccyx, coccygeal	*kokkyx, kokkygos* Greek, the cuckoo bird, and by analogy its beak; in medicine, the human tailbone
cochlea	*cochlea* Latin, snail shell, a bony tunnel structure in the inner ear < *kochlias* Greek, spiral snail shell < *kochlos* land snail
colic	*kolikos* Greek, a pain in the intestines
coll, col	*kolla* Greek, glue, and compare its Medieval Greek synonym *glia*

colo, colon	*kolon* Greek, the large intestine
colpo	*kolpos* Greek, vagina
com	*com* Latin, assimilated form of *cum* with, together
con	*con* Latin, assimilated form of *cum* with, together
condyle	*kondylos* Greek, knuckle; in medicine, a spheroid bump on a bone where it articulates with another bone
contra	*contra* Latin, against, opposite, counter to
corona, coronary	*corona* Latin crown, wreath, garland
corpus, corporal	*corpus, corporis* Latin, body; in medicine, a corpus is the main part of an organ, or some specialized tissue or mass
cortex, cortico	*cortex, corticis* Latin, bark, rind, any outer covering; in medicine, the outer layer of an organ or structure
cost, costa	*costa* Latin, rib
crani	*cranium* Latin, skull < *kranion* Greek, skull
crepit	*crepitare* Latin, to rattle, creak, rumble < *crepitus* a pop, a rattle, a rumble
crin, crine	*krinein* Greek, to secrete, to separate
crine, crino	*krinein* Greek, to separate
crisis, critical	*krisis* Greek, separation, moment of separation, judgment point
crista	*crista* Latin, ridge, crest, comb of a rooster
cryo	*kryos* Greek, very cold
curette	*curette* French, scraper, cleaner < *curer*, to clean
cut, cutis	*cutis* Latin, skin. The cutis, skin, is the outer covering of the body, made up of the dermis and the epidermis.
cyan	*kyanos* Greek, dark blue
cyst	*kystis* Greek, sac, bladder
cysto	*kystis* Greek, sac, bladder; usually in medicine, the urinary bladder
cyte	*kytos* Greek, cell
D	
dacryo	*dakryon* Greek, tear, akin to Latin *lacrima*
dactylo	*daktylos* Greek, digit, finger, toe
de	*de* Latin negative prefix indicates lack of, not, down from
debride	*débrider* French, to unbridle, then in medicine, to remove adhesions + *-ment* French < *mentum* Latin noun suffix
delirium	*de* away from + *lira* Latin, furrow in a field + *ium* Latin noun ending, hence *delirium*, a going off the ploughed track, thus a madness

delt, deltoid	*delta*, the letter *d* + *eides* Greek, form, shape; hence *-oid* means 'formed like, similar to'; deltoid means triangular because the Greek capital letter delta – Δ – was shaped like a triangle
demic	*demos* Greek, town, populace; then people, whole population
dendro, dendrit	*dendrites* Greek adjective, branching like a tree < *dendron* tree
dent	*dens, dentis* Latin, tooth; akin to *odous, odontos* Greek, tooth
derm, dermato	*derma, dermatos* Greek, skin
desis	*desis* Greek, fusion, a binding together
di	*dis* Greek, two, twice, double; akin to Latin *bis, bi-*
dia	*dia* Greek, through, throughout, apart, between, across, very
diabetes	*dia* through + *betes* Greek, passing; the word itself refers to a chief symptom of some of the many forms of diabetes, the 'passing through' of excessive urination
didym	*hoi didymoi* Greek, 'the twins', i.e. the two testicles
diplo	*diploos* Greek, double, twin
dis	*dis* Latin negative prefix, not, apart, absence of
distal	a scientific coinage of the 19th Century, from *dist*-ance + *al*, which is a common adjectival ending. In anatomy, distal means remote from the point of attachment.
dolor	*dolor* Latin, pain
donor	*donor* Latin, one who gives blood, organs, etc.
dors, dorsal	*dorsum* Latin, the back
dorsal, dorsum	*dorsum* Latin, the back; *dorsalis* adjective, of the back
duct	*ductus* Latin, canal, channel, any hollow tube which conveys liquids < *ducere* to carry
dys	*dys* Greek negative prefix indicates difficult or disordered function

E
ec	*ek, ex* Greek, out, out of
ecto	*ektos* Greek, outside, outer
ectomy	*ek* out + *tome* a surgical cutting + *y* noun ending
edema, edemato	*oidema* Greek, fluid-filled swelling
em	*em* short for *haima*, Greek, blood; most commonly in medical words ending in -emia, pathologic blood conditions like anemia and uremia
embol	*embolos* Greek, plug, stopper

embryo	*en > em* Greek, in + *bryon* something that grows in another body < *bryein* to grow
emphysema	*emphysema, emphysematos* Greek, inflation < *en* in + *physan* to blow + *ema* noun ending
en	*en* Greek, in
endo	*endon* Greek, within, inside
endothel	endothelium is epithelial tissue, composed of flat and scale-like cells that line the internal organs of the body like the heart, as well as the veins and arteries
entero	*enteron* Greek, gut
entia	*entia* noun ending
epi	*epi* Greek, on, on top of, above, upper, upon
episio	*epision* Greek, the pubic area
epithel	epithelium is the varied, external tissue that covers the body, the outer layer of the skin
erg, ergy	*ergos* Greek, work; *ergeia* a working
erythro	*erythros* Greek, red
escent, escence	this common suffix to nouns and adjectives derives from the present infinitive form, -*escere*, of what are called inchoate verbs in Latin (*inchoare* to begin). The basic meaning of the suffixes -*escent* and -*escence* is 'just beginning to, starting the initial stage of'.
esis	*esis* Greek noun ending, 'action of'
esthes, esthet	*esthesia* sensing, feeling
etio	*aitia* Greek, cause
eu	*eu* Greek, well, easy, normal, good
ex	*ex* Latin, out of, away from, former, outside
exo	*exo* Greek, outside, away from, on the surface of
extra	*extra* Latin, additional, beyond, outside, on the surface of

F

fascia	*fascis* Latin, a bundle of sticks, firewood tied up to take back to the fire; in medicine a fascia (plural *fasciae*) is a band of fibrous connective tissue that wraps protectively around muscles and some organs
fecal, feces, feco	*faex, faecis* Latin, dung, dregs, stool
femoral, femur	*femur, femoris* Latin, the thigh
fetal, feto, fetus	*fetus* Latin noun, offspring, spawn, brood
fibro	*fibra* Latin, thread, fibrous tissue
fibula	*fibula* Latin, the needle or pin of a brooch; plural *fibulae*; the fibula is the smaller bone of the lower leg

fimbria, fimbrio | *fimbria* Latin, lacy fringe

fiss, fissure | *fissura* Latin, a rip, split, groove

fistula | *fistula* Latin, waterpipe, tube

flatus | *flatus* Latin, a blowing, a wind, flatulence

flavi | *flavus* Latin color adjective, straw-yellow

flex, flexion | *flexio, flexionis* Latin, a bending

follicle | *folliculus* Latin, little bag < *follis* bag + *iculus* diminutive ending meaning 'small'

foramen | *foramen* Latin, hole, aperture

fossa | *fossa* Latin, ditch, trench

fract, fracture | *fractura* Latin, a breaking, a splintering

frenulum | *fraenulum* Latin, a little bridle < *fraenum* bridle, brake, thing that stops an action + *ulum* small. A frenulum is a small fold of ligament that limits movement of a body part.

G
galacto | *gala, galaktos* Greek, milk

ganglion | *gagglion* Greek, encysted tumor on leg, head, etc. The Greek-speaking Roman physician and medical writer Galen (AD 129–199) first compared these knots of nerve tissue to tumors. Ganglia are masses of nervous tissue lying outside the brain and spinal column.

gastro | *gaster* Greek, stomach

gen | *gen* Greek root particle, making, producing

genu | *genu* Latin, knee, or any structure resembling a knee

geri, geronto | *geron, gerontos* Greek, old person

gingiv | *gingiva* the gums

glio, glia | *glia* Medieval Greek, glue

glosso, glott | *glossa* or *glotta* Greek, tongue

gluteal, gluteus | *gluteus* Latin spelling of *gloutos* Greek, buttocks

glutin, gluten | *gluten* Latin, glue; compare *glia* Greek, glue

glyco, gluco | *glykys* Greek, sweet

gnatho | *gnathos* Greek, jaw

gnosis, gnostic | *gnosis* Greek, a knowing, knowledge, telling what is known

gonad, gonado | *gonas, gonadis* New Latin, sex gland, based on *gonos* Greek, seed, offspring

gono | *gone* Greek, seed, offspring, sex organs

gram | *gram* Greek root part, something written or recorded

graphy | *graphe* Greek, a drawing, a picture, a recording of

gyn, gyno, gyny | *gyne* Greek, female

gyr, gyro, gyrus	*gyros* Greek, circle

H

hal	*halare* Latin, to breathe
hallex, hallus, hallux	*hallux, hallucis* Latin, big toe
hallucin	*alucinari* to wander in the mind
hem, hema, hemato, em	*haima, haimatos* Greek, blood
hemi	*hemi* Greek, half
hepat, hepato	*hepar, hepatos* Greek, the liver
hernia, hernio	*hernia* Latin, a rupture, a protruding
herpes, herpet	*herpes* Greek, literally 'the creeps', shingles, from *herpein* to creep
hetero	*heteros* Greek, different, opposite
hiatus	*hiatus* Latin, a gap, a yawning hole < *hiare* to gape, to yawn, to open
hidro	*hidros* Greek, sweat, perspiration
histo	*histos* Greek, something woven, a web, a tissue
homo, homeo	*homoios* Greek, similar, the same, alike
humerus	*humerus* Latin, bone of the upper arm, akin to *omos* Greek, shoulder
hyal	*hyalos* Greek, glass
hydatid	*hydatis, hydatidis* Greek, cyst filled with watery fluid < *hydor, hydros* water
hydro	*hydor, hydros* Greek, water
hymen	*hymen* Greek, any body membrane, also Hymen, ancient Greek god of marriages; the hymen is a fold of mucous membrane, skin and fibrous tissue partly covering – or more rarely totally covering – the vaginal orifice
hyper	*hyper* Greek, over, above, akin to Latin *super*
hypno	*hypnos* Greek, of sleep
hypo	*hypo* Greek, under, below, beneath, less than, akin to Latin *sub*
hysteri, hystero	*hystera* Greek, uterus

I

ia	medical condition
iasis	*-iasis* Greek noun suffix indicating a pathologic condition, similiar to *-osis*
iatro, iatric	*iatros* Greek, doctor + *ikos* adjective ending

ic	*ikos* adjective ending
icter	*ikteros* Greek, a yellow bird, an Hellenic species of oriole or golden thrush whose yellow feathers resembled the yellow skin discoloration of jaundice
idio	*idios* Greek, of an individual, peculiar to one person; compare *idiotes* a private person
ileo, ileum	*ileum* 17th Century medical Latin, the lower part of the small intestine < *eileos* Greek, twisted, because first used to describe a pathological bowel condition like colic
ilia, ilio, ilium	*ilium* Medieval Latin, hipbone < Classical Latin, *ilia* flanks, soft parts < *ilis*, soft
immune, immuno	*in* > *im* not + *munis* Latin, serving, defending; medical meaning: safe from or resistant to disease and infection because of the body's production of antibodies
in	*in* common noun ending for organic chemical compounds
in situ	Latin 'in its *situs*', original position, normal site
in vitro	*in* Latin, in, on + *vitrum* Medieval Latin, glass; literally, in or on glass; modern meaning 'in a glass laboratory container or apparatus' like a test tube, a flask, or a glass slide
in vivo	*in* Latin, in + *vivus* Late Latin, a living person, the living body
infra	*infra* Latin, inside, within, inferior to, beneath, below
inter	*inter* Latin, between, among
intra	*intra* Latin, inside, within
ion	*ion* Greek, a diminutive suffix, that is, a noun ending meaning 'little'
ischio, ischium	*iskion* Greek, rump bone < *iskys* strength, hence strong bone; borrowed by Latin as *ischium*
ism	*ismos* Greek noun ending that indicates action, abstract state, doctrine, moral practice; in medicine, the suffix -*ism* often denotes an abnormal condition brought on by excess, e.g. alcoholism
ism	*ism* noun suffix indicating a condition or a theory
iso	*isos* Greek, equal, the same
ist	*istes* Greek agent noun suffix, one who does, who makes, one who performs an action
itis	*itis* inflammation of
ium	*ium* Latin noun suffix 'thing containing or related to'

J

jejuno, jejunum	*ieiunus* Latin, empty; the jejunum is the middle portion of the small intestine

K

kerat, kerato	*keras, keratos* Greek, horn, cornea of the eye, horny body tissue

L

labia, labio	*labium* Latin, a lip or lip-like structure; plural *labia*; the labia are folds of skin at the vaginal opening
lacrima, lacrimal, lacrimo	*lacrima* Latin, tear, pertaining to tears in the eyes
lact	*lac, lactis* Latin, milk; akin to *galas, galaktos* Greek, milk
lalia	*lalia* Greek, talking, speaking
laparo	*lapara* Greek, loins, flank; the combining form often refers to surgical procedures done through the abdominal walls
lapse	*lapsus* Latin, a slipping, a falling of an organ or structure, equivalent to the Greek word used in medicine, ptosis
laryngo, larynx	*larynx, laryggis* Greek, the upper part of the windpipe; the larynx is an organ that contains the vocal cords
lateral	*lateralis* Latin, of a side, on the side < *latus* side
lesion	*laesio, laesionis* Latin, damage, injury; lesion is a general word in medicine for any abnormal change in the structure or function of tissue because of injury or disease
leuco	*leukos* Greek, white
levator	*levator* Latin, lifter; in medicine, a muscle that lifts or elevates a structure
lig	*ligare* Latin, to tie up, wrap, bind, constrict, pull tight ; as in ligament, ligate, ligation
lip, lipid	*lipos* Greek, fat
lith	*lithos* Greek, stone
logy	*logos* Greek, word, reason, study of
lumbar	*lumbus* Latin, loin; the adjective is lumbar, pertaining to the loins
lumen	*lumen, luminis* Latin, light, or an opening that light comes through, then the hollow part of any tube
lymph, lympho	*lympha* Latin, clear water; cognate with or derived from Greek *nympha*, any of several minor water goddesses; lymph is the thin, watery, extracellular fluid that bathes most body tissues
lysis	*lysis* Greek, a breaking up of

M

macro	*makros* Greek adjective, wide, big, of abnormal bigness

macula	*macula* Latin, spot, blemish; *maculatus* spotted
mal	*male* Latin adverb, badly, poorly, not normally
malacia, malaco	*malakos* Greek, soft, weak > *malakia* softness
malleus	*malleus* Latin, hammer; in medicine, the malleus is a hammer-like little bone of the middle ear
mamma, mammo	*mamma* Latin, breast
mandible, mandibul	*mandibulum* Late Latin, the lower jaw, literally 'the little chewer' < *mandare* to chew
mast	*mastos* Greek, breast
maxilla, maxillo	*mala* Latin, jaw + *illa* diminutive suffix of feminine nouns, little = *maxilla*, one of the two large bones that form the upper jaw
meatus	*meare* Latin, to go, to pass > *meatus* a passageway, a channel, a hole
median, medio	*medianus, medius* Late Latin, in the middle
medulla	*medulla* Latin, the marrow of a bone, but literally, the little part in the middle
meg	*megas, megalos* Greek, big, large
megaly	*megale* enlargement, from the Greek adjective *megas* large, big, great
melan	*melas, melanos* Greek, black in color
membrane	*membrana* Latin, thin skin, any tissue that covers a body part, skin, sheet of parchment < *membrum* limb of the body, penis, a part of something
men, meno	*men, menos* Greek, a month, hence English phrases like 'the monthlies' and Latin terms like *menstrualis*
mening	*meninx, meningis* Latin from *menigx* Greek, membrane. Hippocrates used the word to refer to the dura mater. Three meninges or membranes wrap around and protect the brain and spinal cord.
mere	*meros* Greek, part
meso	*mesos* Greek, middle
meta	*meta* Greek, over, across, indicating change, beyond
metr, metry	*metron* Greek, device that measures
metri	*metra* Greek, literally mother-thing, mother-essence, hence the womb, the uterus
micro	*mikros* Greek adjective, small, of abnormal smallness
mis, miso	*misos* Greek, hatred
mitral	*mitralis* Late Latin, having two points like a *mitra* Latin, bishop's hat

mono	*monos* Greek, one, sole, single
morph	*morphe* Greek, form, shape
mortal	*mors, mortis* Latin, death
muco	*mucus* Latin, slime, phlegm, mucus
mut	*mutare* Latin, to alter, to change
my, mye, myo	*mys, myos* Greek, muscle
myco, myceto	*mykes, myketos* Greek, mushroom, fungus
myelo	*myelos* Greek, spinal cord, confusingly *myelo-* also means bone marrow
myxo	*myxa* Greek, mucus, and akin to the Latin *mucus*

N

nano	*nanos* Greek, dwarf; *nano-* is one of the numerical prefixes of metric measurement used widely in scientific calibration to mean 'one billionth of'. The prefix *nano-* also refers to abnormal smallness of body structures.
narco	*narke* Greek, originally, numbness of an extremity, then, a stupor, a torpor
naris	*naris* Latin, nostril > *nasalis* of the nose, nasal
natal	*natalis* Latin, relating to birth
necro	*nekros* Greek, dead, as in necrosis of tissue
neo	*neos* Greek, new
nephro	*nephros* Greek, kidney
neuro	*neuron* Greek, nerve
nodule	*nodulus* Latin, a little knot, diminutive of *nodus*, a knot; a nodule is a small, firm swelling or node of tissue, larger than a papule, and detectable by touch
noxious	*noxiosus* Late Latin, poisonous, full of harm
nucha, nuche	*nukha* Arabic, spinal marrow; but in Medieval Latin, the Arabic word acquired the same meaning it has in modern medical English, where the nucha is the nape or the back of the neck
nucleo, nucleus	*nucleus*, a contracted form of *nuculeus* Latin, kernel, nutmeat, literally, little nut < *nux, nucis* nut, literally, the part that nourishes; a nucleus is the control structure inside a living cell
nulli	*nullus* Latin, not < *nil* nothing

O

ob	*ob* Latin preposition and prefix, facing toward, against, upon, completely

occipital, occiput	*ob > oc* at the back of + *capitalis* of the head
ocul	*oculus* Latin, eye
odonto	*odous, odontos* Greek, tooth
oid	*-oid,* formed like > *eides* Greek, form
ol	*ol* biochemical suffix indicating an alcohol
ole, ola	*ola* noun suffix indicating smallness
oligo	*oligos* Greek adjective, few, not many, a small quantity of, fewer than normal
oma	*oma* Greek noun ending indicating tumor or swelling
oment	*omentum* Latin, fat, bowels; an omentum is a fold of the peritoneum, like a large purse of tissue that partially encloses, attaches and supports the stomach and nearby viscera
omphalo	*omphalos* Greek, navel, belly button, umbilicus
onco	*ogkos* Greek, mass, bulk, tumor, cancer
onycho	*onyx, onychos* Greek, claw, talon, fingernail, toenail
oo	*oon* Greek, egg, a synonym of and akin to the Latin *ovum*. In English medical words with this root, both *o*'s are pronounced.
oophor	*oon* ovum + *phoros* Greek, carrying, bearing = *oophoron* Greek, egg-bearer, ovary
ophthalmo	*ophthalmos* Greek, eye
opia	*-opia* scientific Latin and Greek, disordered condition of sight < *ops, opos* Greek, eye
opsy, optic	*opsis* Greek, vision, seeing, looking at, and *optikos* Greek, pertaining to sight
or	*or* Latin agent noun ending as in operator, similar to English *-er* as in worker
orchi, orchid, orchio	*orchidion* Greek, single testicle < *orchis, orchios* testicles
orexia	*orexis* Greek, appetite
orifice	*orificium* Latin, making a mouth or a mouth-like opening < *facere* to make, an orifice is a mouth-like opening, an aperture, an entrance, an exit
ortho	*orthos* Greek, straight, correct, upright, erect
os, oral	*os, oris* Latin, mouth
os	*os, oris* Latin, mouth, plural *ora*; os is a formal anatomical name for a mouth-like opening, thus, os uteri is the mouth of the uterus
os, ossa, osseo, ossi	*os, ossis* Latin, bone; *osseus* Latin, bony

379

ose	*-ose* chemical suffix for names of sugars like glucose, sucrose, fructose, lactose
osis	*osis* Greek noun suffix indicating diseased condition
osteo	*osteon* Greek, a bone
osus	*osus* Latin adjectival ending meaning 'full of, abounding in'
ot, oto	*ous, otos* Greek, ear
ous	*ous* English adjective ending, from Latin *-osus*

P

pachy	*pachys* Greek, thick
palpate	*palpare* Latin, to stroke with the palm of the hand < *palpus* palm of the hand
palpebra	*palpebra* Latin, eyelid, literally 'the part that flutters'
pan	*pan* Greek, all
papule	*papula* Latin, pimple, a skin lesion that is small, hard and raised up
para	*para* Greek, outside of, beside, beyond what is normal, hence with a sense of abnormal
partum	*partus* Latin, birth
patella	*patella* Latin, saucer, small pan; in anatomy, the patella is the kneecap
patency, patent	*patens, patentis* Latin, standing wide open, clear, unobstructed (of passages)
patho, pathy	*pathos* Greek, feeling, disease
pector, pectoral	*pectus, pectoris* Latin, chest, thorax
pelvis	*pelvis* Latin washbasin, wide bowl; the pelvis looks like a bowl of bone. It includes the lower part of the backbone and the two hipbones.
pepto, pepsis	*pepsis* Greek, digestion
per	*per* Latin, through
peri	*peri* Greek, around, surrounding
pexy	*pexis* Greek, a fastening to, a fixation
phage, phagy	*phagos* Greek, eater, glutton
phalang	*phalagx, phalangos* Greek, a line of battle; plural *phalanges*. Aristotle first named the bones of the toes and fingers *phalanges* because they were arranged in rows like an ancient Greek infantry battalion.
phasis	*phasis* Greek, power of speech
phleb	*phleps, phlebos* Greek, a vein
phobia	*phobos* fear + *ia* medical condition

photic, photo	*phos, photos* Greek, light
phylaxis	*phylaxis* Greek, protection
physic, physical, physis	*physis* Greek, growth, nature, natural quality > *physikos* Greek, natural, but with the implication of human nature
pili, pilo	*pilus* Latin, hair
plasia	*plasia* Greek, a forming (of cells)
plasty	*plastia* new scientific Greek, a shaping, a forming, with later implication of 'forming by means of surgery'
pleur	*pleuron* Greek, rib, but its plural *pleura* referred to the membrane covering the lungs
plexus	*plexus* Latin, a braid, a plait; plural *plexus*; a plexus is a tangle or intermingling of blood vessels or nerves or lymph vessels, for example the solar plexus
plexy	*plexia* Greek, a striking
pnea	*pnoe* Greek, breathing
pneum	*pneumon* Greek, the lungs < *pneuma* air, gas, spirit < *pnein* to breathe
poly	*polys* Greek, many
post	*post* Latin, after
praxia	*praxis* Greek, action, doing something
pre	*prae* Latin, before, in front of
presby	*presbys* Greek, old
pro	*pro* Latin and Greek, in front of, in favor of, on behalf of, on account of
procto	*prokton* Greek, anus
proximal	*proximus* Latin, the nearest
pruri, pruritus	*pruritus* Latin, itching
pseudo	*pseudos* Greek, false, fake
psyche, psycho	*psyche* Greek, soul, spirit, the breath of life, mind < *psychein* to breathe; echoic in origin, that is, it imitates the sound of an outward breath
ptosis	*ptosis* Greek, a falling down, a drooping, a dropping; adjective is ptotic
ptyal	*ptyalon* Greek, saliva, synonym for the Latin *saliva*
pubes, pubic	*pubes* Latin adjective, grown-up, able to reproduce. In medicine it first meant the pubic area, then the pubic bone. Pubes is still used to refer in general to the genital area of the body.
pulmo, pulmon	*pulmo, pulmonis* Latin, lung > *pulmonarius* Late Latin, of the lung, pulmonary

purul, pus	*pus, puris* Latin, pus. It is akin to *pyon*, the Greek word for pus.
pyelo	*pyelos* Greek, the pelvis
pyo	*pyon* Greek, pus
pyr, pyro	*pyr* Greek, fire, fever

Q

quadri	combining form of *quattuor* Latin, four

R

rachi, rachio, rachis	*rhachis* Greek, backbone, spine; rachis is a medical term for the spinal column
radial, radius	*radius* Latin, a rod, a ray of light, the spoke of a wheel; the radius is the shorter forearm bone that early anatomists thought resembled the spoke of a wheel
radio	*radio-* a combining form of *radius*, with the developed meaning of 'radioactive' or 'of radio waves'
raphe, rrhaphy	*rhaphe* Greek, a suture, a seam, a sewn-up wound
re	*re* Latin prefix, again, back, repeated
rect, rectum	*rectum* Latin, straight, from the old medical Latin phrase *rectum intestinum* 'the straight portion of the great intestine'
ren, renal	*ren, renis* Latin, kidney
reticul	*reticulum* Latin, network, little net < *rete* net
retro	*retro* Latin, backward, situated behind
rheum, rheumat	*rheuma, rheumatos* Greek, a discharge, a flow < *rhein* to flow; rheum is any watery discharge from mucous membranes of the head and throat
rhin, rhino	*rhis, rhinos* Greek, nose
rhythmo	*rrhythmos* Greek, timed beat in music
rrhag	*rrhagia* Greek, bursting, gushing forth
rrhaphy	*rrhaphe* Greek, seam, surgical suture
rrhea	*rrhoia* Greek, a flowing through, a discharge
rrhexis	*rrhexis* Greek, rupture of an organ, tissue, or vessel
rub	*ruber* Latin adjective, red. The Latin noun is *rubor* redness.
rupt	*ruptus* broken

S

sacral, sacro, sacrum	*os sacrum* Latin, holy bone, a translation of a Greek phrase that meant great bone; the sacrum is the largest bone of the spinal column, a fused triangle at the base of the spine composed of five vertebrae at birth, which fuse together in the child

sagittal	*sagitta* Latin, arrow
sal, saline	*sal, salis* Latin, salt
salivary	*saliva* Latin, spittle, akin to *sialon* Greek, saliva
salping	*salpigx, salpingos* Greek, a trumpet, refers in medicine to the Fallopian tube or the Eustachian tube
sarco	*sarx, sarkos* Greek, flesh
scapula	*scapula* Latin, shoulder blade
schisis	*schisis* Greek, a splitting < *schizein* to split
schisto	*schistos* Greek, split, cleft, divided
schizo	*schizein* Greek, to split, to divide
sciatic	*sciaticus* Low Latin corruption of *ischiadikos* Greek, of the *ischion* Greek, hip and loin area; sciatica is an inflammation of the sciatic nerve
sclero, sclerotic, sclerosis	*skleros* Greek, hardened
scopy	*skopein* to look at, to examine + *y* noun ending
sebaceous, sebum	*sebum* Latin, originally, hog fat, lard, fat; sebum is the oily secretion of the sebaceous glands in the dermis layer of the skin
sepsis	*sepsis* Greek, rotting, decaying, infection of a wound
sept, septum	*saeptum* Latin, fence, wall
septic	*septikos* rotten
serous, serum	*serum* Latin, last, late; serum is the fluid that separates from clotted blood; a serous fluid is viscid
sino, sinus	*sinus* Latin, fold, cavity, hollow channel
skeleton	*skeletos* Greek, dried up < *skellein* to dry up. Ancient Greeks used *skeleton* to refer to a mummy, a dried up body. Not until the 16th Century was the term applied to the framework of bones that support the human body.
somn	*somnus* Latin, sleep
speculum	*speculum* Latin, a looking glass, a mirror; in medicine a speculum is an instrument to examine a body cavity that opens on the surface, such as the nose, throat, rectum, or vagina
sphincter, sphincto	*sphinkter* Greek, squeezer, constrictor
spire, spirate	*spirare* Latin, to breathe, akin to *spiritus* 'the breath of life' then 'the divine breath'
splen, spleno	*splen* Greek, spleen
spondyl	*spondylos* Greek, bone of the spine; its Latin translation is *vertebra*

squam	*squama* Latin, a scale on a fish or a snake; squamous is consisting of thin, plate-like structures or squamae; for example the squamous epithelial cells that make up the outer layer of the skin
staped, stapes	*stapes* Latin, stirrup on the saddle of a horse, structure shaped like a stirrup; the stapes is one of the three ossicles (little bones) of the middle ear. It resembles a little stirrup.
staphylo	*staphylos* a bunch of grapes, said of bacteria so shaped
stat	abbreviation of *statim*, Latin, immediately
sten	*stenos* Greek, narrow
ster, stereo	*stereos* Greek, hard, solid, with the developed meaning of 'especially realistic' or 'three-dimensional'
sterno, sternum	*sternum* Late Latin, breastbone < *sternon* Greek, the human chest
stetho	*stethos* Greek, front of the chest
sthen	*sthenos* Greek, strength, seen in asthenia, calisthenics
stomy	*stoma* Greek, mouth
strati, stratum	*stratus* Latin, a flat layer
strepto	*streptos* twisted
sub	*sub* Latin, under, below, less than normal
sudi, sudor	*sudor* Latin, sweat, perspiration
super	*super* Latin, above, over, excessive, akin to the Greek *hyper*
superior	*superior* Latin, more above, higher, on top of
supra	*supra* Latin, above, excessive, more than normal
surgery	*chirurgia* Latin transliteration < *cheir* Greek, hand + *ergos* Greek, work
sym	*sym* Greek, assimilated form of *syn* with, together
syn	*syn* Greek, with, together
syncope	*synkope* Greek, *syn* with + *kope* a cutting, hency *synkope* was 'a cutting short'; a syncope is a fainting spell, due to temporary loss of cellular oxygen in part of the brain
syringe, syrinx	*syrigx, syringos* Greek, any hollow tube, hence a reed pipe, a whistle; syringitis is inflammation of the auditory tube in the ear, also called the syrinx
systole, systolic	*systole* Greek from *syn* > *sys* together + *stole* Greek, a putting, a drawing; systole is the contraction of the ventricles of the heart, when blood is pumped out. Diastole (*diastole* a drawing apart of the ventricles of the heart) is the relaxing and expanding of the ventricles, when blood flows into the heart.

T

tabes, tabetic	*tabes* Latin noun, a wasting away; in medicine the wasting away of body tissue during the course of certain chronic diseases
tachy	*tachys* Greek, swift, quick; tachycardia is a high rate of contraction of heart muscle
talipes	*talus* Latin, ankle + *pes, pedis* Latin, foot; in combination talipes means 'clubfoot'
tarsal, tarsus	*tarsos podos* Greek, Hippocrates' term for the flat of the foot between the heel and the toe; a tarsus is one of the seven bones of the ankle, the tarsi, permitting articulation between the foot and the leg
taxi, taxis, taxo	*taxis* Greek, arrangement, but with the developed sense of 'motion toward or away from'
temple, temporal	*temporalis* Latin, pertaining to the side of the head < *tempus* time, but it also meant the temple of the head
tendon	*tendo, tendinis* Medical Latin, a sinew < *tenon* Greek, a stretched band, a sinew
tense	*tensus* Latin, stretched out, hence narrowed
teras, terato	*teras, teratos* Greek, a wonder, a marvel, a fetal monster
tetanus	*tetanos* Greek adjective, stretched; a bacterium grows at the site of surface lesions to produce this severe infectious disease
therapy	*therapeia* Greek, healing the sick
thermo	*thermos* Greek, hot, warm
thoraco, thorax	*thorax, thorakis* Greek, breastplate of armor, then chest
thrombo, thrombus	*thrombos* Greek, lump, blood clot
thymo, thymus	*thymos* Greek, thyme, the sweet-smelling herb; the thymus gland is found at the bottom of the neck in the chest behind the breastbone
thyroid	*thyreo-eides* Greek, like a door-shaped shield; the thyroid cartilage was named first. It shields the vocal cords of the larynx. The thyroid gland was named after the thyroid cartilage.
tibia, tibio	*tibia* Latin, a flute, any musical pipe; the tibia is the larger bone of the lower leg
toc, tocia	*tokos* Greek, birth, childbirth
tomy	*tome* Greek, a cutting, a dissection; in medicine a surgical incision
ton	*tonos* tension, stretching

tone	*tonos* Greek, quality of being stretched, like a muscle < *teinein*, to stretch
tor	*tor, ator, itor* Latin agent noun suffix indicating the doer of an action, the device that performs an action, akin to English noun suffix *-er*
torq, tors, tort	*torsio, torsionis* Latin, an act of twisting
trachea, tracheo	*tracheia* Greek, rough, then windpipe
trans	*trans* Latin, across, through
trauma	*trauma* Greek, wound, plural traumas, traumata
tri	*tris* Latin, in threes < *tres* three
trich	*thrix, trichos* Greek, a hair
trophy	*trophe* Greek, nourishment, feeding
tropic	*tropikos* Greek, turning toward
tropo	*tropos* Greek, a turning, a changing, an affecting of
tumor	*tumor* Latin, swelling, neoplasm, cancer
tympano, tympanum	*tympanon* Greek, a broad drum made of skin, then eardrum
typh	*typhos* Greek, high fever

U

ulcer	*ulcus* Latin, a sore, an ulcer
ulna	*ulna* Latin, elbow; the ulna is the larger of the two main bones of the forearm
ultra	*ultra* Latin, beyond, in excess of normal
ulus, ulum	*ulus* Latin, diminutive suffix indicating smallness
umbilicus	*umbilicus* Latin, navel, belly button
uni	*unus* Latin, one, single
uria	*ouron* Greek, urine + *ia* medical condition
uterus, uterine	*uterus* Latin, womb

V

vagina, vagino	*vagina* Latin, sheath for a sword, hence the human vagina, based on a pun in Latin where *gladius* was a name for a short army sword and was also widely used as a colloquial word for penis
valve, valvi, valvo	*valva* Latin, the leaf of a folding door < *volvere* to roll up, to fold up
varix, varicose	*varicosus* Medical Latin, full of varices. A varix is a dilated, twisted vein, artery, or lymphatic vessel.
vas, vaso	*vas* Latin, vessel, conduit, duct
vascular	*vasculum* Latin, little blood vessel

vector	*vector* Latin, carrier (of a disease), transporter < *vehere* to carry
veni, veno	*vena* Latin, vein
ventr	*venter* Latin, belly, stomach
ventral	*ventralis* Latin, of the stomach < *venter* stomach, belly
verruca	*verruca* Latin, wart
vertebra	*vertebra* Latin, a turning place, a pivot, a joint < *vertere* to turn; one of the 33 bones of the spinal column, the back bones or joints that permit flexibility of the vertebral column
vesica	*vesica* Latin, bladder, a diminutive form of *vas* bladder, dish, little container
vesicle	*vesicula* Latin, a little sac, a little bladder-like object, a small bag
villi	*villus* Latin, fine hair; plural *villi*
virus, viral	*virus* Latin, poison, venom
viscera	plural of *viscus* Latin, soft flesh, vital organ, entrails, innards
vulva	*vulva* Latin, a covering, a wrapping < *volvere* to roll, to turn. The vulva is the external female genitalia including the labia, mons pubis, clitoris and the openings of the urethra and vagina.

X

xantho	*xanthos* Greek, yellow
xeno	*xenos* Greek, stranger
xero	*xeros* Greek, dry

Y

y	*y* English noun ending derived from various French and Latin noun suffixes

Z

zona, zone	*zona* Latin, belt < *zone* Greek, a girdle
zoo	*zoon* Greek, animal, living thing < *zoe* life
zygo	*zygon* Greek, a yoke for oxen, a pair, a set of twins
zygomatic	*zygoma* Greek, the cheekbone, literally 'the yoke or pair swelling'
zygote	*zygotos* Greek, joined, yoked. The zygote is the cell that results from the union of two sex cells, sperm and egg.

Index

Notes:
1. This index lists words, and phrases defined in the text under single words, as well as a few Latin and Greek roots if they occur in the text out of alphabetical order.
2. Note that Latin and Greek terms that have become familiar in medical English are not italicized. Thus, most terms from Nomina Anatomica (*see* introduction) are not in italics.

A
a as a negative prefix, 1
A&P repair, *see* anterior, 36
ab origine, 4
ab initio, 4
ab ovo, 4
abdominal aorta, *see* celiac artery, 83
abdominal cavity, 83
abducens, 4
abduct, abductor, 4
aberrant, 4
ABG or arterial blood gases, 44
ablactation, 4, 205
abnormal bleeding, *see* hemorrhage, 174
abnormal cell growth, *see* -plasia words, 287
abnormal, 4
abortion, 5
abrade, abrasion, 5
abreaction, 5
abreagieren, German verb, 5
abrupt, 5–6
abruptio placentae, 6
abscess, 6
absorb, 6
abstainer, 6
abstinence, 6
a.c. or ante cibum, 35
acantha, 7
acanthion, 7
acanthocyte, 7
acanthocytosis, 7
acanthoma, acanthomata, 7
acanthosis, 7

acanthosis nigricans, 7
Acanthus spinosus, acanthus leaves, 8
accessory nasal sinus, 318
acetabulum, 8
acetic acid, 8
acetone, 8
acetylcholine, 9; *see also* neurotransmitter, 247
Achilles' tendon, 335
achromatic lens, 95
achromatin, 95
achromatism, 95
achromatophil, 95
acid, 9
acid-base balance, 9
acidemia, 9
acidosis, 9–10
acoustic meatus, 223–224
acquired immunodeficiency syndrome, *see* HIV, 178
acroagnosis, 10
acroanesthesia, 10
acromegaly, 10, 225; *see also* dactylomegaly, 120
acromion, 10
acromphalus, 10–11
acromyotonia, 11
acronym, 11
acrophobia, vi, 11
'across' words, *see* meta-, 231–232; and trans-, 343
actinic rays, 11
actinogenic, 11

actinology, 11
actinotherapy, 11
acupuncture, 12
acute, 12; see also chronic, 96
AD or auris dexter, 49
ad hoc, 12
ad lib, ad libitum, 12
ad nauseam, 12
Adam's apple, see thyroid, 339
adduct, adductor, 13
adenitis, 15
adenocarcinoma, 16
adenoidectomy, 16
adenoids, 16
adenoma, 16
adenomatosis, 16
adenosine monophosphate or AMP, 16
adenosine triphosphate or ATP, 17
adenosine, 16
adenovirus, 17
adhesion, adhesive, 13
adipokinesis, 17
adipokinin, 17
adipolysis, 18
adipose, adiposis, 17
adnexa, 13
adrenal cortex, 13–14
adrenal medulla, 13–14, 225
adrenaline or epinephrine, 14, 144
Aesculapius, see caduceus, 69
affect, 14
afferent neuron, 247; see also efferent, 136
affidavit, 13
after meals, see post cibum, 290
'after' words, see post-, 290
agglutinate, 14
agglutination test, 14
agglutinin, 14
AIDS, 11; see also HIV, 178; infection, 194
air embolism, 137
air sac, 310
air saccule, 310
alb, 19
albescent, 19
albinism, 19
albino, 19
Albion, 19
album, 19
albumen, 19
albumin, 19
albuminuria, 19
alcohol, ethyl, 8

alcohol hallucinosis, see delirium tremens, 122
alcohol withdrawal syndrome, see delirium tremens, 122
algophobia, 20
alimentary canal, 161
'all' words, see pan-, 272
allergen, 21
allergic response, 21
allergy, 21
allesthesia, 22
alloeroticism, 22
alloplasia, see dysplasia, 287
allotrope, allotropic, 22
alpha privative, 1
ALS or amyotrophic lateral sclerosis, 315
alveolar membrane, 22
alveolar pyorrhea, 299
alveolar ridge, 22
alveolar sac, 310
alveoli, see emphysema, 138
alveolus, 22
amble, 23
amblyopia, 261
ambulance, 23
ambulatory, 23
amebic or amoebic dysentery, 132, 141–142
amebicide or amoebicide, 97
amenorrhea, 308
amine, see histamine, 178
amnesia, 1
amnesic apraxia, 3
amniocentesis, 24, 85
amnion, 24
amniorrhexis, 24
amniotic fluid, 24; see also amniocentesis, 85
amniotic sac, 24–25, 310
amniotomy, 25
amorphous, 236
amygdaloid fossa, 157
amyl, 25
amyl nitrite, 25
amylase, 25
amylogen, 26
amylopectin, 25–26
amylopsin, 26
amylose, 26
amyotrophic lateral sclerosis or ALS, 315
anabolic, anabolic steroids, anabolism, 26, 62
anachronism, 27

anaerobic, 1
anal, 29
anal fissure, 29, 154
anal fistula, 29, 154
anal impotence, 29
anal sphincter, 30, 321–322
analgesia, analgesic, 20
analog, 27
analogous, 27
analogue, *see* homologue, 179
analogy, 27
analysis, 27, 215
anaphylactic shock, 28
anaphylaxis, 28
anaplasia, 287
anastomosis, arteriovenous, 27, 45
anatomy, 28, 340
androglossia, 31
androgynoid, 168–169
androgyny, 31
android, 31
androphobia, 32
androsterone, 31
anemia, 1
anemia, aplastic, 287
anemia, hemolytic, *see* schistocyte, 314
anemia, macrocytic, 216
anemia, pernicious, 248
anesthesia, caudal, 82; epidural, 132
anesthetic, 2
aneurysm, 28; *see also* cerebral hemorrhage, 88–89
anger, 32
angina pectoris, 32, 277
angioblastoma, 34
angiocardiogram, 33
angiocardiography, 33
angiofibroma, 34
angiogram, 33
angiolipoma, 34
angiolith, 33
angiolithiasis, 33
angioma, 34
angiomatosis, 34
angionecrosis, 34
angiopathy, 34, 275
angioplasty, 34, 288
angiospasm, 35
angiostenosis, 35, 324
angiotensin I and II, 35
angle, 32
Anglo-Saxon, 32
angostura bitters, 33

angst, 33
anhidrosis, 177
anhydrous, 2
animal starch, *see* glycogen, 166
ankle, 33
ankle bones, *see* tarsus, 333
ankylosing spondylitis, 323
ankylosis, 323; artificial a. *see also* arthrodesis, 126
anodyne, 2
anodynia, 2
anomalous structure, 2
anomaly, 2; congenital, 102
Anopheles mosquito, *see* malaria, 219
anorectal, 305
anorexia nervosa, 2
anorexia, 2, 263
ante cibum or a.c., 35
anteflexion, 35
ante mortem, 36
antepartal, 36
ante partum, 36
antepartum hemorrhage, 36
anterior, 36
anterior chamber, 36
anterior nares, 36
anterior nasal spine, 7
anthrax, *see* bacillus, 52
anti-embolism hose, 137
antiarrhythmic, 3
antiarthritic, 38
antibacterial, 38
antibiotic, 37, 58
antibody, 37; *see also* immunoglobulin, 191
anticoagulant, 38
anticonvulsant, 38
antidepressant, 38
antidiabetic, 38
antidiarrheal, 38
antidote, 38
antiemetic, 38
antiflatulent, 38
antigen, 37
antigen-antibody reaction, 37
antihemorrhagic, 38
antihistamine, 178; *see also* antipruritic, 38
antiinflammatory, 38
antimutagen, 38
antipruritic, 38
antipyretic, 38, 300
antisepsis, 37, 317
antiserum, *see* sero-, 317
antispasmotic, 38

antitoxin, *see* tetanus, 336
antitubercular, 38
antitussive, 38
antiviral, 38
anus, 29
aorta, 38–39; coarctation of a., 102
aortic aneurysm, 39
aortic sinus, 318
aortic stenosis, 39, 324
aortic valve, 39
apathy, 2, 275
apertura sinus frontalis, 39
aperture, 39
apex, apex beat, apical, apices, 40
Apgar score, 40
aphasia, 3
apheresis, 41
aplasia, 287
apnea, 3
apocrine sweat glands, 41, 110; *see also* hidradenitis, 177
apogee, 41
aponeurosis, lingual, 41
apophysis, 42
apoplexy, 42
apostle, 40
apothecary, 42
appendectomy, 134, 340
appendicitis, 42–43, 319; *see also* obturator sign, 252
appendicular skeleton, 319
appendix, 42; *see also* retrocecal, 307
apraxia, apraxic, 3
Arabic versions of Greek medical texts, *see* pia mater, 223
arachnidism, 43
arachnoid meninx, 228
arachnoid membrane, 43
arachnoid sheath, 43
arachnoid villi, 43
arachnoid, 43
arachnoidism, 43
arachnophobia, 43
arch, zygomatic, 363
areola mammae, 44
areolar glands, 44
arm muscles, *see* biceps, triceps, 85
armpit, *see* axilla, 51
'around' prefix, *see* circum-, 98; and peri-, 280–281
arrhythmia, 3
arterial blood gases or ABG, 44

arteries, carotid, 77; coronary, 106; occipital, 75
arteriogram, 45
arteriola, arteriole, 44
arteriosclerosis, 45
arteriovenous anastomosis, 45
artery, 44; coronary a., 32, *see also* coronary thrombosis, 338;
celiac, 83
arthritides: as formal plural of arthritis, 45
arthritis, 45; rheumatoid, 307
arthrocentesis, 46, 85
arthrodesis, 46, 126
arthroendoscopy, 46
arthrosclerosis, 46
arthroscopy, *see* arthroendoscopy, 46
articular, 46
articulate, 46–47
articulation, 47
artificial ankylosis, *see* arthrodesis, 126
AS or auris sinistra, 50
ascending colon, 104
ascites, 47
asepsis, 3, 317
aseptic, 3
asexual, 1
asphyxia, 30
aspirate, 47, 322
aspirating syringe, 47
aspiration of vomitus, 47
aspiration pneumonia, 289
associative neuron, 247; *see also* efferent, 136
asthenia, 326
asthma, 47
astrocyte, *see* glioma and neuroglia, 164
astrocytoma, *see* glioma, 164
astroglia, *see* neuroglia, 164
asymptomatic, 1
ataxia, 333
atheroma, atheromatosis, 48
atherosclerosis, 28, 32; as cause of angio-necrosis, 34
Athlete's foot, *see* tinea pedis, 339
atlas, 48
atonia or atony, 341
atrial fibrillation, 153
atrioventricular node, *see* sinoatrial node, 49
atrium, 48
atrophic vaginitis, 353
atrophy, 346

atypical, 1
auditory tube, *see* syrinx, 331
auditory hallucination, 172
auricle, 49
auricula, 49
auris, 49
auris dexter or AD, 49
auris externa, 49
auris interna, 50
auris media, 50
auris sinistra or AS, 50
auscultate, *see* stethoscope, 326
autism, 51
autoclave, 99
autoeroticism, 22
autoimmune response, 50
automatic, 50
autonomic nervous system, 50
autopsy pathology, 276
Avicenna or Ibn Sina, Persian physician
    and author, *see* cephalic vein, 86
axial skeleton, 319
axial, 51; *see also* computerized axial
    tomography, 79
axilla, axillary, 51
axis, 51
axon, 51
azygos vein, 363
azygous, 363

B
B cell, *see* lymphocyte, 214
b.i.d., 57
B.U.N. test, 350
bacillemia, 52
bacilluria, 52
bacillus, 52
bacillus anthracis, 52
back of the head, *see* occiput, 253
bacteria, 52; necrophilic b., 245
bacterial blood poisoning, *see* septicemia,
    317
bacterial food poisoning, 53
bactericide, 53, 97
bacteriology, 53
bacteriolysin, 53
bacteriolysis, 53
bacteriolytic agent, 53
bacteriophage, 53–54
bacteriostat, bacteriostasis, 54
bacterium: *Streptomyces erythreus*, 145
bad breath, *see* halitosis, 171
bad humor, 6

'bad' words, *see* mal-, 218–219
bag, ileostomy, 190
bag of waters, 25
balloon angioplasty, 34
balloon catheter, 80
balloon dilatation, prostatic, 55–56
balloon valvuloplasty, percutaneous, 114
bandage, scapulary, 313
bariatrics, 54
Barnes' dilator, *see* colposcopy, 105
baroreceptor, 54
barotrauma, 55
Bartholin's abscess, 55
Bartholin's cyst, 55
Bartholinitis, 55
Barton forceps, 252
basal, 55
basal body temperature, 55
basal cell carcioma, 55
basal cell epithelioma, 145, 337
bedsore or decubitus ulcer, 121, 348
'before' words, *see* pre-, 290; and pro-, 291–
    292
benign, 55–56
benign prostatic hypertrophy, 55–56
beta, 56
beta blocker, 56
beta cells, 56
beta rays, 56
beta rhythm, 56
beta waves, 56
biceps brachii or biceps muscle, 56, 85; *see
    also* triceps, 344
Bichat, M.F.X., French anatomist, *see*
    membrane, 227–228
bicuspid tooth, 56
bicuspid valve, 56, 354; *see also* mitral valve,
    234
bifid tongue, *see* schistoglossia, 165
bifocal, 56
big toe, *see* hallux, 172
'big' words, *see* mega- and megalo-, 225–226
bilateral, 57, 208
bilateral carotid artery, 57
bilateral symmetry, 57
bile, 57
biliary ducts, *see* duct, 131
biliary tract, 57
biliousness, 58
bilirubin, 58, 184
binary, 57
binary fission, 57
binasal hemianopia, 172

bioethics, 58–59
biology, 59
bionics, 59
biopsy, 59
biped, 56
bipolar disorder, 57
birth control method, *see* vasectomy, 355
birth hormone, *see* oxytocin, 340
birth trauma, 343
'birth' words, *see* natal, 243–244; and -toc-,
    339–340
bis in die, 57
bisexual, 56
black eye, *see* circumorbital hematoma, 257
'black' words, *see* melano-, 226–227
blastocele or blastocoele, *see* blastula, 60
blastochyle, *see* blastula, 60
blastocyst, 59–60
blastoderm, *see* blastula, 60
blastoma, 60
blastomere, 60
blastula, 60
bleb, 61
bleed to death, *see* exsanguinate, 148
bleeder's disease, *see* hemophilia, 174
bleeding, arterial and venous, 44
blepharectomy, *see* blephar-, 61–62
blepharism, 62
blepharitis, 62
blepharoptosis, 62, 295–296
Bleuler, Eugen, *see* schizophrenia, 314
blind intestine, *see* caecum, 70
blind spot of the eye, *see* punctum caecum,
    298
blindgut, *see* caecum, 70
blister, *see* bulla, 68, and vesicle, 358
blood cancer, *see* leukemia, 209
blood clot, *see* thrombus, 338
blood, occult, 253
blood platelets, *see* thrombocytopenia, 278
blood pressure, *see* systole, 331
blood urea nitrogen test, 350
blood vessel surgery, *see* angioplasty, 288
'blood vessel words', *see* angio-, 33;
    hemangio-, 173; and vaso-, 355–356
'blood' words, *see* hem-, 173–174
blue dome cyst, 115
BMPs or bone morphogenic proteins, 236
body temperature, normal adjustment of,
    see thermotaxis, 337
body types, *see* mesomorph, 230

bone marrow, lining of, *see* endosteum, 140
bone morphogenic proteins or BMPs, 236
'bone' words, *see* osseo-, osteo-, 267–268
bones, parietal, 274
borborygmus, *see* flatus, 155
botulinus neurotoxins, 63
botulism, 63
bow-legged, *see* genu varum, 162
bowel, 64
brachial, 64
brachial artery, 64
brachial plexus, 64
brachialis muscle, 64
brachioradialis muscle, 64
brachycephalic, brachycephaly, 65
brachydactylous, brachydactyly, 65
bradycardia, 65
bradyglossia, 65
bradylalia, 65
bradyphasia, 65
bradytachycardia, 64
brain, *see* encephalon, 139
brain surgery, stereotactic, 324
brainstem, *see* medulla oblongata, 225
breast, *see* mammary gland, 220–221
'breast' words, *see* mammo- 220–221; and
    mast-, 221–222
breastbone, *see* sternum, 325
'breath words', *see* hal-, 171–172
bregma, *see* occiput, 253
bronchiole, 66
bronchitis, 66
bronchodilator, 66
bronchopneumonia, 66, 289
bronchoscope, bronchoscopy, 66–67, 208, 316
bronchus, *see* rale, 304
bruise, *see* hematoma, 257
bruxism, 208
bubo, *see* lymphogranuloma, 214
bucca, 67
buccal cavity, 83
buccal fat pad, 67
buccal glands, 67
buccal smear, 67
buccinator muscle, 67
bulimia, 68; *see also* sitomania, 319
bulla, 68
bullae, emphysematous, 138–139
Bundle of His, 49
bursa, 68
bursitis, 68

C

caduceus: carried by Hermes or Mercury, 69; cult symbol of Asklepios, 69; meaning of snake symbol on caduceus, 69–70

caecum, 70

calcaneus, 70; *see also* talipes, 332

calcar, 70–71

calcar femorale, 70–71

calcar pedis, 70–71

calciferol, 71

calcitonin, 71

calcitonin, *see* thyroid, 339

calcium, 71

calcium, loss of, *see* osteoporosis, 268

calculus, 71–72

calculus, renal, 305; *see also* nephro-, 246

calculus, salivary, *see* ptyalolithotomy, 296

calculus, ureteral, *see* ureterolith, 350

calisthenics, 326

calor, 72; *see also* inflammation, 154–155

calorie, calorimeter, calorimetry, 72

cAMP, 16

canaliculus, lacrimal, 204–205

cancer jargon and medical euphemism, 73

cancer, 72; *see also* carcinoma, 257

Candida, *Candida albicans*, 73

candidiasis, 73

cannula, 74; *see also* trocar, 344

capillary, 74

capitate bone, 75; *see also* carpus, 78

capitulum, 75–76

capitulum humeri, 76

caput costae, 74

caput femoris, 75

caput humeri, 75

carcinoma, 257

carcinoma, verrucous, 357

cardiac arrest, *see* cardi-, 76

cardiac arrhythmia, 3

cardiomegaly, 225

cardiomyopathy, 77, 275; idiopathic c., 190

cardiopulmonary resuscitation, 76

carotid arteries, 77

carpal tunnel syndrome or CTS, 78–79

carpoptosis, 79

carpus, with origin of the names of the wristbones, 77–78

cartilage, articular, 46

cartilage, hyaline, 180

cartilage, palpebral, 272

cartilage softening, *see* chondromalacia patellae, 274

cartilage, thyroid, 339

cartilaginous, *see* chondroid, 256

CAT scan or computerized axial tomography, 79; *see also* tomograph, 341

catabolism, 26, 62–63

catalysis, 81, 215

catalyst, 81, 215

catamenia, 229

cataract, 81

catarrh, 81

catatonia, 81–82

catharsis, 5; physiologic and psychiatric, 79–80

cathartic, 80; saline c., 311

catheter, with list of types, 80

cauda, 82

cauda equina, 82

cauda pancreatis, 82

caudad, *see* crani-, 108

caudal anesthesia, 82

caul, 24

cause, *see* etiology, 146

cavity, medullary, *see* endosteum, 140

cavity, pleural, 288–289

cavity, tympanic, *see* auris media, 50

cavity, with list of body cavities, 82–83

cecofixation, *see* cecopexy, 70

cecopexy, 70

cecum, *see* retrocecal, 307

celiac artery, 83

celiac disease, 84

celiac plexus, 84, 288

cell, 84

cell nucleus, 84, 249

cell membrane, 84

Celsus, Roman medical writer, author of De Medicina, 6, 70, 83

centesis, 84

central vision, *see* macula lutea, 217

cephalad, 15, 86

cephalic, 86

cephalic vein, with note on how badly named it was, 86

cerebellum, 88

cerebral adiposis, 17

cerebral cortex, 88

cerebral edema, 88

cerebral hemiplegia, 173

cerebral hemisphere, 173

cerebral hemorrhage, 88–89

cerebral palsy or CP, 89

cerebrospinal fluid or CSF, 89

cerebrovascular accident or CVA, 89–90; *see also* apoplexy, 42

cerebrum, 89
ceroma, 87
cerumen or earwax, 87
ceruminosis, 88
ceruminous glands, 87
cervical cap, 90
cervical or neck adenitis, 15
cervical vertebrae, 90; *see also* odontoid
    process, 255
cervix or cervix uteri, 90
Chamberlen forceps, 157
cheilitis, cheilitis actinica, cheilitis venenata
    or 'cosmetic lips', 90
cheilognathopalatoschisis, 91, 271
cheiloplasty, 91
cheilorrhaphy, 91
cheiloschisis, 91, 313
cheilosis, 91
chemotaxis, 333
chest area, *see* thorax, 338
'chest' words, *see* expectorate, 148; and
    pector-, 277
chiasm, optic, 262
chickenpox, *see* papule, 273
childbirth labor, normal, *see* eutocia, 340
Chlamydia, *see* lymphogranuloma, 214
chlorine, 92
chlorquine, *see* malaria, 219
cholecystectomy, 92, 134,
cholecystitis, 92, 116
cholecystostomy, 93, 327
choler, *see* melancholy, 93, 226
cholesterol, 93, 324
chondroblast, 93
chondroblastoma, 93
chondroid, 256
chondrolipoma, 256
chondromalacia patellae or runner's knee,
    94, 218, 274
chondromucin, 94
chondrosarcoma, 94
chorion, 25
choroid layer, *see* retinopexy, 281
chromatic, 95
chromatin, 95
chromatophil, 95
chromosome, 95
chronic, 12, 96
chronic fatigue syndrome, *see* asthenia, 326
chyle, 96
chyloderma or scrotal elephantiasis, 96
chylopericardium, 96
chyloperitoneum, *see* chylorrhea, 96

chylopneumothorax, 96–97
chylorrhea, 96
chyme, 97; *see also* gastric, 161
chymosin, 97
chymotrypsin, 97
cilia, 98
ciliary body, 98
ciliary muscle, 98
ciliary process, 291
ciliary zonula, *see* zonule of Zinn, 362; *see*
    also vii
cinema, 17
circumambient, 23
circumcision, 98
circumcorneal, 98
circumlental, 98
circumorbital hematoma, 257
circumrenal, 98
cirrhosis, 99; *see also* hepatomegaly, 225
clamp forceps, 157
clavicle, 99
clavicle, *see* sternocleidomastoid muscle,
    325–326
claw toe, *see* hallux, 172
cleft, 99
cleft palate, 99–100, 271; *see also*
    palatoschisis, 313
cleft tongue, *see* glossoplasty, 288;
    schistoglossia, 165
climax, sexual, *see* orgasm, 264
clinic, 100
clinical diagnosis, 100, 167
clinical thermometer, 337
clitoral prepuce, 290
clitoriditis or clitoritis, 100
clitoris, 100; *see also* circumcision, 98
clitoromegaly, 100
clone, 101, 234–235
clonic spasm, *see* clonus, 101
clonism, *see* myoclonus, 101
clonospasm, *see* myoclonus, 101
clonus, 101
closed fracture, 157–158
Clostridium botulinum, *see* bacterial food
    poisoning, 53;
botulism, 63
Clostridium tetani, 336
clubfoot, *see* talipes, 332
clysis, *see* proctoclysis, 292
clysma, *see* proctoclysis, 292
clyster, *see* proctoclysis, 292
coarctation of the aorta, 102
coccobacillus, 53

coccyx, 103; see also ischiococcygeal, 198
cochlea, 103
cochlear implant, 103
cofactor, 102
coherent, 13
cold sore, see herpes, 176
colectomy, see ileostomy, 190
colic, 104
colitis, see dysentery, 141–142
collagen, 103
collateral, 102, 209
colloid, colloid bath, colloidal suspension, 103
colon, 104; see also rectum, 305
colostomy, 104, 327
colporrhaphy, 104
colposcopy, 105
colpostat, see colposcopy, 105
comminuted fracture, 157–158
common bile dict, see duct, 131
compound fracture, 157–158
computerized axial tomography or CAT scan, 79, 341
conceptus, 102
conchae, inferior, 194
condom, see gonorrhea, 168
condyle, 105; see also mandible, 221
condyle, femoral, 152
condyle, mandibular, see temporomandibular joint, 334
condyloid process, 105
condyloma, 105; see also venereal wart, 359
condyloma acuminatum, 105
congenital, 102
conjunctiva, 105
conjunctivitis, 106
connecting neuron, 247
contact dermatitis, see eczema, 136
contraceptive devices: cervical cap, 90; diaphragm, 128
convalescent, 146
cords, vocal, see glottis, 165
cornea, see photorefractive keratectomy, 283
'cornea' words, see kerato-, 202–203
corneal inflammation, see dendritic keratitis, 124
corona dentis, 106
corona radiata, 106–107
coronal suture, 106
coronary artery, 32, 106
coronary thrombosis, 338
coroner, 107

corpus callosum, 107
corpus cavernosum, 107
corpus luteum, 107; see also lutein, 213
corpus spongiosum, 107
corpus, 107
corpuscle, red, see erythrocyte, 145
corpuscle, white, see leukocyte, 209
corrupt, 5
cortex, 107
cortex, adrenal, 13–14
cortex, olfactory, 255
cortex, renal, 305
corticoafferent, 108
corticoefferent, 108
corticosteroid, 14, 108; see also antipruritic, 38
coruscation, see entoptic, 142–143
costa, costal, 108
costectomy, 108
costotome, 108
costotomy, 108
cowpox, see vaccine, 353
CP or cerebral palsy, 89
CPR or cardiopulmonary resuscitation, 76
craniad, 108
cranial cavity, 83
cranial nerves, see crani-, 108
cranioclasis or cranioclasty, 109
craniomalacia, 218
craniotome, 109
cranium, 108; see also parietal, 274
crepitant rale, 109
crepitation or crepitus, 109
crisis, 111
crista galli, 111
cristae cutis, 111
critical, 111
Crohn's disease, see jejunoileitis, 200
crown of a tooth, see corona dentis, 106
cryobank, 112
cryogen and cryogenics, 112
cryolesion, 113
cryonics, as pseudo-medical scam, 112
cryoprobe, 112
cryosurgery, 112–113
cryptorchidism, 262
CSF or cerebrospinal fluid, 89
cum, Latin preposition and prefix, 101–102
cure-all, see panacea, 272
curettage, 113
curette, 113
cuticle, 113
cutis, 113

cutis vera, *see* derma, 125
CVA or cerebrovascular accident, 89–90
cyanide, 115
cyanobacteria, 115
cyanophilous, 115
cyanopsia, 115
cyanosis, cyanotic, 115
cyclic adenosine monophosphate or cAMP, 16
cyst, 115
cyst, pathologic, 285
cyst, pilonidal, 286
cyst, sebaceous, 316
cystic duct, 116; *see also* duct, 131
cystic fibrosis, 116
cystic mastitis, 222
cystitis, 116
cystocele, 83; *see also* cystopexy, 116
cystopexy, 83, 116
cystoscope, 116–117, 316
cystostomy, 117, 327
cytology, *see* cell, 84
cytopenia, 278
cytoplasm, *see* cell, 84
cytotoxic, 118

D
D&C or dilatation and curettage, 113
dacryocyst or lacrimal sac or tear sac, 119; *see also* cyst, 115
dacryocystitis, 119
dacryocystoblennorrhea, 119
dacryocystocele, 119
dactylitis, 120
dactylomegaly, 120
daub, 19
de: uses of prefix in English words, 120
dead words, *see* necro-, 245
débride, débridement, 120
decidua, *see* endometrium, 140, 232
decrepit, 109
decubitus ulcer or bedsore, 121, 348
deep fascia, 151
defecate, 121
defecation, 151
defect, congenital, 102
defibrillate, defibrillator, 121, 153
delirium, 122
delirium tremens or 'the d.t.'s', 122
delta rhythm, 122–123
deltoid muscle, 123, 256
dementia praecox, *see* precocious, 290
demyelination, 121, 239

dendrite, 123–124
dendritic keratitis, 124
dens in dente, 124
dental alveolus, 22
dentia, 124
dentifrice, *see* dent-, 124
dentin, 124; *see also* odontoblast, 61
dentition, precocious, 290
dentulous, *see* edentia, 125
derma or dermis, 125; *see also* cutis, 113
dermatitis, 125; *see also* eczema, 136
dermatoglyphics, 125
dermatome, 125
descending colon, 104
desquamation, 122, 323
desquamative exfoliation, 122
detached retina, *see* retinopexy, 281
Dhobie itch, *see* tinea cruris, 339
diabetes mellitus, 8, 127–128
diabetic retinitis, 305
diagnosis, 128, 167
diagnostics, 167
dialysis, 128, 215
diaphragm, 128; *see also* phrenic nerve, 284
'diaphragm' words, *see* phren-, 284
diarrhea, 128
diastole, 128; *see also* systole, 331
diastolic, 129
dicentric, 127
dicoria, 127
dicyclic, 127
diencephalon, 127
differential diagnosis, 128, 167
difficult labor, *see* dystocia, 133
digestive system, 161
digital subtraction angiography or DSA, 33
diglossia, 127
dilatation and curettage or D&C, 113
dilator, Barnes', *see* colposcopy, 105
dimorphic, 127
diphasic, 127
diplegia, 127
diplococcus, 53
diploid cell, 127
diplopia or double vision, 127
diplopiometer, 127
'discharge' words, *see* -rrhea, 308–309
disease, infectious, 194
'disease' prefix and suffix, *see* patho- and -pathy, 275–276
disorder, factitious, 150
disorder, psychosomatic, 295
dissociation, 129

distal, 129–130
distal phalanx, 282
distress, fetal, 153
disuse atrophy, 346
diuretics, use of, *see* hypochloremia, 92
dolor, 130; *see also* inflammation, 154–155
donor, 130
dorsad, 15, 130
dorsal, 130
dorsocephalad, 15, 130
dorsum, 130
double-channel catheter, 80
double pneumonia, 289
draining sinus, 318
dromomania, 130
dropsy, *see* edema, 136
drug abuse, aspiration, 47
dry mouth, pathologic, *see* xerostoma, 361
dry clinic, 100
DSA or digital subtraction angiography, 33
duct, 4, 131; lacrimal, 204–205; sebaceous, 316
ductus deferens, 131; *see also* vas deferens, 354–355
duodenum, *see* enteron, 141
dupp, 131
dura mater, 132, 223; *see also* pachyleptomeningitis, 270
'dwarf' words, *see* nano-, 241
dwarfism, *see* nanism, 241
dysentery, 132, 141–142
dysmenorrhea, 132, 229, 309
dyspepsia, *see* eupepsia, 147
dysplasia, 133, 287
dyspnea, 133; *see also* eupnea, 147
dystocia, 133, 340
dystonia, 133, 342
dystonia musculorum deformans, 133
dystrophy, 133, 346

E
ear drum, *see* tympanum, 346; *see also* stapes, 323
'ear' words, *see* auris, 49–50; and oto-, 268–269
earwax, *see* cerumen, 87
eccentric, 134
ecchymosis, 97
eccrine, 110; *see also* hidradenitis, 177
ECG or electrocardiogram, 76
eclampsia, 134
eclectic, 134
ecstasy, 134

ectoderm, 125–126
ectomorph, 230
ectopia, ectopic, 135–136
ectopic pregnancy, 135–136
eczema, 136
edema, 136
edentia, 125
edentulous, *see* edentia, 125
EEG or electroencephalogram, 87
efferent, 136
efferent neuron, 136, 247
effusion, *see* ascites, 47
'egg' words, *see* oo-, 259–260; and ovum, 269
elbow, 137
elbowed catheter, 80
electrocardiogram, 76
electroencephalogram or EEG, 87
elephantiasis, 188; scrotal elephantiasis, *see also* chyloderma, 96
Elliot forceps, 252
embolectomy, 137
embolism, 63, 137
embolus, 63, 137
embryo, 137; *see also* blasto-, 59
embryology, 137
embryoma, 138
emesis, emetic, 138
emesis basin, 138
emmenagogue, 18
emphysema, 138
emphysematous bullae, *see* bulla, 68
empyema, 139, 299
encephalitis, 86
encephalomyelitis, 139
encephalomyelopathy, 139, 276
encephalon, 86, 139
encephalosclerosis, 139
encysted or saccate, 117
endemic, 123
endoblast, 60
endocrine, 110
endocrinology, 110
endocyst, 117
endoderm, 126
endometrium, 140, 232, 351–352; *see also* menstruation, 230
endomorph, 230
endorphin, 140
endoscope, endoscopy, 140, 316; *see also* bronchoscope, 66–67
endoscopic gastrostomy, percutaneous, or PEG, 114
endosteum, 140, 267

endothelium, 141, 336; see also RES, 306
endotracheal, 141
endotracheal tube, uses of, 141
enema, see proctoclysis, 292
enema, saline, 311
England, English, 32
ensiform process, see sternum, 325
enteric coating of tablets, 141
enteritis, 142
enteritis, necrotizing, 245
enteron, 141
Enterovirus, 142
entoptic, 142
entropion, see trichiasis, 344
enucleation, 249
enzyme, see amylase, 25
enzyme, salivary, see ptyalin, 296
EOM or extraocular muscles, 149
ephedrine, see vasoconstrictor, 355
epiblast, 60
epidemic, 123
epidemiology, 123
epidermis, 143; see also cutis, 113
epidermis, layers of, see stratum, 327
epididymis, 129
epidural, 132
epiglottis, 143
epilepsy, 143–144
epilepsy, photic, 283
epinephrine or adrenaline, 14, 144; see also
    medulla, 225; vasopressor, 355–356
epiphysis, 144
epiploic foramen, see omentum, 257
epiploon, see omentum, 257
episiorrhaphy, 305; see also episiotomy, 144
episiotomy, 144; see also episiorrhaphy, 305
epispadias, 321
epithelial tissue, see endothelium, 141
epithelioma, 145, 337
epithelium, 144–145, 336–337
Epstein-Barr virus, see mononucleosis, 235
equinus, see talipes, 332
erase, 5
erasure, 5
erogenous zone, 362
errant, 4
erythrism, 145
erythroblast, 61
erythroblastoma, 61
erythrocyte, 7, 145
erythromycin, 145
-escent and -escence, their meaning as
    suffixes, 145–146

esophagus, 146, 281
essential, its special meaning in medicine,
    146
estrogen therapy, see menopause, 229–230
ESWL or extracorporeal shock-wave
    lithotripsy, 212
Ethics, treatise by Aristotle, 58–59
ethyl alcohol, 8
etiology, 146; see also idiopathic, 190
etiotropic, 146
eupepsia, 147
euphoria, 147
eupnea, 147
eurhythmia, 147
Eustachian tube, see salpinx, 312; see also
    nasopharynx, 243
euthanasia, 147
eutocia, 340; see also dystocia, 133
excise, 148
excrement, 151
excreta, 151
exfoliation, see squam-, 323
exhalation, 171
exhale, 171
exocrine, 110; see also hidradenitis, 177
expectorant, 148
expectorate, 148
expire, see -spir-, 322
exsanguinate, 148
extensor muscles, see carpoptosis, 79
external auditory meatus, 49, 223–224
extracorporeal, 148–149
extraocular muscles or EOM, 149
extravasate, extravasation, 149
exudate, exudation, 148
'eye' words, see oculus, 254; ophthalmo-,
    260–261; -opia, 261–262
eye surgeon, see ophthalmologist, 260–261
eye, structures of, see uvea, 352
eyeball, see sclera, 315
eyelashes, see cilia, 98
eyelid, see blephar- entries, 61–62
eyelid, see palpebra, 272

F
facies, 150
facies abdominalis, 150
facies gastrica splenis, 150
factitial, 150
factitious, 150
fainting spell, see syncope, 331
falling sickness, see epilepsy, 143–144
Fallopian fimbriae, 154

Fallopian tube, 150; *see also* oophoro-
    salpingectomy, 260
'Fallopian tube' words, *see* salpingo-, 312
Fallopio, Gabriele, 150
false pregnancy, *see* pseudocyesis, 294
'false' words, *see* pseudo-, 294
FAS or fetal alcohol syndrome, 152
fascia, 151
fascicle, 151
fasciculation, 151
fasciculus, 151
fasciitis, 151
fasciitis, necrotizing, 245
fat, *see* lipid, 211
fat cell, *see* lipocyte, 211
fat embolism, 137
'fat' words, *see* lipo-, 211
fecal impaction, 151–152
fecalith, 152
fecaloma as inappropriate medical word,
    152
feces, 151
feeding tube, jejunal, 200
female circumcision as cruel mutilation, 98
female gonad, 167
'female' words, *see* -gyn-, 168–169
femoral condyle, 152
femur, 8, 152
fertilization, in vitro, 192
fetal alcohol syndrome, 152
fetal anomaly, 2
fetal distress, 153
fetal hydrops, 182
fetal nuchal chord, 249
fetal monster, *see* terato-, 335
fetometry, 153
fetotoxic, *see* terato-, 335
fetus, 152
fever, *see* pyrexia, 300
'few' words, *see* oligo-, 255–256
fiber, *see* fascia, 151
fibril, 153; collagen fibril, 103
fibrillation, 153; *see also* defibrillate, 121
fibrin, *see* sero-, 317
fibrinogen, *see* sero-, 317
fibrosarcoma, odontogenic, 255
fibrosis, 116
fibrous membrane, 227
fibula, 153
fimbria, 154
finger and toe bones, *see* phalanges, 282
'finger and toe' words, *see* dactyl-, 120;
    phalang-, 282

fingernail biting, *see* onychophagy, 259
fingerprint comparison, *see*
    dermatoglyphics, 125
fingerprints, *see* cristae cutis, 111
firebug disorder, *see* pyromania, 300
fissure, 154
fissure, anal, 29
fissure of Rolando, 29, 154
fissure of Sylvius, 29, 154
fistula, 154
fistula, anal, or fistula in ano, 29, 154
fistula, arteriovenous, 45
flatulence, 155; *see also* crepitation and
    crepitus, 109
flatus, 155
flavedo, 155
flavin, 155
flavivirus, 155
Flavobacterium, 155
flavone, 155
flavoprotein, 155
'flesh' words, *see* sarco-, 312
flexor, 156
flexure, hepatic, 156
flexure, splenic, 156
floating kidney, *see* nephroptosis, 296
flora, intestinal, 197
flu, *see* influenza, 195
Foley catheter, 80
Foley, Frederick, American urologist, 80
follicle, 156
follicular tonsillitis, 156
foot bones, *see* metatarsal, 232
footprints, *see* cristae cutis, 111
foramen, 156
foramen, infraorbital, 195
foramen magnum, 156; *see also* occiput, 75;
    see also occipital bone, 253
foramen, mental, 157
foramen, obturator, 252
forceps, 157
forceps delivery, 157
forceps, obstetric, 252
forearm bone, *see* radius, 303
forensic pathology, 276
foreskin, *see* prepuce, 290; *see also*
    circumcision, 98
forty days of quarantine, origin of, 301
fossa, 157
fossa, temporal, *see* temporomandibular
    joint, 334
fovea centralis, *see* macula lutea, 217
fracture, 157–158

freckle, *see* macula, 217
frenulum, 158
frenzy, *see* phren- and phrenology, 284
fresh-eating disease, *see* necrotizing fasciitis, 245
front of the head, *see* bregma under occiput, 253
functional disease, 158
functional psychosis, 158
fungicide, 97
fungus, *see* Candida, 73
funic presentation, 158
funic souffle, 158
funis umbilicalis, 158
fusing joints, *see* arthrodesis, 46

G
gait, tabetic, 332
galactagogue, 18, 159
galactase, 159
galactocele, 159
galactopoetic, 159
galactorrhea, 160
galactostatic, 159
Galen, Greek-speaking Roman doctor, *see* cancer, 72
gallbladder, 160; *see also* cholecyst- words, 92–93
ganglion, 160
gangrene, 160–161
gastric, 161
gastric artery, left, *see* celiac artery, 83
gastroenteritis, 142
gastroesophageal reflux, *see* hiatus hernia, 175
gastrogavage, 161
gastrointestinal tract, 161
gastrolavage, 161
gastrostomy, 161
genetic anomaly, dental, *see* dens in dente, 124
geniculate ganglion, 162
geniculate neuralgia, 21
genital herpes, 176
genital wart, *see* condyloma, 105
genu recurvatum, 162
genu valgum, 162
genu varum, 162
genuflect, 162
geriatric, 163
German measles, *see* rubella, 308
gerontology, 163
GI series, *see* gastrointestinal, 161

gingiva, 163
gingivectomy, 163
gingivitis, 163; severe gingivitis, *see also* pyorrhea, 390
girdle, pelvic, 277
GISA or gastrointestinal system assessment, 161
gladiolus, *see* sternum, 325
gland, areolar, 44
gland, ceruminous, 87
gland, lacrimal, 204–205
gland, preputial, 290
gland, salivary, 311
gland, sebaceous, 44, 316
gland, sudoriferous, 328
glaucoma, 164
glenoid cavity, *see* caput humeri, 75
glenoid fossa, 157
glial cell, *see* neuroglia, 164; *see also* optic glioma, 262
glioma, 164
glioma, optic, 262
glomerulus, *see* nephron, 246
glossal, 164
glossoplasty, 164–165, 288
glossorrhaphy, 165
glottal stop, *see* glottis, 165
glottis, 165
glucose, 165
glucose tolerance test or GTT, 166
glucosuria, 165–166; and *see also* glycosuria, 167
gluteal tuberosity, 166
gluten-induced enteropathy, *see* celiac disease, 84
gluteus: maxiumus, medius, minimus, 166
glycemia or glycosemia, 167
glycogen, 166
glycoprotein, *see* mucin, 237
glycosuria, 167
gnosis, 10
goiter, *see* thyroid, 339; colloid goiter, 103
gonad, 167–168
gonadotropin, 168
gonococcal ophthalmia of the newborn, 260
gonococcus, 168
gonorrhea, 168
good humour, 6
gooseflesh, *see* cutis anserina, 113
gout, false, 294
grafted tissue, *see* transplant, 343
grand mal seizure, *see* epilepsy, 143–144

granuloma, fibrous, *see* nodule, 248
gravid, 244
great toe, *see* hallux, 172
great saphenous vein, 312
greater omentum, 257
greenstick fracture, 157–158
GTT or glucose tolerance test, 166
gullet, *see* esophagus, 146, 281
'gum' words, *see* gingiva, 163
gustatory hallucination, 172
gynander, 169
gynandrism, 169
gynandry, 31
gynecology, 169
gynecomastia, 168
gynephobia, 32, 169
gyniatrics, 169
gyri cerebri, 170
gyrus, 170

H

h.s. or hora somni, 171, 320
hair cyst, *see* pilonidal cyst, 286
hair follicle, 156
hair muscles, *see* pilomotor reflex, 286
'hair' words, *see* pili-, 285–286; and tricho-, 344
'half' words, *see* hemi-, 172–173
halitosis, 171
halitus, 171
hallucination, 172
hallucinogen, 172
hallux flexus, 172
hallux or hallex or hallus, 172
hamate bone, *see* carpus, 78
hammertoe, *see* hallux, 172
hand bones, *see* metacarpal, 231
hard palate, 271
harelip, *see* cheiloschisis, 91, 313
heart attack, *see* myocardial infarction, 76, 194
heart beat, rapid, *see* tachycardia, 332
heart muscle, 237; *see also* myocardium, 239
heart muscle disease, *see* cardiomyopathy, 275
heart sac, *see* pericardium, 280
heart valves, *see* bicuspid and mitral, 354
'heart' words, *see* cardi-, 76–77
heebie-jeebies, *see* delirium tremens, 122
heel bone, *see* calcaneus, 70; os calcis, 266
hemangioma, 34, 173
hematemesis, 173
hematocrit, 173

hematoma, 257
hematoma, circumorbital, v, 257
hemianopia, 172
hemianopsia, 172
hemifacial, 173
hemiplegia, 173
hemisphere, cerebral, 89, 173
hemodialysis, 128, 215
hemoglobin, 22, 174; *see also* erythrocyte, 145
hemoglobinuria, 174
hemolysis, 174; *see also* schistocyte, 314
hemolytic anemia, 174
hemophilia, 174
hemorrhage, 174
hemorrhage, antepartum, 36
hemorrhagic blood, *see* ecchymosis, 97
hemostasis, 174
hemostat, 174
hepatic adiposis, 17
hepatic artery, common, *see* celiac artery, 83
hepatic flexure, 156
hepatitides: as formal plural of hepatitis, 45
hepatitis, 175
hepatomegaly, 175, 225
hermaphrodite, 31
hernia, 175
hernia, umbilical, 349
hernia, ventral, 357
herniorrhaphy, 176, 304
herpes, 176
herpes simplex virus, 176
herpes labialis, 176
herpes zoster, 176
heterogeneous, 176 (Note different spelling and meaning of the next word.)
heterogenous, 176
heterograft, 176
heteroplasia, *see* dysplasia, 287
heterosexual, 176
hiatus, 176
hiatus aorticus, 176
hiatus esophageus, 176
hiatus hernia, 175
hidradenitis, 177
hidrosis, *see* anhidrosis, 177
high blood pressure, *see* hypertension, 184
hipbone, part of, *see* ilium, 190–191
Hippocrates, 139, 177; *see also* caduceus, 69; pneumonia, 289; quarantine, 301
Hippocratic oath, 177
histamine, 178

histocompatibility, 178
histology, 178
HIV, 178
holocrine glands, 110
homeostasis, 178
homograft, *see* hetero-, 176
homologous, *see* analog, 27
homologue, 179
homosexual, 179
hordeolum, 179
hormone, 179–180
hormone replacement therapy, *see*
    menopause, 229–230
'hot tubes', *see* salpingitis, 312
HSV-1, HSV-2, *see* herpes, 176
human immunodeficiency virus or HIV, 178
humerus, 180
humors, theory of, *see* abscess, 6
humpback, *see* kyphosis, 203
hunchback, *see* kyphosis, 203
hyalin, 180
hyaline body, 180
hyalitis, 180
hyaloid membrane, 180
hyaloiditis, 180
hydatid cyst, 117, 181
hydradenitis, 177
hydrocele, 181; *see also* hydrocelectomy, 83
hydrocephalus, 87, 181
hydrometer, 181
hydronephrosis, 181–182
hydrophobia, 182; *see also* rabies, 302
hydrops, 182
hydrosalpinx, 182
hymen, 182
hymenotomy, 183
hyoglossus muscle, *see* hyoid, 183
hyoid bone, 183, 256
hyperactive, 183
hyperalgesia, 20
hyperbaric, 54–55
hyperbetalipoproteinemia, 183–184; *see also*
    beta, 56
hyperbilirubinemia, 58, 184
hyperchloremia, 92
hypercyanosis, 115
hyperemesis gravidarum, 138
hyperglycemia, 167
hyperkeratosis, *see* pachyonychia, 270–271
hyperkinesis, *see* hyperactive, 183
hyperlipoproteinemia, *see* beta, 56
hyperplasia, 185, 287
hyperplastic sinusitis, 318

hypersensitivity, 184
hypertension, 184; *see also* arteriosclerosis, 45
hypertrophy, 184–185, 346
hypertropia, 345
hyperventilate, 185
hypnagogue, 18
hypnodontics, 186
hypnosis, 185
hypnotherapy, 185–186
hypo, *see* hypodermic, 186
hypochloremia, 92
hypochondria, 94
hypochondriasis, 94
hypodermic, 186
hypodermic syringe, 330
hypoglycemia, 167, 186–187
hypospadias, 321
hypotension, 186
hypothermia, 186
hysterectomy, 187
hysteria, 187

I
IM or intramuscularly, 198
iatric, *see* geriatric, 163
iatrogenic, 188–189
IAV or intermittent assisted ventilation,
    196–197
icteroanemia, 189
icterohepatitis, 189
icterus, 189
icterus neonatorum, 189
idiopathic, 190
idiopathic cardiomyopathy, 77
idiosyncrasy, 190
idiot, 189
ileostomy, 190
ileum, 190; *see also* enteron, 141
ileus, 190
iliac muscle or iliacus, 191
ilium, 190–191
imaging techniques, *see* ultrasonic, 349
immune, 191
immune system, 191
immunoglobulin, 191; *see also* antibody, 37
impaction, fecal, 151–152
impetigo, 191
impotence, 191
in situ, 192, 319
in utero, 192
in vitro, 192
in vivo, 192
incompetence, 193

incontinence, 102, 193
incontinence of milk, *see* galactorrhea, 160
incudectomy, *see* incus, 193
incudomalleal, *see* incus, 193
incudostapedial, *see* incus, 193
incus, 193
induced abortion, 5
induration, 193
indurative myocarditis, 193
indwelling catheter, 80
infarct, 194; *see also* myocardial infarction, 76, 194
infection, 194
inferior, 194
infibulation, 153–154
inflammation, 154–155
influenza, 195
infra, 195
infraorbital, 195
infrared, 195
infusion pump, intravenous, 198
inguinal hernia, 175
inhalation, 171
inhalator, 171–172
inhaler, 171–172
inherent, 13
inoculate, 254
inoculum, 254
insomnia, 320
insufficiency, vascular, 355
insulin, 196
interatrial septum, 49
intercostal muscle, 196
intercristal diameter, 111–112
intermittent, 196–197
intermuscular, 198
interosseous membrane, 227
interrupt, 5
interstice, 197
interstitial fluid, 197
interstitial lung disorders, 197
interstitium, 197
interval, 197
interventricular septum, 49
intestinal absorption, 6, 218–219
intestinal flora, 197
intestine, 197; *see also* bowel, 64
intestine, large, *see* colon, 104
intramuscular, 198
intrauterine, 198
intravenous or IV, 198
intravenous pyelography, *see* pyelo-nephritis, 246–247

intravenous pyelogram, 299
ischemia, *see* syncope, 331
ischiococcygeal, 198
ischium, 198
islets of Langerhans, *see* insulin, 196
isobar, isobaric, 55
isocaloric, 199
isodontic, 199
isometric, 199, 341
isotonic, 199, 341
-istes, Greek suffix for agent nouns in English words, *see* note under catalyst, 81
-itis, origin of the medical suffix, 199
IUD or intrauterine device, 198
IV or intravenous, 198
IVF or in vitro fertilization, 192
IVP or intravenous pyelography, *see* pyelonephritis, 246–247

J
jaudice, 189; *see also* hyperbilirubinemia, 58
jawbone, *see* mental foramen, 157
jejunal feeding tube, 200
jejunoileitis, 200
jejunostomy, 200
jejunum, 200; *see also* enteron, 141
joint, sacroiliac, 311
jugular vein, 200–201
juices, gastric, 161
JVP or jugular venous pressure, 201

K
karyogenesis, *see* nucleus, 249
karyokinesis, *see* nucleus, 249
karyomegaly, *see* nucleus, 249
karyon, *see* nucleus, 249
keloid, 202
keratectomy, photorefractive, 283
keratin, 202; *see also* cutis, 113; pachyonychia, 270–271
keratitis, *see* dendritic keratitis, 124
keratomalacia, 202
keratoscopy, 202
keratosis, 203
'keyhole' surgery, *see* cholecystectomy, 135; laparoscopy, 206
kidney, *see* nephron, 246
kidney stone, *see* lithotripsy, 212
'kidney' words, *see* nephro-, 246–247; and renal, 305
Kielland forceps, 252
knee jerk, *see* patellar reflex, 274–275

'knee' words, *see* genu-, 162
kneecap, *see* patella, 274
knock-kneed, *see* genu valgum, 162
kyphosis, 203

L
L-shaped, *see* lambdoid, 256
labia majora, 204
labia minora, 204
labial, 204
labial frenulum, 158
labiodental, 204
labium, 204
labor, difficult, *see* dystocia, 340
laboratory diagnosis, 167
labyrinth, 228
lac, lactis, and 'milk' words, 5
'lack' or 'deficiency' suffix, *see* -penia, 278
lack of period, *see* amenorrhea, 308
lacrimal apparatus, 204–205
lacrimal duct and sac, *see* punctum, 298
lactase, 5, 205
lactiferous duct, 5, 206
lactose, 5, 205
Laennec, René, French physician, *see*
    cirrhosis, 99
lambdoid suture, 256
laparoscopic cholecystectomy, 92
laparoscopy, 206
lapsus linguae, 207
lapsus calami, 207
large intestine, *see* colon, 104
laryngectomy, 207
laryngismus, 208
laryngopharynx, 243
laryngospasm, 208
larynx, 207
LASER, 11, 208
laser-beam keratectomy, 283
lateral, 208
laterality, 208
left, *see* oculus sinister, 254
left colic flexure, 156
left cardiac atrium, *see* pulmonary
    circulation, 297
left eye, *see* oculus sinister, 254
leprosy, *see* Mycobacterium, 238
lesion, 209
lesion, skin, *see* papule, 273
lesser omentum, 257
leucocyte, 118
leukemia, 209
leukemia, leukopenic, 278

leukoblast or leukocytoblast, 61
leukocyte chemotaxis, 333
leukocyte, 209
leukocytopenia, 278
leukocytosis, 209
leukopenia, 278
leukoplakia, *see* pachyleptomeningitis, 270–
    271
leukorrhea, 210
levator anguli oris, 210
levator muscles, 210
levator palpebrae superioris, 210
levator scapulae, 210
LH or luteinizing hormone, 214
LHRH or luteinizing hormone-releasing
    hormone, 214
ligament, 210; *see also* tendon, 335
ligament, collateral, 102, 209
ligament, nuchal, 249
ligation, 211
'light' words, *see* photo-, 283–284
light-touch palpation, 271–272
lingua bifida, *see* schistoglossia, 165
lingual frenulum, 158
lipase, 211
lipid, 211
lipocyte, 211
lipolysis, 18; *see also* lipase, 211
liposuction, 211–212
lithotripsy, 149, 212
lithotriptor, 149
'liver' words, *see* hepato-, 175
livid, 212
lividity, 212
livor mortis, 212
lobe, occipital, 75
lobe, temporal, 334
locomotor ataxia, *see* tabes, 332
longitudinal arch of the foot, *see* metatarsal
    arches, 232
lordosis, 212
Lou Gehrig's disease or ALS, 315
low blood pressure, *see* hypotension, 186
low blood sugar, *see* hypoglycemia, 186–187
lower small intestine, *see* ileum, 190
lower jawbone, *see* mandible, 221
lower-back ache, *see* lumbago, 213
lubb, *see* dupp, 131
lumbago, 213
lumbar, 212
lumbar puncture, 213; *see also* cerebrospinal
    fluid, 89
lumen, 6, 213

lumpectomy, *see* mastectomy, 135
lunate bone, *see* carpus, 78
'lung' words, *see* pneum-, 289; and
    pulmono-, 297
lutein, 213–214
luteinizing hormone, 214
lymph follicle, 156
lymph, 214
lymphangiofibroma, 34
lymphangioma, 34
lymphoblast, *see* follicle, 156
lymphocyte, 214; *see also* follicle, 156;
    thymo-, 338
lymphogranuloma venereum, 214
lymphoid cells of immune system, *see* T-
    cell, 334
lymphoma, 215

M

ma as root of 'mother' words, 220
macrocephaly, 216; *see also* megalocephaly,
    226
macrocyte, macrocytosis, 216
macrodrip, 216
macroglossia, 216
macrophage, 216–217
macroscopic, 217
macula, 217
macula lutea retinae, 217
macular degeneration, 217
maculate, 217
MAF or macrophage activating factor,
    216–217
magna cum laude, 101
maidenhead, *see* hymen, 182
malabsorption syndrome, 218–219
malacia, 218
malacosis, 218
malacosteon, *see* osteomalacia, 218
malaise, 219
malaria, 219
male gonad, 167
malignant, 219
malleable, 220
malleolus, 220
malleolus, medial, *see* tibia, 339
malleus, 220; *see also* incus, 193
malocchio, 'the evil eye', 254
malocclusion, *see* occlusal, 253
mamma, 220
Mammalia, 220
mammary gland, 220–221
mammogram, 221

mammoplasty, 221, 228
mammothermography, 221
mandible, 221
mandibular condyle, *see* temporo-
    mandibular joint, 334
manubrium, *see* sternum, 325
'many' words, *see* poly-, 289
mass, atheromatous, *see* atherosclerosis, 48
masseter muscle, 221
mastalgia, 222
mastectomy, 135, 222
mastectomy, radical, 303
mastitis, 222
mastoid bone, 222
mastoid process, 325–326
mastoidectomy, 222
mastoiditis, 222
masturbate, 223
mater, 223
maxilla, 7, 223
maxillary bones, *see* mandible, 221
meatus, 223–224
meatus, external auditory, 49
medial, 224
median phalanx, 282
median, 224
medical imaging process: *see* DSA, 33
medical bioethics, 59
medical euphemism, 73
medicine, 224
medulla oblongata, 225
medulla, 225
medulla, adrenal, 13–14
medulla, renal, 305
medullary cavity, *see* endosteum, 140
megabladder, 225
megacardia, 225
megacolon, 225
megaloblast, 61
megalocardia, 225
megalocephaly, 226
megalocyte, 226
megalomania, 226
megalosyndactyly, 226
megarectum, 225
megaureter, 225
meibomian glands, *see* blepharitis, 62
melancholia, melancholy, 6, 93, 226
melanin, 227
melanocyte, 227
melanoma, 227
melatonin, 227; *see also* pineal, 286
membrane, 227

membrane, arachnoid, 43
membranous labyrinth, 228
meninges, 228
meningitis, 228
meningocele, 229
meninx, *see* dura mater, 132; pia mater, 223
menopause, 229–230
menstruation, 230
mental foramen, 157
mental as adjective pertaining to the chin, 157
mercy killing, *see* euthanasia, 147
merocrine glands, 111
mesentery, 230
mesocolon, 230
mesoderm, 126
mesomorph, 230
meta-, meaning of prefix, 231
metabolism, 26, 63, 231; *see also* catabolism, 62–63
metacarpal, 78, 231
metamorphosis, 231
metastasis, 231
metatarsal, 232, 333
metatarsal arches, 232
microbiology, 59
microcephaly, 87; *see also* macrocephaly, 216
micrococcus, 53
microdrip, 216
microorganism, 233
microscope, 233
microscopic anatomy, 27
microsurgery, 233
micturate, 233; *see also* urin-, 351
middle ear bones, *see* ossicle, 267
middle ear, *see* auris media, 50
'middle' words, *see* median, 224; meso-, 230
midwifery, *see* tocology, 339
migrainous neuralgia, 20
milia, 233–234
'milk' words, *see* galacto-, 159–160; and lac-, 205–206
milk sugar, *see* lactose, 205
milker's nodules, 248
'mind' words, *see* psycho-, 295
misandry, 32; *see also* misogyny, 169
misogyny, 32, 169, 234
mitral valve, 234, 354; *see also* cuspid, 56
MMIF or macrophage migration-inhibiting factor, 217
mobile caecum, *see* cecopexy, 70
mole, *see* macula, 217

moniliasis, *see* candidiasis, 73
monoclonal, 234–235
monocyte, 235
mononucleosis, 235, 250
mons pubis, 235, 297
mons Veneris, 297
monthly period, *see* catamenia and menorrhea, 229
Moore's lightning streaks, *see* entoptic, 142–143
morning sickness, *see* nausea gravidarum, 244
morphine, 236
morphogenesis, *see* BMPs, 236
mosquito forceps, 157
motor neuron, 247
motor neuron, *see* efferent, 136
motor apraxia, 3
MS or multiple sclerosis, *see* demyelination, 121, 239
mucin, 237
mucociliary clearance, pulmonary, 297
mucopurulent, 237, 298
mucosa, 237
mucus, 236
multip, multipara, 250, 274
multiple sclerosis, *see* demyelination, 121, 239
Munchausen's syndrome, 150
murmur, mitral, 354
muscae volitantes, *see* entoptic, 142
muscle, 237
muscle, abducens, 4; abductor, 4
muscle spasm, *see* dystonia and myotonia, 342
muscle tone, 341
muscle weakness, *see* myasthenia, 326
'muscle' words, *see* my-, myo-, 238–239
muscular dystrophy, 238
mushroom poisoning, *see* mycotoxicosis, 238
musicians' 'chops', *see* buccinator muscle, 67
mutagen, 38, 238
mutant, 238
muton, 238
myalgia, 20
myasthenia, 326
Mycobacterium, 238
mycology, 238
mycosis, 238
mycotic aneurysm, *see* myco-, 238
mycotoxicosis, 238

myectomy, *see* torticollis, 342
myelin, 239; *see also* demyelination, 121
myelin sheath, *see* demyelination, 121
myelography, 240
myeloma, 240
myocardial infarction, 76–77, 194, 239
myocardium, 239
myoclonus or myoclonia, 101
myoma, 239
myometrium, 232, 351–352
myopathy, 276; *see also* cardiomyopathy, 77
myope, 261
myopia, 261
myotonia and myotonus, 239, 342
myxadenitis, 240
myxedema, 136
myxoma, myxomatosis, 240
myxovirus, 240

N

naeval angioma, 34
naevus, 34
nail refill test or nail blanch test, *see* capillary, 74
nanism, 241
nanocephaly, 241
nanocormia, 241
nanocurie, 241
nanogram, 241
nanoid, 241
nanomelia, 241–242
nanosecond, 241
nanosoma, 241
nanosomia, 241
nanosomus, 241
nanus, 241
nape of the neck, *see* nucha, 249
narcohypnosis, 242
narcolepsy, 242
narcosis, 242
narcotic, 242
naris, 243
'narrow' words, *see* -sten-, 324
nasal, 243
nasal mucosa, *see* rhino-, 307
nasal septum, 243
nasal speculum, 243, 321
nasopharynx, 243
natal, 243–244
nates, *see* gluteus, 166
nausea, 244
nausea gravidarum, 244

nausea navalis or seasickness, 244
navel hernia, congenital, *see* omphalocele, 258
'navel' words, *see* omphalo-, 257–258; and umbilicus, 349
nearsightedness, *see* myopia, 261
nebulizer, 172
necrophilia, 245
necrosis, 245; *see also* gangrene, 160–161
necrotizing enteritis, 245
necrotizing fasciitis, 245
Neisseria gonorrhoeae, *see* gonococcus and gonorrhea, 168
neologism, 245
neology, 245
neonatal, 244
neonatology, 244
neoplasm, 245–246
neoplasty, 245–246
nephrolith, 246
nephron, 246
nephropexy, 281
nephroptosis, 296
nephrosis, 246
nephrostomy, 246
nephrotic syndrome, *see* nephrosis, 246
nerve, abducens, 4
nerve cell, *see* neuron, 247
nerve, median, 224
nerve pain, *see* neuritis, 247; neuralgia, 247–248
nerve, radial, 303
nerve, sciatic, 315
'nerve' words, *see* neuro-, 247–248
nervous system, autonomic, 50
neuralgia, 20, 247–248; *see also* neuritis, 247
neuritis, 247
neurocirculatory asthenia, 326
neuroglia, 164
neurology, 248
neuron, 247; *see also* efferent, 136
neuropeptide, *see* endorphin, 140
neurosurgery, 248
neurotransmitter, 247
neurotropism, 345
'new' words, *see* neo-, 245–246
newborn's rash, *see* milia, 233–234
nexus, 13
night blindness, *see* nyctalopia, 261
nil per os or NPO, 248
nipple pain or thelalgia, *see* epithelium, 144–145
nipple, inflamed, or thelitis, *see* epithelium, 144–145

nipple, *see* areola mammae, 44
NMR or nuclear magnetic resonance, 250
noctambulate, 23
node, atrioventricular, 49
node, axillary, 51
node, lymphatic, 214
node, sinoatrial, 49
nodule, 248
Nomina Anatomica, definition of, iii-iv, *see also* cervix, 90
Non-Hodgkin's lymphoma, 215
non-pitting edema, 136
non-specific immune response, *see* RES, 306
nose job, *see* rhinoplasty, 307
'nose' words, *see* nasal, 243; and rhino-, 307–308
nosotropic, *see* etiotropic, 146
nostalgia, 20
nostril, *see* naris, 243
noxious, 248
NPO or nil per os, 248
nucha, 249
nuchal chord, 249
nuchal ligament, 249
nuclear magnetic resonance or NMR, 250
nucleus, 249
nucleus pulposus, 249
nulligravida, 244
nullipara, 250, 274
nyctalopia, 261

O
O.B., *see* obstetrics, 252
ob: meanings of the prefix, 251
oblique, 251
oblique bandage, 151
oblique presentation, 251
obliquus externus abdominis muscle, 251–252
obliquus internus abdominis muscle, 251–252
obliquus muscle, 251–252
obsolescent, 146
obstetric forceps, 157, 252
obstetrics, 252
obturator, a prosthetic device, 252
obturator externus muscle, 252
obturator internus muscle, 252
obturator muscle, 252
obturator sign, 252
occipital bone, 75, 253
occipitobregmatic, *see* occiput, 253
occipitofrontalis muscle, 253

occiput, 75, 253
occlusal, occlusion, 253
occult, 253
oculus, 254
OD or oculus dexter, 254
odontoblast, 61
odontogenic, 254
odontoid process, 255, 291
odontology, 254
-oid, as medical suffix, 256
'old' words, *see* geri-, 162–163; and presby-, 290–291
'old age' words, *see* geri-, geronto-, 162–163
olfaction, *see* osmesis, 266
olfactory, 255
olfactory hallucination, 172
oligodactyly, 255
oligospermia, 255–256
-oma as medical suffix, 256
omentoplasty, 257
omentum, 257
omphalocele, 258
omphalos or navel, 257
omphalotomy, 258
onco-RNA-virus, 258
oncogenic, 258
oncology, 258
onychogryphosis or onychogryposis, 259
onycholysis, 259
onychophagy, 259
oocyte, 259
oocytin, 259
oogonium, 259
oophorocystectomy, 260
oophorosalpingectomy, 260
ootid, 259
open fracture, 157–158
ophthalmia neonatorum, 260
ophthalmologist, 260–261
ophthalmoscope, 261
opportunistic infection, 194
optic, 261
optic chiasm or chiasma, 262
optic glioma, 262
optician, 261
optometrist, 261
orad, 15
oral muscosa, 237
oral, 264
orbicularis oris muscle, 264
orbital cavity, 83
orchidopexy, 263
orchitis, 263

orexia, 263
orexigenic, 263
organ, 264
organelle, 264
organic, 264
orgasm, 264
orifice, 265
oropharynx, *see* nasopharynx, 243
orthodontist, 265
orthopedics, 265
orthopnea, 265
OS or oculus sinister, 254
os calcis, 266; *see also* calcaneus, 70
os or bone, 266
os or mouth, 265
os pubis, 297
os uteri, 265
oscillate, 266
oscilloscope, 266
osculate, 266
osmesis, 266
osmesthesia, 266
osmoreceptor, 266
osmosis, *see* osmoreceptor, 266–267
osseous, 267
ossicle, 267; *see also* incus, 193
ossification, 267
ostealgia, 21
osteomalacia, 218, 267; *see also* rickets, 302
osteopath, 276
osteoporosis, 268
osteotome, 268
otalgia, 21
otitis, otitis externa, otitis interna, otitis
    media, 268
otorhinolaryngology, 268, 308
ovarian, 269
ovarian cyst, 115; *see also*
    oophorocystectomy, 260
ovarian follicle, *see* lutein, 213–214
ovary, 269; *see also* oophor- words, 260
ovary, polycystic, 289
'over' words, *see* hyper 183–185; and super,
    328–329
oviduct or Fallopian tube, 269
ovulate, 269
ovule, 269
ovum, 269
oxytocin, 340

P
p.c. or post cibum, 290
P.U.O. or pyrexia of unknown origin, 300

pachyderma vesicae, 270
pachyleptomeningitis, 270
pachyonychia congenita, 270–271
palatal myoclonus, *see* myoclonus, 101
palate, 271
palatine bone, *see* palat-, 271
palatoplasty, 271; *see also* cleft palate, 99–100
palatorrhaphy, 271; *see also* cleft palate, 99–
    100
palatoschisis, 271, 313; *see also* cleft palate,
    99–100
Pall Mall, 220
palpate, 271–272
palpatory percussion, 271–272
palpebra, inferior and superior, 272
palpebrate, 272
palpitate, palpitation, 272
panacea, 272
pancreas, 272; *see also* cauda pancreatis, 82;
    see also insulin, 196
pancreatic enzyme, *see* amylopsin, 26;
    chymotrypsin, 97;
pandemic, 123
papilla, 273
papilloma, 273
papovavirus, *see* verruca, 357
papule, 273
para-, meaning of prefix, 273
-para, meaning of suffix, 274
paracentesis, *see* ascites, 47
parainfluenza, *see* para-, 273
paralysis of arms and legs, *see* quadriplegia,
    301
paralysis, 215, 273
paramedic, 273
parametrium, 351–352
paranasal sinus, 318
paranoia, *see* para-, 273
paraplegia, 273
parasite, 318–319
paratyphoid, *see* para-, 273
parietal, 274
parietal bone, 275
parietal lobe, 274
parietal pleura, 288–289
Parkinsonian facies, 150
parorexia, 263
parotid, 273
parotid gland, 269, 311
Pasteur, Louis, *see* hydrophobia, 182;
    rabies, 302
patella, 274; *see also* chondromalacia
    patellae, 94

patellar reflex, 274–275
patency, patent, 275
patent medicine, 275
patent, see transluminal, 213
pathogen, pathogenesis, 276
pathology, 276
pathos, 2; for Greek meaning, see patho-
and apathy, 275
pectin, 25
pectoral muscle, 277
pectoralis major and minor, 277
pelvic cavity, 83
pelvic inflammatory disease or PID, see
gonorrhea, 168; salpingitis, 312
pelvic socket, 8
pelvimetry, 277
pelvis, 277
pelvis, renal, 305
penile frenulum, 158
penis, 278–279; see also circumcision, 98
pepsin, 279
peptic ulcer, 279
per anum, 279
per rectum, 279
per vaginam, 279
per vias naturales, 279
perambulator, 23
percutaneous, 114
percutaneous nephrostomy, 246
percutaneous transluminal coronary
angioplasty, 213
perfusion, 279–280
pericardial sac, 310
pericarditis, 280
pericardium, 280
perimeter, 280
perimetrium, 232
perinatal, 244
period, painful, see dysmenorrhea, 309
period, see catamenia and menorrhea, 229
periosteum, 268
perisylvian slope, see fissure, 154
peritoneal folds, see mesentery and
mesocolon, 230
peritoneum, 280; see also omentum, 257
peritonitis, 280–281
perliche, see cheilosis, 91
permeable membrane, 228, 279
pernicious anemia, 248
perone, Greek word for fibula, 153
peroneus longus, see fibula, 153
perspiration, see sudor, 328
petit mal seizure, see epilepsy, 143–144

phage, see bacteriophage, 53–54
phagocyte, 282; see also RES, 306
phalanges, phalanx, 282
phallus, 278–279
phantom pregnancy, see pseudocyesis, 294
pharynx, 282
pheresis, see apheresis, 41
phimosis, see circumcision, 98
phlebitis, 282
phlebotomy, 283
photic epilepsy, 283
photopsia, see entoptic, 142–143
photorefractive keratectomy, 283
photoretinitis, 283
phototaxis, 284; see also chemotaxis, 333
phototropism, 284, 345
phrenic nerve, 284
phrenology as quackery, 284
physical, 284
physician, 285
physikoi, Greek philosophers, 285
physiology, 285
physiotherapy, 285
physique, 285
pia mater, 223; see also
pachyleptomeningitis, 270
picornavirus, see Enterovirus, 142
PID, acute, see gonorrhea, 168
pigmentosa, see xeroderma, 360
pilar cyst, 285
pilomotor reflex, 286
pilonidal cyst, 286
pilonidal sinus, 286
pineal gland, 286
pinealoma, 286
pinkeye, see conjunctivitis, 106
pinna, 49
pisiform bone, see carpus, 78
pitting edema, 136
placenta, 6
plane, sagittal, 311
plantar wart, 286, 359
plasia, 287
plastic surgery, 287
-plasty, meaning of suffix, 288
pleura, 288–289
pleurisy, 288–289
pleuritis, 288–289
plexus, 288
plicae vocales, see glottis, 165
Pliny, Roman encyclopedist, 8
PMC or pulmonary mucociliary clearance,
297

pneumococci, *see* bronchopneumonia, 66
pneumonia, 289
pneumonia, aspiration, 47
pneumonitis, 289
poison, *see* toxin, 342
polio or poliomyelitis, 240
polycystic ovary, 117
polycystic, 289
polycythemia, *see* phlebotomy, 283
polydactylism, 289
polyodontia, 289
popliteal vein, *see* saphena, 312
post cibum or p.c., 290
post mortem, 36, 290
post mortem lividity, 212
post partum, 290
posterior, 36
posterior chamber, 36
posterior nares, *see* anterior, 36
postnatal, 244
postoperative, 290
Pott's curvature, *see* kyphosis, 203
preamble, 23
precancerous, 290
precocious, 290
precursor, 290
prefix, 23
pregnancy, ectopic, 135–136
pregnancy, tubal, 135–136
pregnant, *see* nausea gravidarum, 244
premature aging, *see* progeria, 163
prenatal, 36, 244
prepuce or preputium, 290; *see also*
    circumcision, 98
preputial gland, 290
presbyacousia, 291
presbyopia, 261, 291
Presbyterian, 290–291
pretzel, *see* brachial plexus, 64
prickle-cell layer of the skin, 7
primary lesion, 209
primigravida, 244
primip, primipara, 250, 274
process, 291
proctectomy, 293
proctoclysis, 292
proctology, 292
proctoscope, 293
proctosigmoidectomy, 293
prodrome, 130
progeria, 163, 291
prognosis, 167, 291
prolactin, 206

prolapse, 207, 292; *see also* carpoptosis, 79;
    ptosis, 295–296
prolapse, mitral valve, 234, 354
pronation, *see* supine, 329
pronator, *see* supine, 329
prone, *see* supine, 329
prostate, 292
prostatectomy, 292
prostatic catheter, 80
prosthetic device, *see* obturator, 252
protocol, 104
protoplasm, 293; *see also* cell, 84
proximal, 293; *see also* distal, 129–130
proximal phalanx, 282, 293
prurient, 293
prurigo, 294
pruritus, 294
pruritus ani, 30
pruritus vulvae, 294
pseudocyesis, 294
pseudogout, 294
pseudohermaphrodite, 31
pseudohermaphrodite, female, 169
pseudosarcomatous fasciitis, 151
psoriasis, 7, 294
psyche, *see* superego, 328
psychiatry, 189, 295
psychoanalysis, 295
psychology, 189, 295
psychoneurosis, 295
psychosis, 295
psychosomatic, 295
ptosis, ptotic, ptosed, 295–296; *see also*
    carpoptosis, 79
ptyalin, 296
ptyalism, 296
ptyalolithotomy, 296
puberty, precocious, 290
pubes, pubic, 296
pubic symphysis, *see* mons pubis, 235; os
    pubis, 297
pubic bone, *see* os pubis, 266, 297
pulling out one's hair, *see* trichotillomania,
    344
pulmonary alveoli, 22
pulmonary circulation, 297
pulmonary edema, 297
pulmonary embolism, 63, 137; *see also*
    phlebitis, 282
pulmonary fibrosis, idiopathic, 190
pulmonary mucociliary clearance or PMC,
    297
pulse, jugular, 200–201

pulse, radial, 303
pumping out the stomach, *see* gastrolavage, 161
punctum, 298
punctum caecum, 298
punctum lacrimale, 205, 298
puncture, lumbar, 213
pupil, 298
pupillary sphincter, 30, 321–322
purulence, 298–299
pus, 298
'pus' words, *see* pur-, 298–299; and pyo-, 299–300
pustule, 298
pyelitis, 299
pyelogram, 299; *see also* pyelonephritis, 246–247
pyelography, intravenous, *see* pyelonephritis, 246–247
pyelonephritis, 246–247
pyloric stenosis, 324
pyonephrosis, 299
pyorrhea, 299, 309
pyothorax, *see* empyema, 139
pyrexia, 300
pyrimethamine, *see* malaria, 219
pyrogen, 300
pyromania, 300
pyuria, 300

Q
quadriceps femoris, 85, 301
quadriplegia, 301
quarantine, 301
quinine, *see* malaria, 219

R
rabies, 302; *see also* hydrophobia, 182
rachiometer, 302
rachis, 302
rachischisis, 302
rachitic rosary, *see* rickets, 302
rachitis, 302
radial, 303
radiate, 303
radiation, ultraviolet, 349
radical mastectomy, 135, 222
radical, 303
radicle, 303
radiculitis, *see* radicle, 303
radio-, meaning of prefix, 303
radioactive, 303
radiology, 303

radiolucent, 304
radiopaque, 304
radiopaque contrast medium, *see* arteriogram, 45
radius, 303
rale, 109, 304
ramble, 23
raphe, 304
rays, actinic, 11
razor, 5
re-, meaning of the prefix, 305
reaction, antigen-antibody, 37
receptor, olfactory, 255
recovery score, *see* Apgar, 40
rectal speculum, 321
rectum, 305
rectum, prolapse of, 292
rectus femoris muscle, 301
red blood cell, *see* erythrocyte, 145; megalocyte, 226
'red' words, *see* erythro-, 145; rub-, 308
red corpuscle, *see* erythrocyte, 145
red-hairedness, *see* erythrism, 145
reductive mammoplasty, 221
reflex incontinence, 193
reflex, quadriceps, 301
reflex, *see* re-, 305
reflex, scapulohumeral, 313
reflux, *see* aortic valve, 39; *see also* hiatus hernia, 175
reflux, *see* re-, 305
refraction, *see* photorefractive keratectomy, 283
rehydration, *see* dysentery, 132, 141–142
relapse, 207
REM sleep, 23
remedy, *see* re-, 305
remission, *see* re-, 305
renal, 305
renal calculus, *see* nephro-, 246
renal pelvis, *see* pyelo-, 299; pyelonephritis, 246–247
rennin, obsolete name for chymosin, 97
RES or reticuloendothelial system, 306
resection, prostatic, 292
respirator, *see* -spir-, 322
respiratory, 305–306
respiratory distress syndrome of the newborn, 305–306
response, allergic, 21
response, autoimmune, 50
rete, 306
reticular, 306

reticuloendothelial system or RES, 306
retina, 306; *see also* retinopexy, 281
retinitis, 306
retinopexy, 281
retrocecal, 307
retrograde pyelogram, 299
Rh factor or rhesus factor, 307
rhesus factor, 307
rheumatic fever, *see* aortic stenosis, 39
rheumatism, 307
rheumatoid arthritis, 45
rhinitis, 307
rhinoplasty, 307
rhoncus, *see* rale, 304
riboflavin, 155
rickets, 302
rickets, adult form of, *see* osteomalacia,
    218, 267
Rickettsia, *see* typhus, 347
right cardiac ventricle, *see* pulmonary
    circulation, 297
right colic flexure, 156
right eye, *see* oculus dexter, 254
right, *see* oculus dexter, 254
rima glottidis, *see* glottis, 165
ringworm, *see* tinea, 339
rubella, 308
rubeosis, 308
rubor, 308; *see also* inflammation, 154–155
rump bone, *see* ischium, 198
runner's knee, 218, 274; *see also*
    chondromalacia patellae, 94
rupture, 5; *see also* inguinal hernia, 175–176

S

sac, 310; *see also* bursa, 68
sac, amniotic, 24–25
sac, lacrimal, 204–205
saccular aneurysm, 310
sacral, 310
sacroiliac, 311
sacrum, 310
sagittal, 311
sal ammoniac, 311
sal soda, 311
saline, 311
saline IV, *see* hypochloremia, 92
saliva, 311; *see also* buccal glands, 67
'saliva' words, *see* ptyalo- and sialo-, 296;
    and saliva, 311
salivary calculus, *see* ptyalolithotomy, 296
salivary gland, *see* parotid, 269
salivation, excessive, *see* ptyalism, 296

Salmonella, 53
Salmonella typhi, *see* typhoid fever, 346
salpingitis, 312
salpingogram, 312
salpingostomy, *see* salpingogram, 312
salpinx, 312
salpinx auditiva, 312
salpinx uterina, 312
'salt' words, *see* sal-, 311
saphena, 312
sarcinae bacteria, 53
sarcoma, 312–313
satyriasis, 188
scalpel, 313
scaphoid bone, *see* carpus, 77
scapula, 313
scapulohumeral reflex, 313
scar tissue, *see* keloid, 202
schistocyte, 314
schistocytosis, 314
schistoglossia, 165
schistosomiasis, 314
schistothorax, 314
schizoid, 314
schizophrenia, 314
sciatica, 315
sclera, 315
sclerosis, 315
scrotal raphe, 304
scrotum, *see* testis, 335; *see also*
    cryptorchidism, 262
scybalum, *see* fecal impaction, 151–152
seasickness or nausea navalis, *see* nausea,
    244
sebaceous cyst, 115, 316; *see also* atheroma,
    48; wen, 359
sebaceous gland, 316; *see also* follicle, 156
seborrhea, 316–317
seborrheic dermatitis, 316–317
sebum, 316
sebum, *see* blepharitis, 62
secretagogue, 18
secundipara, 250, 274
*see also*ing pink elephants, *see* zoopsia, 363
self-mutilation to gain medical attention,
    150
seminal vesicle, 358
senescent, 145
sense of balance, *see* membranous
    labyrinth, 228
sense of smell, *see* osmesis, 266
sense of well-being, *see* euphoria, 147
sensory neuron, 247; *see also* efferent, 136

sepsis, septic, 37, 317
septicemia, 317
septum, interatrial, 49
septum, nasal, 243
sequela, *see* glaucoma, 164
serotonin, *see* pineal, 286
serous, 318; *see also* pericardium, 280
serum, 317
sexual climax, *see* orgasm, 264
'shakes, the', *see* delirium tremens, 122
sheath, arachnoid, 43
sheath, myelin, 239
shin bone, *see* tibia, 339
shock, anaphylactic, 28
shock-wave lithotripsy, extracorporeal, 149
short-headedness, *see* brachycephalic, 65
shoulder cap muscle, *see* deltoid, 256
shoulder blade, *see* scapula, 313
shunt, arteriovenous, 45
sialogogue, *see* saliva, 311
sialolith, *see* saliva, 311
sialorrhea, *see* ptyalism, 296
sickle cell anemia, 84
sickle cell dactylitis, 120
SIDS (Sudden Infant Death Syndrome), 11
sign, *see* symptom, 330
simple fracture, 157–158
Simpson forceps, 252
sinciput, 75
sinew, *see* tendon, 335
sinoatrial node, 49
sinus, 318
sinus, front: *see also* aperture, 39
sinus, pilonidal, 286
sinus, sphenoid, 321
sinusitis, 318
site, 319; *see also* in situ, 192
sitomania, 319
situate as adjective, *see* in situ, 192
skeleton, 319
skeleton, visceral, 358
'sleep' words, *see* hypno-, 185–186
sleep apnea, 3
sleepwalking, 23; *see also* somnambulism, 320
slip of the tongue, *see* lapsus linguae, 207
small saphenous vein, 312
'small' words, *see* micro-, 233
small intestine, middle, *see* jejunum, 200
small intestine, *see* enteron, 141
smile muscle, *see* levator anguli oris, 210
smooth muscle, 237
socket, pelvic, 8

sodium chloride or common salt, *see* chlorine, 92
soft palate, 271
solar plexus, 288, 320; *see also* celiac plexus, 84
solution, saline, 311
somnambulism, 23, 320
space, pleural, 288–289
spastic paralysis, *see* cerebral palsy, 89
speculum, 321
speculum, nasal, 243
speculum, vaginal, *see* colposcopy, 105
sperm bank, *see* cryobank, 112
spermatic duct, *see* vas deferens, 354–355
spermicide, 97
sphenoid bone, 321
sphincter, 321–322
sphincter, anal, 30
sphincter, pupillary, 30
sphinx, 30
sphygmometer, 30
sphygmoscope, 30
spina bifida, *see* rachischisis, 302
spinal cavity, 83
spinal column, *see* cervical vertebrae, 90; vertebra, 357
spinal fusion, *see* spondylosyndesis, 126
spinal tap, *see* cerebrospinal fluid, 89; lumbar puncture, 213
spirilla, 53
spirochete, 53
spleen, 322; *see also* splenectomy, 135, 322
splenic artery, *see* celiac artery, 83
splenic flexure, 156
split lip, *see* cheiloschisis, 91
split tongue, *see* schistoglossia, 165
'split' words, *see* -schisis, schisto-, schizo-, 313–314
spondyl- and vertebra-, 323
spondylosis, 323
spondylosyndesis or spinal fusion, 126
spontaneous abortion, 5
sprue, *see* celiac disease, 84
squamous, 323; *see also* desquamation, 122
stapedius muscle, 323
stapes, 323; *see also* incus, 193
staphylococcus, 53
starch, *see* amyl-, amylase, 25; amylopectin, 25–26; amylopsin, amylose, amyluria, 26
stat, 323
stenosis, aortic, 39
stenosis, mitral valve, 234, 354

stereotaxis, 324
sternocleidomastoid muscle, 325–326; *see also* torticollis, 342
sternum, 325
steroid, 325
steroid, anabolic, 26
stethoscope, 326
stoma, 327; *see also* colostomy, 104
'stomach' words, *see* gastri-, 161
stone, vesical, *see* vesicle, 358
stool, 151
strabismus, form of, *see* hypertropia, 345
strain, sacroiliac, 311
stratum, 327
stratum corneum, 327
stratum germinativum, 327
stratum granulosum, 327
stratum lucidum, 327
streptobacillus, 53
streptococcus, 53
Streptomyces erythreus, *see* erythromycin, 145
striated muscle, 237
'stupor' words, *see* narko-, 242.
stye, *see* hordeolum, 179
subarachnoid space, 43
subclavian artery, 328
subconscious, 328
subcutaneous, 114, 328; *see also* hypodermic, 185
subdeltoid bursae, *see* bursitis, 68
subliminal, 328
sublingual salivary gland, 311
submandibular salivary gland, 311
sudamen, 328; *see also* milia, 233–234
sudatorium, 328
sudomotor nerve, 328
sudor, 328
sudoriferous gland, 328
sudorific, 328
'sugar' words, *see* glyco-, 166–167
suicide, 97
sulcus, 170
superego, 328
superficial fascia, 151
superficial wound, 328
superior, 329
supernumerary digit, 328
supination, 329
supinator muscle, 329
supine, 329
suppuration, 298–299
suppurative sinusitis, 318

suprarenal, 329
surfactant, *see* respiratory, 305–306
surfer's nodules, 248
surgery, origin of term, *see* cryosurgery, 112–113
surgical fixation, *see* -pexy, 281
suture, sagittal, 311
swayback, *see* lordosis, 212
sweat glands: apocrine, 110; eccrine, 110; exocrine, 110; *see also* hidradenitis, 177
sweat, *see* sudor, 328
sympathy, 276–277
symphysis, 329
symphysis, pubic, 235; *see also* os pubis, 297
symptom, 330
synapse, 330; *see also* neurotransmitter, 247
syncope, 331
syndrome, 131, 330
synovial fluid, *see* bursa, 68; *see also* arthrocentesis, 85
synthesis, 330
syphilis, *see* tabes, 332
syringe, 330
syringe, aspirating, 47
syringitis, 331
syrinx, 331
systole, 331; *see also* diastole, 128
systolic, 129

T
T cell, 334; *see also* lymphocyte, 214
tabes dorsalis, 332; *see also* dorsum, 130
tabescent, 146
tachycardia, 332; *see also* bradycardia, 65
tailbone, *see* coccyx, 103
talipes, 332
tarsal, 232, 333
tarsal bones, *see* calcaneus, 70
tarsus, 333
taxis, 333; *see also* phototaxis, 284
taxonomy, 334
tear sac or lacrimal sac, *see* dacryocyst, 119
technician, radiologic, 303
teeth, extra, *see* polyodontia, 289
temperature, axillary, 51
temperomandibular joint, 221
temperomandibular joint syndrome, 334
temporal, 334
temporal bone, 334
temporal lobe, 334
tendon, 335
tendonitis, *see* tennis elbow, 137
tennis elbow, 137

tensor tympani muscle, *see* stapes, 323
teras, 335
teratism, 335
teratogenic, 335
teratology, 335
test, agglutination, 14
test, lipid, 211
testes, descent of, *see* inguinal hernia, 175–176; cryptorchidism, 262
'testicle' words, *see* orchi-, 262–263
testis, 335
testosterone, 31
tetanus, 336
tetany, 336
thelalgia, *see* epithelium, 144–145
thelarche, 337
thelitis, *see* epithelium, 144–145
theory of humors: 6; *see also* eczema, 136; melancholy, 226; myocardial infarction, 76, 194
therapy, 337
thermometer, 337
thermotaxis, 337
'thick' words, *see* pachy-, 270–271
thigh bone, 152
thigh muscle, *see* obturator, 252; quadriceps femoris, 86
thoracentesis or thoracocentesis, 338
thoracic cavity, 83
thorax, 338
throat, three areas of the, *see* nasopharynx, 243
thrombocytopenia, 278
thrombosis, 338
thrombus, 338
thrush, *see* candid-, 73
thymosin, 338
thymus gland, 338
thyroid hormone, *see* calcitonin, 71
thyroid, 339
thyroxine, 339
tibia, 339
tibiofemoral, 339
tinea, 339
tinea cruris, 339
tinea pedis, 339
tinnitus, *see* hallucination, 172
tissue, indurated, 193
tissue, reticular, 306
tissue transplant, *see* histocompatibility, 178
'tissue' words, *see* histo-, 177
tocology, 339

'together' words, *see* co-, 101–102; and sym-, syn-, 329–330
toilets, Roman: sociological note, 29
tomograph, tomography, 79, 341
tone, 341
'tongue' words, *see* glossa- and glossal, 164–165
tonic spasm, 11; *see also* clonus, 101
tonsillitis, follicular, *see* follicle, 156
tonus, 341
'tooth' words, *see* dent-, 124–125; and odonto-, 254–255
toothlessness or edentia, 125
torsion, 342
Torti, Francisco, *see* malaria, 219
torticollis, 342
towel forceps, 157
toxic, toxin, 342
toxicology, 342
toxicosis, 342
tracer study, in vivo, 192
trachea, 343
tracheotomy, 343
transfusion, 343
transhepatic cholangiography, percutaneous, or PTC, 114
transluminal, 213
transplant, 343
transurethral prostatectomy, 292
transverse arch of the foot, *see* metatarsal arches, 232
transverse colon, 104; *see also* flexure, 156
trapezium bone, *see* carpus, 78
trapezoid bone, *see* carpus, 78
trauma, 343
trench mouth, *see* gingivitis, 163
triangular or triquetral bone, *see* carpus, 78
triangular, *see* deltoid, 256
triceps, 85
triceps muscle, 344
trichiasis or trichoma, 344
trichotillomania, 344
triple-lumen catheter, 80
trocar, 344; *see also* cannula, 74
trocar cystostomy, *see* cannula, 74
trochanter, 344–345
tropomysin, 345
true cartilage, 180
tubal ligation, 211
tubal pregnancy, 135–136
tuberculosis, *see* antitubercular, 38 and Mycobacterium, 238
tumor, 346; *see also* inflammation, 154–155

'turn' words, *see* trop-, 345
TURP (transurethral prostatectomy), 11
tympanic cavity, *see* auris media, 50
tympanostomy, *see* otitis, 268
tympanum, 346; *see also* meatus, 223–224
typhoid fever, 346
typhus, 347

U

U-shaped, *see* hyoid, 256
ulcer, 348; *see also* decubitus ulcer, 121
ulcerative colitis, 348
ulna, 348
ultrasonic, 349
ultrasonic lithotripsy, percutaneous, 114
ultraviolet or UV, 349
umbilical cord, cutting of, *see*
    omphalotomy, 258
umbilical hernia, 11
umbilical prolapse, occult, 253
umbilicus, 349; *see also* omphalo-, 257
'under' words, *see* hypo-, 186–187; and sub,
    328
undescended testicle, *see* cryptorchidism,
    262; testis, 335
unicellular, 349
unilateral, 350
unipara, 250, 274, 349
upper arm bone, *see* humerus, 180
upper jaw, *see* maxilla, 223
urea, 350
uremia, *see* B.U.N. test, 350
ureter, 350; *see also* pyelonephritis, 246–247
ureterectasis, 351
ureterolith, 350
ureterostenosis, 351
urethra, 351
urethral meatus, *see* orifice, 265
urethral orifice, external, 265
urinaria, *see* vesica, 357
urinary bladder, thickened lining of, *see*
    pachyderma, 270
urinary meatus, 223–224
urinary stress incontinence, 102, 193
urinary system, 351
urine, 351
uterine cervix, 90
uterine linings, 232
uterus, 351–352
uterus, inner lining of, *see* endometrium,
    140
uterus, prolapse of, 292
'uterus' words, *see* hystero-, 187

UV or ultraviolet, 349
uvea, 352
uveitis, 353
uvula, 352

V

vaccine, 353; *see also* poliomyelitis, 240
vagina, 353
vaginal hernia, *see* cystocele, 83
vaginal incision, *see* episiotomy, 144
vaginal speculum, 321; *see also* colposcopy,
    105
vaginitis, 353
valve, 39, 353–354
valve sounds, *see* dupp, 131
varicose vein, 354
varicosis, 354
vas deferens, 354–355
vascular, 355
vasectomy, 355
vasoconstrictor, 355
vasodilator, 355; *see also* amyl nitrite, 25
vasopressin, 355–356
vasopressor, 355–356
vasotomy, 355
vastus muscle, 301
vectorcardiogram, *see* vector, 356
vector, 356
'vein' words, *see* phleb-, 282–283; veno-, 356
vein, 356
vena cava, 356
vena cava, inferior and superior, 194–195
venereal wart, 359
ventilate, ventilator, 356
ventrad, 15, 357
ventral, 357
ventricle, 357
ventricle of the heart, *see* systole, 331
ventricular fibrillation or VF, 153
vermiform appendix, 42–43
verruca, 357; *see also* plantar wart, 286
vertebra, 357
vertebra, cervical, 90
vertebra, coccygeal, *see* coccyx, 103
vesica, 357
vesicle, 358; *see also* bulla, 68
vesicovaginal fistula, 154
vessel, collateral, 209
vessel, lymphatic, 214
VF or ventricular fibrillation, 153
viable, *see* nullipara, 250
vibrio, 53
vinegar, *see* acetic acid, 8

virion, 358
virus, 358
viscera, 358
visceral pleura, 288–289
visceral, *see* parietal, 274
vitamin B$_2$, *see* riboflavin, 155
vitamin B$_{12}$, *see* pernicious anemia, 248
vitamin D deficiency, *see* rickets, 302
vitamin D$_2$, *see* calciferol, 71
vitamin megadose, 225
vocal folds, *see* glottis, 165
vomitus, *see* emetic, 138
vulva, 358
vulval pruritus, 294
vulvitis, 358
vulvovaginitis, 358

W

wart, 359
wart, plantar, 286, 359
wasting away, *see* atrophy, 346
'water' words, *see* hydro-, 181–182
water on the brain, *see* hydrocephalus, 87, 181
weal, *see* papule, 273
weaning, 5; *see also* ablactation, 205
webbed fingers or toes, enlarged, *see* megalosyndactyly, 226
wen, 359; *see also* sebaceous cyst, 115
white blood cell, *see* leucocyte, 118; macrophage, 216–217
white corpuscle, *see* leukocyte, 209
'white' words: *see also* alb-, 19; candid-, 73; leuko-, 209–210
whitehead, *see* milia, 233–234
windpipe, *see* trachea, 343; *see also* endotracheal, 141

'womb' words, *see* hystero-, 187; and uterus, 351–352
wound, *see* trauma, 343
wrist drop, *see* carpoptosis, 79
wrist, *see* carpus, 77–78
wrist stress, *see* CTS, 78–79
wryneck, *see* torticollis, 342

X

X-ray scan, *see* tomograph, 341
X-ray, *see* mammogram, 221; myelography, 240
xanthoma, 360
xenophobia, 360
xeroderma, 360–361
xerostoma, 361
xiphoid process, *see* sternum, 325

Y

yeast infections and *Candida albicans*, 73
yellow enzyme, *see* flavoprotein, 155
yellow spot, *see* macula lutea, 217
'yellow words', *see* flavi-, 155; and xantho-, 360

Z

zona, 362
zona glomerulosa, 362
zonule of Zinn, vii, 362
zoograft, 362
zoopsia, 363
zootoxin, 363
zygomatic bone, 363
zygomaticus muscle, 363
zygote, 363